IT DOESN'T HAVE TO HURT

ALSO BY SANJAY GUPTA

World War C

Keep Sharp

Monday Mornings: A Novel

Cheating Death

Chasing Life

IT DOESN'T HAVE TO HURT

YOUR SMART GUIDE TO A PAIN-FREE LIFE

Sanjay Gupta

The information in this book may not be suitable for everyone and is not intended to be a substitute for medical advice or medical treatment. You are advised to consult a doctor on any matters relating to your health, and in particular on any matters that may require diagnosis or medical attention. Any use of the information in this book is made on the reader's good judgement after consulting with his or her doctor and is the reader's sole responsibility.

First published in the United States in 2025 by Simon & Schuster

First published in the United Kingdom in 2025 by Headline Home
An imprint of Headline Publishing Group Limited

1

Cataloguing in Publication Data is available from the British Library

Trade Paperback ISBN 978 1 0354 3589 0
ebook ISBN 978 1 0354 3585 2

Offset in 11.84/16.48pt Arno Pro by Six Red Marbles UK, Thetford, Norfolk

Interior design by Joy O'Meara

Printed and bound in Great Britain by Clays Ltd, Elcograf S.p.A.

MIX
Paper | Supporting responsible forestry
FSC® C104740
FSC www.fsc.org

Headline's policy is to use papers that are natural, renewable and recyclable products and made from wood grown in well-managed forests and other controlled sources. The logging and manufacturing processes are expected to conform to the environmental regulations of the country of origin.

Headline Publishing Group Limited
An Hachette UK Company
Carmelite House
50 Victoria Embankment
London EC4Y 0DZ

The authorised representative in the EEA is Hachette Ireland, 8 Castlecourt Centre, Dublin 15, D15 XTP3, Ireland (email: info@hbgi.ie)

www.headline.co.uk
www.hachette.co.uk

For my three daughters, Sage, Sky, and Soleil.
Every word in this book is dedicated to you. One of our greatest fears is seeing the people we love in pain, and with this book I hope to prevent that from happening for you. Having parents who live a pain-free life is the gift I aim to give you, so that your mother and I may always be present, active, and engaged.

For my dear wife, Rebecca.
You, like too many others, have lived with physical pain. Yet during those times when I felt powerless to help, you inspired me to dig deep into what is possible and put what I learned in this book. Thank you for always taking the time to listen, encourage, and offer stellar suggestions for how to make this book the best it could be.

And for the millions of people out there with chronic pain.
I know it presents you with profound challenges, often invisible to others. I wrote this book for you, to share your stories and my confidence that together we can chart a path beyond pain—a path of action, hope, and healing.

Contents

IT DOESN'T HAVE TO HURT

Introduction

Bess Talbot feared she was going crazy.

At age forty-seven, she was having debilitating migraine headaches. She'd had her first one two decades earlier while she was in law school, and for a while the migraines happened only occasionally. But after she had children, they "came back with a vengeance," she told me. Now she was suffering from them every day.

The near-constant pain was affecting every part of her life. Drugs prescribed by various doctors made her woozy and dizzy, fogging her brain. She forgot grocery lists and once left her keys in a fitting room at a department store. Not able to focus until she made her way to the parking lot, she fought back tears, trying to orient herself. *Where am I? Where are my things? Where is my car?* "It puts you in a very dark place," she says.

Even when her migraines were less frequent, they could last for days and still dominated her life. "At times I thought, 'Am I going crazy? Is this something more than a migraine? Do I have a tumor?' At one point I was even wishing that they would find something like that just so they could operate and alleviate the issue."

After years of trying, and failing, to find relief for her migraines, Talbot was at the end of her rope. That's when her neurologist, stymied by her condition, recommended she travel from her home in Alabama to the Michigan Headache and Neurological Institute (MHNI) in Ann Arbor to see a physician he'd heard about named Joel Saper. Desperate, Talbot decided to make the trip. Maybe, just maybe, *he* could help.

Even before arriving in Ann Arbor, Talbot had phone conversations and evaluations with the team Dr. Saper had assembled. She spoke with neurologists and psychologists—doctors of the brain and the mind. She was evaluated by other specialists to fine-tune her treatment with physical and occupational therapy, as well as nutritional and pharmaceutical strategies. But the most important member of the treatment team was Talbot herself.

As simple as it sounds, this is Dr. Saper's most revolutionary concept: treating the patient not as a passive participant but as an active investigator working shoulder to shoulder with the experts. By focusing on not only the "what" of treatment but also the "who"—a patient's history, outlook, and expectations—he created an optimal healing environment. He helped people believe they could drive their own care.

In the course of her weeklong hospitalization for treatment, Talbot told Saper about a high school cheerleading accident from decades earlier. The team had been practicing a challenging new formation, and as a "flier"—the cheerleading daredevil who perches atop the human pyramid—Talbot had taken a steep plunge to the floor when the formation suddenly crumbled. She landed hard on her tailbone and felt a stab of pain in her back. Then the formation next to hers toppled too, and Talbot felt her head slam as a flier in that group crash-landed on her.

The team members disentangled, practice was canceled, and Talbot slumped home in excruciating pain. She had to skip the Guns N' Roses concert she'd planned to see that weekend with a friend, and when her doctor prescribed a bulky back brace, her mother had to alter her prom dress to accommodate it. But eventually the episode receded into the backdrop of her active life: College. Law school. Running, including marathon training and entering races as a way to manage stress.

A few years later, when she began to experience occasional migraine headaches, she did wonder if there might be a connection to her old injury. But even as the headaches worsened over time, whenever she brought up that idea with new doctors, they dismissed the link as too flimsy to pursue.

Then she sat down with Saper.

He was the first doctor to really dig into the aftermath of her fall. He learned that a few hours after the accident, her mother had insisted on taking her to the hospital emergency department. A workup with scans revealed hairline fractures in three upper thoracic vertebrae. Though none were considered serious enough to require surgery, she was admitted for a short hospital stay, followed by wearing that rigid back brace for six months. To Saper, these layers of detail were a significant part of the story—a history that held clues to her current condition.

A deeper investigation revealed a family history of migraines, which likely also increased the risk for Talbot. Without the cheerleading accident, however, that risk might never have manifested. Saper describes a person's propensity for migraines as a big rock perched on a high hill. "Genetics put the rock near the cliff," he says. And then "whether it's a glass of wine or a menstrual period, a bad emotional time in a person's life, something sort of tips it over the hill and it starts rolling." For Talbot, the cheerleading accident and the trauma to her spine, neck, and the base of her brain had tipped the boulder. Over the years, efforts at pain relief had never addressed that deeper issue.

As Saper described to Talbot how the pieces of her pain puzzle fit together, her misery and confusion gave way to something new—a hopeful sense of possibility. He used Talbot's history to inform her treatment plan, which now included dedicated physical therapy and exercises designed to specifically strengthen her spine and neck. Over the years, she had tried countless medications for migraines, including triptans, opioids, and others to address inflammation and depression, but no one had ever suggested adding a practical rehabilitation of the base of her neck.

The benefits of Saper's approach—the thorough initial evaluation, the continual calibrations of her medications, and the dedicated neck physical therapy—collectively made all the difference. Talbot gained more confidence in reading and responding to her physical and emotional cues for an approaching migraine. What's more, when she began to experience her pain changing as she and Saper fine-tuned the treatments, she felt newly encouraged to focus more at home on exercise, stress management, and meditation. Even when she can't do all of them all of the time, they are an antidote to hopelessness. "It was life changing for me," Talbot says. And she told Saper so. "I said, 'You've given me my life back.' And I wonder, if I'd met him twenty years ago, you know, what a better mother I would have been. What a better wife I would have been. What a better *everything* I would have been but for the migraines."

Talbot's healing journey began simply, with a fresh conversation about pain. Dr. Saper had brought medical precision, multidisciplinary expertise, and a deeply collaborative partnership with his patient to frame her relationship with pain in a new way, rewriting the pain script and providing new options for treatment and prevention. I start with Talbot's story because it offers a sense of optimism for the hundreds of millions of people suffering from chronic pain, and particularly those who have felt forgotten, suffering inside bodies they believe have betrayed them.

There is a very real path forward through pain and beyond. In this book, I walk you through the steps that I am confident will take you there.

A dizzying amount of medical progress has been made since I became a neurosurgeon more than twenty-five years ago. We can remove tumors once considered inaccessible and fuse spines previously thought to be too broken. We have a pretty good idea where certain emotions and addictions lie in the brain and can even tinker with them using deep brain stimulation. Pain, because of its complexity and subjective nature, has presented a larger challenge, and yet even there, we have made important advances.

Over the past few decades, we've learned more than ever about the true nature of pain. We better understand what causes it, what may best relieve it, and what we can do to minimize or even eliminate certain types of pain. Many of those life-changing insights have not yet been made easily available to the public. With this book, I want to change that. Over the past few years, I've placed both my neurosurgeon's and my investigative journalist's lens on the problem of pain, and I am now convinced: *It doesn't have to hurt.*

There is hope. There is help. And there is healing beyond anything we may have imagined.

In these pages, I offer new accessible lessons from doctors and researchers who specialize in pain and have been steadily changing the way we understand and experience it. You will hear directly from patients, many of whom struggled with chronic pain through a broken landscape of health care but found relief through conventional (and sometimes unconventional) tools.

Their consistent message is this: if you are in pain, there are far more effective options than you may have previously realized, as well as important things you should start doing *today* to greatly reduce your chances of suffering pain *tomorrow.* These are strategies I have started incorporating into my life, as well as the lives of my wife, teenage kids, and eighty-year-old parents.

The significance of reducing and even eliminating pain cannot be overstated. Nearly one-quarter of adults (24.3 percent) say they suffer from chronic pain, and nearly one in ten (8.5 percent) report high-impact pain—pain so bad it not only persists but in the previous three months also frequently limited their daily life and work activities. The outlook worsens with age. Among respondents to the 2023 National Health Interview Survey, the percentage of adults who had chronic pain in the past three months increased from 12.3 percent of those aged eighteen to twenty-nine, to 36 percent—more than one-third—of those age sixty-five and older. High-impact chronic pain increased with age too, from 3 percent of those aged eighteen to twenty-nine to 13.5 percent of those age sixty-five and older. Among those who reported chronic pain, almost two-thirds still suffered from it a year later.

New cases of chronic pain have also skyrocketed, and they now occur more often among US adults than new cases of most other common conditions, including diabetes, depression, and high blood pressure. These numbers translate globally. About one in five people around the world experience some form of chronic pain, making it one of the biggest burdens on the global health care system.

We recently got a glimpse of where Americans feel that pain the most.

In its 2022 survey report, "A Chronic Pain Crisis," the US Pain Foundation revealed the most common pain conditions:

- Back pain (67 percent)
- Joint pain due to arthritis (56 percent)
- Neuropathy (nerve pain; 53 percent)
- Neck pain (51 percent)

Also widespread:

- Muscle spasms (38 percent)
- Hip pain (37 percent)
- Headache (36 percent)
- Fibromyalgia (36 percent)
- Osteoarthritis (33 percent)
- Irritable bowel syndrome (28 percent)
- Migraine (27 percent)

Perhaps most striking, only 35 percent of respondents said their pain was a direct result of trauma or injury, such as from a car accident or workplace mishap. The vast majority of people in the survey cited no obvious cause, or entirely separate health conditions, that contributed to their pain. In fact, 20 percent had two to five contributory conditions, 30 percent had six to ten conditions, 24 percent had eleven to fifteen conditions, and 21 percent had fifteen or more contributory conditions. At least one person had a staggering forty-two conditions. Can you even imagine the burden that causes in their lives? Pain carries an enormous amount of physical, social, and emotional baggage, which is why, in part, it has been so hard to treat and too often ignored by doctors.

Pain can be acute or chronic. Acute pain is sudden or urgent, whereas chronic pain is long-standing, typically beyond three months. Acute pain is usually a straightforward response to a discernible injury. It serves a clear function: to grab our attention and teach us a lesson about avoiding potentially harmful stimuli in the future.

Chronic pain, however, can be a misfire of the body's central nervous system (CNS), which can be particularly bewildering because the persistent pain serves no obvious purpose. In some cases, though, the cause may be less a misfire and more a stubborn mystery until scientific understanding advances enough to solve it. Until then, any insights into why a person's system has gone haywire remain buried in complexities that have baffled the best minds in science and medicine since ancient times.

While writing this book, I was reminded of something I learned as a child: humans have a tendency to try and find lessons in awful situations, to try and make sense of them. They search for meaning in misery, a moral to the story that sometimes leads to blaming themselves. Yet when it comes to chronic pain, there's often no lesson to be learned and no blame to be placed. Sometimes pain is just that—pain. Nothing more.

Yet this hasn't kept societies from marginalizing and ignoring those who suffer from pain, in particular due to four chronic conditions: migraine, fibromyalgia, irritable bowel syndrome, and endometriosis. These conditions, among others, are often thought of as "invisible" or "silent," not only because the symptoms aren't always obvious but also because testing often doesn't reveal anything abnormal. For most mainstream medicine, that means there's nothing clear-cut to treat. The unfortunate—and incorrect—inference is that if the best medical minds can't solve the problem, the problem probably "doesn't really exist."

The lack of an objective standard of pain has even given rise to the term *subjective suffering,* which suggests that one person's pain is open to another's interpretation. Too often, this leads to dismissive attitudes toward those suffering from chronic pain. Some people judge them as personally failing or not trying hard enough to get over it. Others might see their complaints as a ruse to get drugs or to get out of work. But for those of us in health care whose aim is to relieve suffering—measurable or not—the fact that pain is subjective does not mean that it isn't real. It's just more enigmatic.

One reason I wanted to write this book is because some members of my own family suffer from chronic pain, and being immersed in their experiences has taught me a lot. For example, I have seen firsthand how challenging it is for them to navigate the health care system, even with my help. I have personally witnessed remarkably talented doctors being dismissive of their symptoms, even after reviewing detailed records of their near-daily pain.

This is problematic, of course, but it's also an indicator of how complicated the problem is. What I've learned from my patients, colleagues, and family members, as well as from my own experience, is that pain and suffering can present in infinite ways, and yet we have tremendous control in choosing how we'll respond. We can not only change our relationship with pain, we can change pain itself.

That's what this book is about.

In the pages ahead, you will learn things you can start doing today—physically, nutritionally, mentally, and behaviorally—that can greatly reduce the chance of developing pain in the future. Some of it may surprise you. For example, you may have heard of rest, ice, compression, elevation treatment, known as RICE, to help with an injury. Increasingly, the evidence is instead pointing us toward MEAT—movement, exercise, analgesia, treatment. This amid a flurry of other tweaks and catchy acronyms over the years, including POLICE (protection, optimal loading, ice, compression, elevation), PEACE (protection, elevation, avoid anti-inflammatories, compression, education), and LOVE (load, optimism, vascularization, exercise). The thing these strategies all have in common is the emphasis on letting your body's natural healing processes work normally, rather than interrupting or rushing to manipulate them.

I will explain later why this is so important, but the headline is that not all inflammation is necessarily bad. And among the most critical tools you will need are muscle-massage foam rollers, which with regular use can diminish your chances of pain, especially after a soft tissue injury. As you will learn, the thin connective tissue called fascia, which surrounds all our muscles, can get painfully stiff and tight throughout your life, so keeping it loose and flexible with those rollers is critically important. There is also new, encouraging data emerging on acupuncture, trigger point injections, and hands-on physical manipulation as well. And what about substances like cannabis and cannabinoids such as cannabidiol (CBD), ketamine, and the broad class of psychedelics? I'll examine the research we have so far on all of these, as well as the case for some natural pain relieving supplements.

With emerging evidence-based science, medical advances, and our own wisdom, we can rewrite the story of pain, as well as our own lifelong potential for managing it—and often preventing it. I'm ready to show you how.

While conducting dozens of interviews for this book, I saw firsthand that experts in pain science and medicine are impatient to see change in the understanding, diagnosis, and treatment of pain. In fact, over the past several years, despite increased spending on pain and new approaches to it, from better imaging technology to new drugs and surgical options, the prevalence and impact of chronic pain have worsened. A consortium pain task force white paper laid out these four reasons why:

1. Both patients and medical practitioners labor under the mistaken idea that most pain problems can be fixed ... with a drug or procedure.
2. Medical school and graduate courses still emphasize ... opioid medications rather than considering other options.
3. The business model of medicine ... has promoted simplistic solutions to complex problems.
4. Patients are often regarded as passive participants, with little emphasis placed on self-care, pain prevention, or therapies that engage self-care strategies, despite demonstrated (lasting) benefit.

These four barriers can be overcome. And I am optimistic that the field of pain is ripe for massive change. Why? Because we—both patients and doctors—are at the dawn of a new era in the way we understand and respond to pain.

Here are some key takeaways I explain in the upcoming chapters:

- The brain "creates" pain, but it also has the capacity to profoundly change our experience of pain, reducing or even eliminating it.

- Because we have unique pain signatures in our own brain waves, highly personalized pain treatments may be possible.
- Your brain responds to sensory nerve signals by activating neural circuitry, which triggers physiological changes throughout the body. This two-way brain-body interaction creates opportunities for changing pain circuitry and chemistry.
- Gender, racial, and other systemic biases and inequities in pain treatment are now in the spotlight. A broad recognition of those biases will pave the way for more effective and individualized care.
- Advances in technology, including AI assists for pain assessment and management, are charting a new path for safer, more precise, and effective treatments.
- There is more evidence than ever before about the benefits of sleep, a healthy diet, exercise, mindfulness-based pain management (MBPM), myofascial therapy, yoga, and specialized psychotherapies, and as a result more doctors are focusing on them.

And most encouraging of all:

- The push is on from all corners to bring a dose of reality to pain research, with new efforts to conduct treatment trials. Instead of pain sufferers being minimized, they are increasingly sought out to share their experiences, including being added to research committees and advisory boards. This is a long overdue acknowledgment that we should always start by listening to patients to understand their unique problems and needs.

If you've read anything about pain over the past twenty years, you have likely been angered by the opioid epidemic, a tragedy fueled by ignorance, arrogance, and greed. Like me, you have probably been saddened at seeing lives destroyed or devastated by addiction. I was a young trainee in neurosurgery at the beginning of the epidemic and followed it closely as a doctor and journalist—but there's an untold part of that story I want to share.

Because opioids have consumed most of the conversation, most people don't even realize there are plenty of other effective options to help relieve pain. While I was writing this book, the FDA approved a new non-opioid pain medication for the first time in more than twenty-five years, and nowadays there are entire emergency room systems that use hardly any opioids. (I'll take you inside one to understand how it was done and what it means for the future of pain management.)

Some elements of pain relief and prevention have actually been around a long time, in the form of ancient healing practices handed down over thousands of years. Despite being effective for many people, they have too often been unfairly dismissed from serious consideration by Western medicine. I will explain how to apply some of these traditions to our daily lives. Finally, there have been breathtaking breakthroughs in pain management that would have been unimaginable only a few years ago. Modern science and ancient wisdom have collectively begun to crack the code on pain. You can too.

As you read the book, remember this. We are the most essential experts on our own pain. If we pay close attention to our own bodies, strategies to address our pain come into clearer focus. Each of us has inner resources that can help prevent or reduce pain now and for the rest of our lives. This begins with connections—between doctor and patient, within families, and among communities of caring. But the most important connection is the one within us, between body and brain.

Prevention is often the most powerful antidote to pain, giving you a range of ways to control your risk for acute and chronic pain. In this book, I'll recommend some tips and strategies that may reduce your vulnerability, strengthen your resilience to pain, and, when it does occur, work with the fullest range of tools to heal more readily.

I'll begin by reframing your understanding of pain, so you and your health care providers can intervene in the way your brain and body process those signals.

PART 1

The New Science of Pain

CHAPTER 1

Pain Comes Home

Not too long ago, I was skiing with my kids on their spring break when my mother called. As a trauma neurosurgeon and medical reporter, I'm always on call, and there are several people who can reach me any time of the day or night—among them, my wife, Rebecca; the chairman of neurosurgery at Emory University Hospital; the breaking-news producer for CNN; and, of course, my mom. She knew I was on the slopes, so I was concerned at seeing her number pop up. I pushed my helmet away from my ear and said hello, and she got straight to the point, no pleasantries. In a completely even tone, she said, "I broke my back."

My eighty-two-year-old mother, who's hardly ever been sick a day in her life, had fallen. It was a simple fall. She had lost her balance while rolling her suitcase and toppled backward, landing in a sitting position. It hurt, and afterward her back felt sore, but she didn't think much of it until the pain persisted. Despite massaging her back, resting it, icing it, and even heating it for a few days, the pain wouldn't go away. So nearly a week after the injury, she went to get an X-ray, which showed a fracture in the lower back, known as the lumbar spine.

The fact that Mom called at all was an indicator of how serious the situation was. She doesn't complain about anything. She wears adversity like a badge of honor, something to brag about later, usually while showing off a scar or a bruise. She declined to use an epidural during childbirth and is surprised that anyone else is surprised by that. When she had breast cancer thirty years ago, she treated it like a blip on the radar. It came and went, and she rarely talked about it. She takes no medications, bounds out of bed in the morning, and regularly outworks her grandkids, rising earlier and staying up later than they do, cleaning the kitchen, cooking meals, and still making it to many of their school performances. Mom is the one regularly urging us to do more. Since I was a child, I envisioned her in constant motion, never sitting still. She has always been a human in a hurry.

I never imagined my mom injured, sick, or frail. So when I got the call that something was wrong and heard a tone in her voice I'd never heard before, it worried me.

I flew straight to Florida to see her, and over the next few days, I reviewed her images, spoke with her doctors, and helped determine the best course of therapy. When I first arrived, she was in so much pain she could barely get out of bed. Up until that point, my mom had barely seemed to age, but now her cheeks were hollowed and the wrinkles around her eyes were more pronounced. She winced with every movement, leading me to jump out of my chair to try and help her, even though I wasn't sure what I could do.

Mom had a fracture of the first vertebra in her lumbar spine. The human spine has three sections. The cervical spine, or neck area, has seven vertebrae. The thoracic area behind the chest has twelve more vertebrae, each one generally corresponding with a pair of ribs. And the lumbar spine, which attaches to the sacrum, situated between the hip bones of the pelvis, has five more.

With the type of injury my mom had, the first branch of the decision tree is typically: surgical versus nonsurgical. Is operating the best option? For some injuries, such as a large collection of blood on the brain or a ruptured appendix, surgery is more clearly warranted. It was a bit more nuanced in my mom's case, however.

In medical parlance, she had an L1 compression fracture, meaning the bone had been compressed or flattened from its normal cube shape to that of a pancake. Luckily, she was "neurologically intact," meaning she had no weakness or numbness and was able to use the bathroom normally. Her predominant symptom was pain, and that generated another set of questions.

- Was the pain so bad that nonoperative pain measures, such as medications or physical therapy, would be inadequate or intolerable?
- How long was the pain expected to last while the fracture healed, and could she tolerate it for that long?
- Might her age and bone health affect that healing time, possibly prolonging it—along with the pain?
- And most important, would an operation actually help alleviate that pain?

My mom left little doubt how she would answer that first question. "I cannot live like this," she told me. I knew the excruciating pain could be expected to last at least a couple of months, which would feel like a lifetime for her. I also knew she wasn't interested in taking high doses of opioid pain medications. She's small and thin, and whenever she has taken such medications in the past, they've left her zombified, complicating her recovery. Finally, she made it clear that she didn't want an aggressive operation, given her age and frailty.

So, along with her doctors, we landed on a relatively new approach to deal with her pain, a minimally invasive procedure known as kyphoplasty. I was very familiar with the procedure and had written scientific papers about how it was performed. This is how I explained it to my mom:

Picture a cardboard box. Now imagine that box crushed from the top down. As you visualize it, you'll realize that two things happen simultaneously: the box loses its height and it gains width. That's what happened to the vertebra in my mom's back, and that's what was causing her pain.

With kyphoplasty, the surgeon inserts a hollow needle through the skin and into the broken bone, then slowly advances a small balloon through the needle's opening. Once the balloon is in the bone, the surgeon inflates it. As the balloon enlarges, the bone starts to regain its normal height. X-rays make it possible to assess when the bone looks close to normal again, and then the balloon can be deflated and removed. The final step is to use that same hollow needle to inject a dollop of hot liquid cement, which quickly hardens and helps the vertebra maintain its normal anatomy.

The data suggested that kyphoplasty would help restore the height and reduce the width of my mom's flattened bone, so after much discussion, we scheduled the procedure for her. "How likely is this to help, Sanjay?" she asked. It was a fair question but difficult to answer. One of the biggest challenges in medicine is trying to insert the highest level of certainty into a probabilistic discipline. The truth was that I had a good feeling about the procedure, but I couldn't be sure about the outcome. She understood.

On the morning of her procedure, as we were driving to the hospital, she looked at me and said, "If this doesn't help with the pain, I think my time here on earth is done." It was devastating to hear. My tough mom, who had lived in refugee camps during her childhood and still went on to become the first woman hired as an automotive engineer at Ford Motor Company, now seemed so weak. And there was no doubt it was the pain that was making her feel this way. That is the thing about pain. When you are in agony, it is all-encompassing, robbing my mom of the ability to simply imagine a future.

Thankfully the procedure, which took about an hour, went well. And, quite remarkably, she felt almost instantaneous relief. In all honesty, it's still not completely clear to me (or to many of the doctors who perform the procedure) why kyphoplasty is so effective at alleviating pain. Is it because the anatomy of the broken bone has been restored? Or is it, as her surgeon suggested, that the warmed cement heats up and dulls the nerve fibers that provide sensation to the bone? It certainly seemed that a significant amount of her pain relief was psychological, because the procedure had provided a much needed dose of hope. Things were finally moving in the right direction for my mom, and that alone likely gave her some comfort.

Whatever the case, she immediately reduced her pain score from "I want to die" to a 3 out of 10. Her mood improved, not only because she was in less pain but also because she no longer needed powerful pain medications. While the narcotics had initially helped with the pain, they had also caused her to become depressed. They made her constipated, which took away her appetite, and because she wasn't eating, she had become lethargic. It was a vicious cycle.

All of that changed when she got the pain under better control. Over the next few days I spent with her, first in the hospital and then at home, I was reminded that everything is connected—her symptoms, her pain, her very self. She was soon like a new woman, with a new lease on life. Even though she had been near suicidal a week earlier, on the day I left her she was whistling in the kitchen as she cooked.

Pain's Complexity Holds Opportunities

Pain is an incredibly elaborate biological process, but it is also mostly a product of the mind.

The stubborn puzzle of pain persists in part because all pain is generated in the brain, and the brain is a complex organ. Even after thirty years of practicing neurosurgery, I am still regularly fascinated, delighted, and bewildered by the human brain.

Here's what we do know: Pain does not start where you might think, at the broken bone in your wrist or your twisted ankle. It begins when your brain scrambles to make sense of the sudden new signals coming from these injured places. Your brain rapidly tethers new information to existing information such as previous similar exposures, corresponding expectations, social norms, and other sensory data. Looking down and seeing blood on your hands, for example, will in all likelihood objectively worsen your pain.

Now imagine your brain trying to decipher all that incoming information in just a split second. On top of that, it has to instantly determine whether the information is accurate, authentic, and noteworthy, or if there's a component of "fake news" (to steal a term from my other field of journalism). It's why a child may not cry out in pain until he sees the look of concern on a parent's face. He's looking to a trusted source to interpret the significance of the sensation.

When you anticipate pain—say, at the first sight of a needle—your brain primes for a pain response, even if whatever follows next might not objectively cause pain. As "danger or distress" signals travel to the brain through nerve fibers in the spinal cord, they're upregulated or downregulated—meaning, given more or less importance. It's as if the brain is scrolling a social media feed, then suddenly comes across something incendiary. If that alarming message comes from a familiar, reliable source the brain trusts, that message gets immediately prioritized—amplified. If it's a garbage source, the message may be minimized or even ignored.

As the brain tries to make sense of all this new information, it may sometimes send out convoluted, imprecise pain signals. Typically, the brain gets it right, but more times than you might realize, it misinterprets pain because it doesn't quite recognize or trust the source.

One example is something known as *referred pain*. This is the response that makes your jaw ache when you're having a heart attack or gives you a "brain freeze" when extreme cold touches the top of your mouth. In that case, the brain's imprecision might cause you to clutch the sides of your head when the better solution would be to press your warm tongue against your cold palate. The brain can even create a very real experience of pain in a body part that no longer exists due to amputation or other loss, a phenomenon called "phantom limb" pain.

Regardless of what's happening in the rest of your body, it is your brain that decides how much to turn up the pain, whether to turn it off completely, or maybe even to create pain for seemingly no reason whatsoever. Your brain's response is dependent partly on your genes, but it might arise from the most surprisingly arbitrary things. What you had for lunch might influence how much pain you suffer by dinnertime. Whether you had a good call with your mom or your boss could do the same thing. If you've lived a life with pain, then you and pain have a history, and for better or for worse, that could affect how much pain you have in the present. For those who've suffered adverse childhood experiences, that can be a setup for a life of increased pain sensitivity.

Interestingly, there are also people with significant pain tolerance at the other end of the spectrum. Some of the same factors described above, including your genetics, can decrease your chances of developing or feeling intense pain. When I was a surgical resident, I once had an equestrian show up in the ER with a badly fractured hip. He wasn't even planning on getting it checked out until his wife insisted. The hip is a ball-and-socket joint, and when we saw his X-ray, the ball was completely out of the socket, which was smashed into several pieces. And yet he was itching to be discharged as quickly as possible.

The point is that the brain creates pain on cue from a vast array of stimuli—biological, psychological, social, emotional, environmental, even cultural. And just as we now understand that the brain can be nurtured, developed, and optimized at any age, there's growing evidence that the brain can also rewire itself in ways that change the neural circuitry for pain, reducing its intensity or duration and potentially eliminating it altogether.

For all these reasons, pain can be hard to predict, measure, diagnose, and treat, and as a result, wildly different approaches may work for one individual versus another. Many treatments fail entirely for reasons no one can explain, and others provide an unanticipated burst of relief. The subjective quality of pain has always been described as the fundamental problem with treating it, but after this experience with my mom, I realized it could also be part of the solution.

Think of it as harnessing the untapped power of your own biology. This may involve a variety of approaches, including medications and procedures, as well as nonmedical ones like exercise, nutrition, and breathing techniques. Additionally, psychological approaches are increasingly being recognized and recommended as a first response rather than a last resort. For example, a visit to a psychologist both before and after surgery is increasingly being used to promote optimal recovery and minimize the risk that acute pain will turn into chronic pain. And with chronic pain patients, psychological therapy has helped manage pain enough so that sufferers can avoid unnecessary surgery, reduce the need for medication, and feel they are living a full life.

The Promise and Possibility of Personalized Pain Treatment

As I write this chapter, my mom is still recovering. She recently ditched her cane, and before that her walker. Now she's back to her brisk morning walks, though she's always clutching my dad's hand while doing so. We talk regularly, and after getting through medical updates, I've asked how the whole episode affected her. I listened intently as my mom, never especially self-reflective in the past, described the loss of control she felt when her pain was calling the shots. I saw someone far more human than the pioneering engineer I grew up with. I saw a vulnerability that was at once frightening and deeply bonding. I don't know what would've happened had the procedure not worked and whether she was serious about wanting to end her life. But I do know that for so many of the people I spoke with for this book, that negotiation is a constant one.

What I can tell you is that in my mom's case, our discussions themselves and the optimism they nurtured became part of her healing experience. Simply talking made her feel better, and my listening validated her pain and reminded her how much she was loved. Through these conversations, she also felt the need to share what was happening as she worked through her pain, and how she had become open to new approaches for its management. Once she was on the mend, she became focused on preventing an episode like this from ever happening again. For example, she wanted to incorporate everyday ways to improve her balance (including better ways to get that suitcase to the car!) and get herself in better shape to weather pain of any kind with greater intention. I was all for it. I'd learned my own lesson from her experience as well, and felt changed by it.

As much as I was able to bring medical expertise to my mother's situation, I realized that when it came to her pain, what I was seeing and hearing from her—the subjective experience so often discounted—provided the most valuable insight. Her personal experience was absolutely essential for me and her doctors to know. To someone who's suffering, pain is an objective fact, but the subjective nature of it makes every person an expert on their own pain.

The human body has a remarkable capacity for healing if we simply let it. This isn't meant to replace medical advice, but to share a perspective encouraging you to think differently about pain. The way to do this is by paying close attention to our unique pain experiences, listening intently to what our bodies are telling us, and intervene only when necessary.

To do this, we need to first understand the language of pain.

CHAPTER 2

Tell Me about Your Pain

HOW WE TALK ABOUT PAIN, HOW WE LISTEN, AND WHY IT MATTERS

The flagstone path that leads from the rear door of Wendy Miller's century-old Maryland house to her backyard studio is typically an easy walk. But lately, Miller's first steps along that path every morning have ignited deep pain where a knee injury has been slow to heal.

A long personal experience of chronic pain has informed Miller's work as an art therapist. On a recent morning, she gently seats herself in a chair across from a table and couch, waiting for a client to arrive for a therapy session. On the table sits an array of waxy, colorful oil pastel sticks and a blank sheet of paper. The client, an accomplished artist in her late forties, will sketch as they talk, conveying through drawings a dimension of the daily pain she suffers.

The woman arrives and takes her seat on the couch. She plucks an oil pastel stick from the tray and reflects for a moment. The idea that you can tap into past experience to express yourself is not news to an artist. In this case, she draws from an inner palette of pain that helps her convey her suffering in ways modern medicine generally does not recognize or appreciate.

As the woman sketches and shades on the paper, Miller occasionally responds and observes the composition take shape. Sometimes the images are similar to those the woman has drawn in previous sessions. Certain elements—animals, shapes, patterns, placements—recur each time.

"She would create a composition and then she would fill it in, the way you would fill in a predesigned coloring book," Miller told me. "As I observed her carefully and quietly, I began to understand that her artworks were intentionally multilayered with a pattern of meaning. Sometimes she was drawing shapes and colors about her physical pain, sometimes about her emotional pain, and sometimes about a past history of traumatic pain. As she talked, I could see which layer she went to, and we would talk about it. Each type of pain was always a certain color."

The roughly sketched blocks, strips, and organic shapes carefully overlaying one another were a reflection of how this woman's chronic pain commanded constant attention and strategic planning in every aspect of her life. She used bold colors and intense lines to represent her irritable bowel syndrome (IBS). Other layers represented her childhood experience and the secrets she had to keep about her parents' alcoholism.

"The intensity of those painful experiences was expressed more through a jagged use of line and color, a crisscrossing of markings which would go in different directions or filled-in shapes," Miller told me. "In other drawings, these sensations from childhood trauma were expressed in threats of wide-opened animals' mouths or teeth juxtaposed toward one another."

I was reminded of the renowned Mexican painter Frida Kahlo, who famously said, "My painting carries with it the message of pain," referring to her self-portraits spanning decades of deteriorating health from massive injuries she suffered in a bus accident when she was eighteen. Just forty-seven when she died in 1954, Kahlo painted her pain in raw, tortured imagery, including the countless operations, orthopedic corsets and contraptions that immobilized her, and other treatments that likely made her pain worse. Kahlo was often described as a surrealist painter, but she rejected the label, saying: "I don't paint dreams or nightmares. I paint my own reality."

Every picture tells a story, especially when it comes to each person's unique pain experience. Not only can art convey the type and intensity of pain someone is suffering, it may also give a sense of the extent to which pain has overwhelmed their life.

"The problem is that most clinicians speak only one language," Miller says. Chronic pain, however, is twisted and tangled, layered with emotions alongside the physical pain, and art therapy, or others such as dance or music therapy, move beyond the confines of the purely clinical conversation. I've often heard the most vivid descriptions of pain from patients when I invite them to use imagery—whatever comes to mind—to describe how their pain feels. Drawing enabled this woman to respond in her own way to the universal question that begins every clinical pain conversation: *Tell me about your pain.*

Taking the Measure of Pain: Conversation Is Key

Medical evaluations usually begin with measurements: height, weight, body temperature, pulse rate, blood pressure, blood work. These data points set the table for assessing the patient's complaints, and sometimes they even reveal issues the patient hasn't yet recognized. They help both patient and physician understand whatever problems we're dealing with and what steps we might take to alleviate them. When pain is the problem, however, how do you even begin to take its measure? How can you assess something that everyone experiences differently?

In many ways, pain remains as inscrutable today as it has ever been. Eavesdropping with a stethoscope, which doctors use to listen to sounds inside the body, yields nothing about the intensity, duration, or location of pain. It provides no clues about what aggravates or relieves that pain or to what extent it impinges on your everyday activity—all considered essential measures for an accurate diagnosis and treatment plan.

It's frustrating that with all the extraordinary medical technology at our fingertips, when it comes to evaluating pain, we often reach for a visual aid based on smiley and frowny face cartoon images. There must be a better way.

So, where to begin?

Questions, Clues, and Other Tools of the Pain Detective

I'm used to reviewing lots of information about my patients. They show up in my office with lab results, imaging studies, detailed medical histories, and full reports of neurological exams. Even observing how they walk in the door—which limb they may favor, whether they stand upright or are stooped over—provides clues. I glean information about their nervous system by observing the strength of their shoulder shrugs and how long they can stand on their toes. I spend a lot of time asking questions, and even more time listening to the answers—not just the words but the tone and the emphasis in their voices.

Almost thirty years ago, Dr. Regina Fink at the University of Colorado took the art of the patient's pain history to a different level. In an attempt to create an objective measurement, she developed a quick-list questionnaire called WILDA, which stands for words, intensity, location, duration, and aggravating and alleviating factors.

WILDA struck a chord because it creates a conversational structure that organizes pertinent information. It uses consistent language as a bridge between clinician and patient and provides carefully designed questions any provider can use as prompts. In my own experience this has meant that every new generation of medical students and residents, as well as established providers in different specialties, can consistently characterize a patient's pain. Many doctors even carry a card-sized copy of it in their white-coat pocket.

It starts with the first words someone uses to describe their pain. These become the initial GPS coordinates as we begin to map our way to the source.

The WILDA Pain Assessment Guide—DIY

Pain Assessment Guide

Tell me about your pain

Words to describe pain

aching	throbbing	shooting
stabbing	gnawing	sharp
tender	burning	exhausting
tiring	penetrating	nagging
numb	miserable	unbearable
dull	radiating	squeezing
crampy	deep	pressure

Pain in other languages

itami	Japanese	dolor	Spanish
tong	Chinese	douleur	French
dau	Vietnamese	bolno	Russian

Intensity (0–10)

if 0 is no pain and 10 is the worst pain imaginable, what is your pain now? . . . in the last 24 hours?

Location

Where is your pain?

Duration

Is the pain always there?
Does the pain come and go? (Breakthrough Pain)
Do you have both types of pain?

Aggravating and Alleviating Factors

What makes the pain better?
What makes the pain worse?

How does pain affect

sleep	energy	relationships
appetite	activity	mood

Are you esperiencing any other symptoms?

nausea/vomiting	itching	urinary retention
constipation	sleepiness/confusion	weakness

Things to check

Vital signs, past medication history, knowledge of pain and use of noninvasive techniques

A pocket card for health care providers summarizes the WILDA approach to pain assessment. Copyright 1996, Regina Fink, University of Colorado Health Sciences Center.

Words: Let Your Body Speak

Choose your words carefully. *Aching* versus *shooting* can be an indication that a person's back pain is due to a muscle spasm rather than a pinched nerve. *Dull* can mean a persistent throb, whereas *numb* may refer to a sensation brought on by cold or a loss of feeling. I often invite my patients to use imagery—for example, "It feels like a wolf has bitten down on my knee," a woman with a large, painful, and infected hematoma once told me. "He bites harder and there's shooting pain. And when I move, he sinks his teeth deeper and grinds."

Intensity: How Bad Does It Hurt?

Intensity remains the most subjective part of the WILDA assessment. Those frowny face cartoons and number scales do have value if context is provided to show what the numbers mean. Asking about the impact of pain on relationships, appetite, mood, and sleep can provide a sense of intensity. The reality is that pain often infringes on your life, even if you don't always recognize it.

Pain that wakes you up from sleep is classified as particularly intense. It is considered worse than daytime pain, because it is able to overwhelm your brain's powerful sleeping circuits.

The most common pain scale has you rate your pain from 0 to 10, with 0 meaning no pain and 10 meaning the "worst pain imaginable." Yes, that's a subjective measure, but it's still a helpful detail that allows you and your health care provider to monitor changes over time to see how effective a treatment is, or how your pain may be changing. Generally, an exact number (1–10) to quantify your pain isn't as essential as identifying the range. Lower numbers indicate lighter pain. I'll often ask patients, "Is the pain nagging but not interfering with your daily life? If you're aware of pain but still able to do the things you enjoy, that might be characterized as mild pain, or levels 1 to 3."

Moderate pain (4–6) is more restrictive. If you find yourself canceling events or social gatherings because of pain, your level is probably at least a 5. If you can no longer reliably concentrate, such as even reading this book, it rises to a 6 or 7.

Level 8 is where we get into severe pain, the type that will wake you up or prevent you from falling asleep in the first place. At level 9, your ability to be physically active is greatly impaired. And the worst pain, level 10, disrupts life entirely, often causing delirium and uncontrollable moaning.

Sometimes a lack of sensation can also be a descriptive clue. In my practice, I've treated patients who didn't even realize they had areas of numbness until I ran a steel instrument along the side of their foot and they couldn't feel it. One time, a patient came in with terribly infected blisters on his pinky toe that he hadn't even noticed.

Location: Where Does it Hurt?

When identifying the source of pain, the most obvious answer is often the correct one. But sometimes it's just one point along a pain signal's circuitous path through the nervous system.

A familiar example is the left arm and shoulder pain that accompanies a myocardial infarction (or heart attack). Although the site of the pain is the left arm, the source is the heart. In experiencing that type of pain, you might not initially think of your heart, but that's the nature of referred pain. It can trick you.

This is especially true of pain that involves the head and neck. Dr. Saper in Michigan once told me about a man who came to him with severe pain behind his right eye. The man had been seen by many ophthalmologists and other specialists, and no one could find the source of his pain. "Everybody had looked, and we did too—what the hell is wrong with his eye or behind his eye?" Saper said. "We eventually found it was coming from a herniated disc in his neck. The disc had triggered these nerve pathways, and the man was very much feeling the pain in his right eye." Confusion around referred pain is one reason so many unnecessary scans are performed as we look for sources of pain in the wrong places.

Different sources can also cause pain in the same region. Sinus pain is often described as head pain. Kidney pain can show up as back pain. And more than you would believe, hip pain is mistaken for generalized abdominal pain—which, as you can imagine, leads to entirely different tests and treatment. To figure out the specific location of my patients' pain, I often have them stop, close their eyes, take a few calming breaths, and then point at what they believe is the source of their pain. My goal is to help them focus directly on their pain while disentangling it from other factors. I've been surprised many times when the places patients point to are different from what's reflected in their medical chart.

But that may also be because some types of pain migrate, moving from one part of the body to another—just one more confounding factor in diagnosing pain. Migratory pain is common in a number of chronic conditions, including arthritis, lupus, and other autoimmune diseases, and it's a signature symptom of fibromyalgia, a chronic condition that causes widespread pain throughout the body or in multiple parts at different times. Migrating pain can also be caused by chronic inflammation or by factors as simple as overexertion, dehydration, and poor sleep, all of which can worsen inflammation in different ways.

Duration: How Long Has it Hurt?

This can be a tricky question. You may have noticed the pain after a specific injury and you can recall the time it occurred. But thinking back you may realize you felt a lesser ache sometime earlier and it has only now become bothersome. Time also can mean very different things to different people. When you're in the throes of pain, time becomes warped, sometimes seeming to slow or even stop. For some people, a burst of pain may mean several minutes, and for others a few hours. It's important to drill down on how long such bursts really last because the answer may help determine whether they're a result of pain medications wearing off, a recurring physical problem, or something else entirely. Questions about duration help to establish whether pain is constant, intermittent, true breakthrough pain that comes and goes, or some combination of all these.

Chronic pain is often defined as pain persisting for three months or more, because that's the point at which acute pain from an injury or tissue damage would ordinarily resolve itself. Another definition sets the timer at six months in which pain has been present for 50 percent or more days. Either way, when pain extends beyond these points, especially if no discernible physical cause has been found, treatment considerations tend to shift to other possible causes, sometimes psychological.

Many pain experts now recommend psychological therapy as a first response rather than a last resort for pain management, the idea being the sooner the better. Because no matter what cause is eventually found, the brain is processing those signals through the full range of neural networks that also process cognitive, emotional, and sensory input—all of which may be creating or coloring the pain experience more intensely. Therapy can alter how you process pain sensations.

Patterns and Types of Pain

Though everyone experiences pain differently, common patterns provide a way to talk about and respond to it based on familiar coordinates: frequency, duration, intensity, and the likely source.

Some of these distinctions continue to be the subject of debate in the international community of pain scientists, but this simple breakdown describes the main types of pain as they're generally described by the National Institute of Neurological Disorders and Stroke, the International Association for the Study of Pain, and American Chronic Pain Association and Stanford Medicine Resource Guide to Chronic Pain Management.

Pain can be acute, chronic, or episodic, based on how long it lasts and its frequency:

- Acute pain is recent, typically starts suddenly, and ends when the cause is resolved. The feeling of acute pain is usually sharp or severe because it tends to act as a warning signal about a threat to the body from an injury, disease, overuse, or other environmental stress. Common causes for acute pain are strained muscles, broken bones, dental work, surgery, childbirth, infections, and burns.
- Episodic or flare-up pain happens from time to time and may come at irregular intervals. It may be associated with a long-term medical condition, such as sickle cell disease or cancer, or a change in treatment. It can also be caused by stress or by emotions such as anxiety, worry, anger, or fear. Chronic migraine and painful menstrual periods are examples of episodic pain. So is gout, a type of inflammatory arthritis that causes joint pain and swelling in flares that last a week or two. Episodic pain may be caused by known triggers but also can arise without an obvious cause.

- Chronic (or persistent) pain is described as pain that continues beyond three months, or past the expected healing time of an injury or other tissue damage or inflammation. In some cases, an acute pain condition might persist and become chronic pain. In other cases, chronic pain happens for no identifiable physical reason. Someone might experience one or more chronic pain conditions, called *co-occurring* or *coexisting* conditions, *comorbidities*, or they might experience chronic and acute pain at the same time.

Pain can also be described in categories based on its most likely source. In many cases, it fits into more than one of these categories:

- Nociceptive pain: Considered the most common type of pain, nociceptive pain has a protective purpose: it's an alarm system to alert us to tissue injury or damage and/or inflammation. Tissue injury may be *somatic* (arising from injury to muscles, skin, bones, and joints) or *visceral*, arising from internal organs. Inflammation is a natural biological response produced by the tissues within our body as a reaction to harmful stimuli and to start the repair process. Pain from inflammation may be chronic or acute; the sensation can be sharp, pricking, dull, or aching, depending on what caused the damage. Examples of nociceptive pain are pain from a paper cut, an infection, a broken bone, burns, or osteoarthritis.
- Neuropathic pain: This is pain caused by abnormal nerve function or nerve damage due to an injury or disease. Neuropathic pain sensations are often described as burning, numbness or tingling, shooting pain, or electric-like shocks. Examples of conditions that cause neuropathic pain are diabetic neuropathy, shingles, sciatica, and complex regional pain syndrome.
- Neuroplastic pain, also called nociplastic, noninflammatory, or nonneuropathic pain: In the case of neuroplastic pain, it is

the brain's processing circuitry that is most likely the culprit. Search as hard as we might, and we are unlikely to find any evidence of a clear injury or tissue damage driving the pain in the first place. Even how the sufferer perceives the pain can vary wildly, from burning to dull, such as someone might have with widespread back pain that changes throughout the day. Of course phantom limb pain would be a clear cut example, but fibromyalgia and irritable bowel syndrome fit the criteria as well.

Aggravating and Alleviating Factors: What Makes It Better (or Worse)?

Equally important are the alleviating and aggravating factors that make pain better or worse—for example, standing, sitting, or reclining. People who have pain due to poor blood flow in their lower extremities feel better when they hang their legs over the side of the bed. A herniated disc in the lower back can cause a blast of pain when raising the leg straight up from a lying position. And if you see someone hunched over a shopping cart in the grocery store, they might be trying to subconsciously create space in their back around a pinched nerve in the lumbar spine. All of these factors can provide hints as to what might be causing the pain.

Figuring out how pain behaves at different times of day can also be important. Sinus headaches tend to be worse in the morning because your sinuses don't drain as well if you've been lying down all night. Evening headaches often result from the consequences of your day—factors such as muscle tension, dehydration, too much caffeine, or skipping meals. There's even something called hypnic headaches, which seem to occur only when people enter certain stages of sleep. They tend to strike between 1:00 a.m. and 3:00 a.m., leading to their nickname: the "alarm clock headache." There's no blood test or imaging study to confirm a diagnosis of hypnic headaches.

Only a detailed history and conversation would lead patient and physician down that path.

We also know that mental, emotional, and physical pain are tightly linked. Patients in the midst of a depressive episode, for example, are likely to report higher pain scores after surgery. As a result, many surgeons have their own predictions on who's likely to do well after an operation and who will probably have more challenges based on factors not directly related to the surgical problem.

As anyone who has had joint problems knows, weather conditions can trigger certain kinds of pain. The theory is that changes in barometric pressure and temperature can expand soft tissue, increase inflammation, and decrease circulation, any or all of which can cause pain. If you're one of the many who experience weather-related aches and pains, don't forget to mention it to your doctor. It may be a useful clue.

Figuring out pain sources can feel like a Sherlock Holmesian whodunit, with Holmes and Watson sifting through clues and notes to find the culprit. While conducting research for this book, I found a pretty consistent predictor for success: a mutual understanding between provider and patients of the pain episodes. While it can be challenging and may take a few attempts, you can achieve this only by finding someone who will listen carefully and taking time to chronicle the story of your pain as fully as you can. WILDA can help you frame that story.

The truth is that conversations about pain have never been the medical profession's strong suit. And it's gotten even worse in recent years as the time available for such discussions has been squeezed ever tighter by mounting administrative demands and the push to see more patients. Reams of paperwork for insurance requirements and increasingly frequent denials cut into time that was once reserved for face-to-face office visits.

"This is one of the reasons pain has not attained the priority as a health condition that it should, given its public health impact," says Roger Fillingim, a clinical psychologist, professor, and founder and director of the Pain Research and Intervention Center of Excellence at the University of Florida. Less time to talk means doctors are often forced to fill in gaps about their patients' pain with their own assumptions or guesstimates, and that's a problem. Studies show that when others try to assess a person's pain, whether they're health care providers or family members and friends, they almost always underestimate it.

This has shortchanged patients in the worst way, leaving them feeling minimized while also limiting critical information that could—and *should*—shape any treatment plan. Especially now, as science has illuminated the biological, psychological, and social factors involved in pain, conversation becomes paramount. The old script simply isn't good enough.

Can We Talk about It?

Dr. Carmen Renée Green, dean of the City College of New York School of Medicine, is a pain medicine physician and professor of anesthesiology with joint appointments in obstetrics and gynecology as well as health management and policy. When I began thinking about this book, Dr. Green was one of the first people I wanted to interview. During my neurosurgery residency, she often gave talks about pain for the residents and faculty, which started to guide my thinking about pain as a far more complicated problem than young surgeons sometimes recognize.

Because Dr. Green supervised the Back and Pain Center at the University of Michigan, we often cared for patients hand in hand. Some had seen several other doctors before coming to us, and we worked to offer them relief. Dr. Green had the rare ability to be empathetic but also relay honest and tough news to her patients.

"Most people are just wanting someone to ask them about their pain," she says. "The number of times that I go into a patient's room, and they say, 'Dr. Green, you're the first person to ask me these questions'—it's astounding." She agrees that assessing pain with numbers is challenging and believes that it becomes even more so because biases often play a role.

For example, it is well documented that Black patients are less likely than white patients to receive pain medications. And even when they *are* given pain medications, they receive lower quantities. In 2016, a University of Virginia research team found that "a substantial number" of white medical students and residents held "false beliefs about biological differences" between Blacks and whites and that those beliefs "predict racial bias in perception and treatment recommendation accuracy." In other words, the study found that white trainees believed Black patients inherently had higher pain thresholds and required fewer pain medications. Again, this was in *2016*.

Racial disparities were found in both the evaluation and treatment process, according to a summary review of patterns of how Black patients report pain and the medical response to it. One study that tracked more than sixteen hundred North Carolina residents with chronic back pain found that even when Blacks reported greater pain than whites, they were still rated by their providers as having less severe pain and were less likely to be offered comprehensive diagnostic and treatment approaches. A review of more than five thousand medical records of patients with degenerative lumbosacral pathology, a disc disease in the lower back, found that ethnicity and gender strongly predicted the type of workup and treatment they received. As an example, minority women were 52 percent less likely than nonminority men to have surgery offered as a treatment option.

Talking Points: How to Talk about Your Pain with Your Provider

Doing a self-assessment before you go to the doctor's office will help you prepare, and it can be used to provide information for any friends or family members who plan to accompany you.

Here are two approaches. Pain stories are by nature detailed and complex, but the WILDA approach (see page 16) offers a simple first step toward better understanding them. The Talking Points questionnaire that follows, based on the Yale Pain Management Collaboratory Coordinating Center guide, offers additional questions expanded with brief tips.

Preparing for a Provider Visit

It's important to share your chronic pain experiences honestly and openly with your providers. Try not to worry about how they'll respond: pain is a universal problem, and most providers have been trained to respond in respectful and appropriate ways to a person's experience of chronic pain, with the goal of working together to develop a treatment plan. It's a good idea to be prepared for questions that providers are likely to ask. In the weeks prior to your appointment, think about the questions that follow. You might also want to jot down notes about your pain experience.

The WILDA questions are designed to help assess your physical pain for purposes of diagnosis and initial treatment options. Other questions, considered part of the "whole person" approach to pain treatment, focus on psychological, social, and emotional aspects of your pain. These are important, too, as you talk with your health care provider about treatment options and how to tailor a plan that prioritizes what's most important to you in everyday life. With that in mind, these questions may help you organize those thoughts.

What factors seem to make your pain better or worse?

Are there situations, activities, foods, or any other variables that make your pain worse? Are there any that make it better? Or even any that make the pain change in other ways—for example, when or where in your body you feel it? The answers to these questions can help guide the discussion between you and your provider about options that might minimize your experience of pain while still maintaining a high level of function.

Are there any factors that have changed recently in your life?
Have you recently had a career shift, loss of job, or retirement? Have you moved or changed living arrangements? Adjustments to life events—even when they're welcome—can be stressful. The same is true for changes in routines or relationships. Have you experienced stressful periods with family, friends, or at work? Any kind of loss? Have your appetite or eating habits changed? All of these factors can influence our moods, our activity levels, social engagement, and how we feel about ourselves, all of which can play a role in our experience of pain.

How do you manage daily activities, work, and other pursuits important to you?
Be prepared to talk about pain strategies that are working well for you and about challenges that call for something different. Is pain keeping you from engaging in activities or interests that matter to you? Think in terms of a plan that supports your involvement in the things that matter most to you and gives you an organized way to adjust those strategies. You want to balance pain management with engagement in activities that are meaningful to you, including work, hobbies, and your involvement with family, friends, and community.

What providers or practitioners are you seeing for pain management?
Be sure that your various health care providers know about each other, as well as any approaches you're trying, so they can think about how they fit into your integrated pain treatment plan. When giving this information to providers, include over-the-counter medications, lifestyle changes, and practices and techniques such as yoga, meditation, and massage.

What goals do you want to accomplish in spite of your pain?
Goals can be extremely helpful to the success of a pain management plan. Setting modest goals each week, or even each day, can lead to

positive behavioral changes, enhancing your quality of life and reducing your pain.

Source: Adapted from the Pain Management Collaboratory, https://painmanagementcollaboratory.org/talking-points-preparing-for-a-provider-visit/.

Sex Differences and Disparities Overlooked for Too Long

A 2021 study revealed that gender played a larger role than previously recognized when it came to perceptions of pain. Some forms of pain are inherently related to fundamental functional differences between the female and male bodies, with childbirth being the most obvious example. But other forms of acute or chronic pain are seen more frequently in women than men as well, including migraine, rheumatological, and musculoskeletal pain, in particular fibromyalgia, according to the study. A recent scoping review covering seventy-eight studies, published in the journal *Pain*, found that of young adults (aged eighteen to twenty-nine) who experience chronic pain—one of the most consistent factors is simply being female. The review, among other studies, notes that anxiety, depression, and sleep issues, all associated with chronic pain, are more prevalent among women.

Fillingim says basic biological distinctions between men and women are routinely overlooked, with women often wrongly dismissed as oversensitive complainers. "It's not that one person is complaining more than the other about the same experience," he says. "It's that these two people are having vastly different experiences." For pain that uniquely belongs to women, attention has been even less forthcoming.

For example, an estimated 70 percent of women will experience musculoskeletal pain due to menopause, a natural midlife stage when estrogen production in the ovaries diminishes and then stops. For one in four, the pain will be disabling. The problem has plagued women but has been overlooked or misunderstood by doctors, who ascribed it simply to aging. Only in 2024 was the constellation of pain symptoms officially recognized with a diagnostic term—*musculoskeletal syndrome of menopause*—legitimizing women's experience and focusing new attention on estrogen replacement or other treatments for the pain.

Some aspects of women's reproductive health procedures, such as insertion of an intrauterine device (IUD), are moderately to intensely painful, yet women haven't traditionally been offered IV sedation for the procedure. In recent years, as increasing numbers of younger women have opted to use IUDs, they've been shocked by the unexpected pain and angered that they weren't warned or given adequate pain medication. No longer willing to suffer in silence, many have gone public, posting videos on TikTok of themselves undergoing the procedure—often in excruciating pain—to warn other women of the potential pain and side effects and to level criticism at providers for ignoring the issue.

This social media campaign caught the attention of Duke University researchers, who analyzed the top #IUD video posts and identified a gap in managing patients' pain that needs to be addressed. The Centers for Disease Control and Prevention followed up in August 2024 with updated guidance on managing pain during IUD insertion. (The new recommendations include counseling patients on pain management before the procedure and expanded options, including topical application of lidocaine gel or spray on the cervical area to numb the tissue and reduce pain.) While the CDC action is helpful, the point is that it should not have taken an organic social media campaign to bring to light the pain.

In another example of gender bias, for years, drug companies and other research programs excluded women from studies due to the belief that their hormonal cycles would skew test results. So male-only drug testing was the norm, with outcomes based solely on male physiology. As a result, many women were overmedicated because drugs and dosing were never properly adjusted for female physiology. It took an act of Congress in 1993 to change federal policy to require the inclusion of women of childbearing age in National Institutes of Health–funded drug trials. Unfortunately, that didn't fix the problem with drugs already in use. One recent study by University of Chicago researchers identified eighty-six drugs for which there is "clear evidence of sex differences" in how the body breaks down the drug, and found that for "nearly all of these drugs, women metabolized them more slowly than men, leading to higher levels of exposure to the drug." As a result, in 96 percent of cases, there were "significantly higher rates of adverse side effects in women." "These drugs are optimized from the beginning to work on male bodies," says Brian Prendergast, a University of Chicago psychologist and coauthor of the study examining the gender gap in research. "We need to immediately reevaluate the widespread practice of prescribing the same doses to men and women."

Numerous studies show that physicians respond to pain differently depending on a patient's sex or race, and their own sex or race can also play a role in how they react and the type of treatment they recommend. The bottom line is that women's pain is taken less seriously than men's (often by men, but also by some women clinicians) and therefore is underdiagnosed or undertreated. Women are also more likely to be told to seek psychotherapy or other behavioral counseling, which can be helpful but may also reflect the provider's doubt that a woman's pain is "real."

"Probably the most important action we can encourage providers to take today is [to] check your biases at the door and help the patient as they are—and address the pain they have as opposed to the pain you think they should have," Fillingim says.

What We Don't Know or Don't Share

"Everybody lies," says the fictional physician in the TV series *House*, reflecting the character's cynical view of patients' candor (or lack of it) when describing how they ended up in his care. It's a great line because it has a kernel of truth: many of us prefer for a variety of reasons not to mention certain things to our doctor.

In two national online surveys of 4,510 US adults in 2015, most participants reported withholding at least one of several types of medically relevant information. The most common reasons included not wanting to be judged or to hear how harmful their behavior is to their body. Other reasons? Not wanting the clinician to think they're a difficult patient and not wanting to take up more of the clinician's time.

Other studies have shown that people are often less than candid about drinking, smoking, substance use (recreational or otherwise), mental health challenges, and sexual problems. Many already feel stigmatized socially; they don't want their doctor to write them off too.

An acquaintance of mine who'd struggled with long COVID symptoms told me that despite ongoing body aches and pain in her chest, hands, and feet (which would suddenly go ice cold), she was reluctant to talk about them with her primary care physician. Why? Because her doctor had brushed off "the whole long Covid thing" when she'd first sought care for it. So now she was reluctant to seem like "a complainer" in her doctor's eyes. Withholding information from a provider can lead to both short- and long-term consequences, particularly when it comes to pain. One major survey found that while nearly half of people over fifty years old said arthritis or joint pain limits their usual activities, many hadn't bothered to talk to a doctor about treatment options.

Sometimes patients don't share information because they don't fully appreciate how important it is. Once, just before the holidays, an older patient showed up in our clinic with persistent headaches and difficulties with balance. His symptoms had seemingly come out of the blue, and initially we were looking at a medical mystery. One day he was fine, walking his dog as usual. The next day, he could barely get out of bed without the room spinning. He had already seen several doctors to evaluate his ears, sinuses, and cardiac function. All those tests turned out normal, and he had been prescribed everything from aspirin to opioids, but the headaches continued to get worse.

As we slowly and methodically worked through the history of his headaches, a clue finally emerged. While hurrying to get into a car a few months earlier, the patient had whacked his head on the door frame. He hadn't thought much of it at the time, but for me, this news was a revelation. The CT scan of his head that I subsequently ordered revealed a blood collection known as a subdural hematoma on top of his brain, which had been slowly growing over the past couple of months.

We were both relieved to find the cause. He consented to surgery, and the next day I took him to the operating room to drill two small holes—called Burr holes—in his skull just above the hematoma. Because several weeks had passed since his injury, the blood had liquefied, so I was able to remove it easily through those tiny openings.

I was pleased that we'd finally been able to get to the bottom of the matter, but one thing was clear: no detail is too small, even if it doesn't seem important at the time.

Why Patients Lie . . . and Why the Truth Matters

Patients commonly withhold medically relevant information from their clinicians, often not aware that doing so may well inhibit the quality of care they receive. As part of a study on this topic, a questionnaire asked whether participants had "ever avoided telling a health care provider" that they

- did not understand the provider's instructions.
- disagreed with the provider's recommendation.
- did not exercise or did not exercise regularly.
- had an unhealthy diet or how unhealthy their diet was.
- took a certain medication.
- did not take their prescription medication as instructed.
- took someone else's prescription medication.

The study resulted in two important findings. First, most patients have withheld medically relevant information from their clinician at least once, especially when they disagree with a recommendation.

Second, survey respondents who were sicker—meaning those who had worse self-reported health and/or chronic conditions—were significantly more likely to withhold information from their clinician. This indicates that the very patients who are in greatest need of high-quality health care may be more likely to compromise that care by withholding important details.

This vicious cycle can be discouraging for both patient and provider. While I certainly can't speak for all physicians, I'm pretty confident that however embarrassing or uncomfortable patients feel, I have probably already heard it all. If you're wondering whether a detail—no matter how small—may be important, write it down ahead of time and share it during your visit. Worst case is that it may not amount to much. Best case is that it might prevent a complication or even provide a shortcut to getting you pain free.

Hidden in Plain Sight: Head Trauma from Physical Abuse

Eve Valera was a graduate student studying neuropsychology in the mid-1990s when she volunteered at a local shelter for battered women and their children, intending to focus on child abuse and prevention. As she spent time with the women and children, she learned horrifying details of how they had landed at the shelter.

"I would hear the stories of some of these women getting clocked in the head, they're getting their head stomped on, they're getting choked, strangled, slammed against door frames—bludgeoned," she recalls. "And they're also reporting a lot of the same symptoms that women suffering from brain injuries experience—what you might call post-concussive symptoms, like something from a fall or an accident. And I was thinking, well this is really interesting. What do we know about this?" An exhaustive search of the literature gave her an unsettling answer: pretty much zero. Why? Often because no one asked. Or when they did, too often these patients were reluctant to disclose their injuries, let alone the manner in which they'd received them.

Valera, now an associate professor in psychiatry at Harvard Medical School and research scientist at Massachusetts General Hospital, decided to fill that gap. She pioneered the field of traumatic brain injury from intimate partner violence (IPV).

Initially, she took advantage of inexpensive and simple-to-use measures to examine the relationship of cognition, psychological distress, and brain injuries sustained from IPV. She then expanded her efforts, using imaging technology to show the unique consequences of brain injuries that women suffer at the hands of abusive partners. Nonpenetrating traumatic brain injuries (TBIs) are essentially invisible from the outside, meaning that the brain is damaged but signs of it are buried. Valera felt that in the same way that TBI in athletes' brains drew public attention to the problem of sports injuries, her research could do the same for abused women.

The evidence of brain injury wasn't surprising, given the terrible physical trauma to the head and neck that the assaults caused. Most striking, however, was a general lack of awareness and interest in IPV-related TBI, even as the condition was being seriously evaluated in cases that involved military veterans and football players.

The Centers for Disease Control and Prevention estimates that nearly one in five women has experienced severe IPV in her lifetime. Think about that: 20 percent of the women you know may be victims of this trauma. Among these women, it's estimated that 60 to 92 percent have experienced facial or head injuries or strangulation. Valera notes that historically, increases in violence against women have corresponded with natural disasters and economic crises, as women find themselves sheltering with abusers and even more cut off from family and friends who might help them. The early years of the COVID pandemic were no exception, as extended lockdowns, economic hardships, and social isolation increased women's exposure and vulnerability to violent partners.

Valera has redoubled efforts to put IPV-related TBI on the radar for health care providers and patients, insisting that medical schools should teach about it, and practicing physicians should bring it up consistently and directly with their patients. Given the potential link between physical abuse and pain conditions, especially headaches and chronic pain, "now we know that we need to consider brain injury as a possible contributor," Valera notes. "As common as these injuries are, they are also some of the least likely to be disclosed to their physicians. If doctors don't ask about partner violence, they may never understand the source of these symptoms."

AI and Other Data-Driven Assessment Tools Promise Greater Precision

Over the past several years, researchers have made enormous strides in creating personalized pain assessments, primarily by merging data from individual patients with those of vast numbers of others. From the National Institutes of Health (NIH) research centers to regional medical centers including Mayo Clinic, Columbia University Medical Center, Stanford School of Medicine, the MIT Center for Precision Cancer Medicine, and others, major studies are mining data about symptoms and lifestyle factors with the goal of developing precision medicine—identifying which pain treatments are likely to work best for which people, based on their shared characteristics. The data will one day be used to develop readily accessible algorithms of patient pain profiles. And as those profiles are refined for general use, providers will have access to that tool as we consider options for pain relief.

"Building that individualized treatment package sometimes is a little bit of trial and error, and what our research trials are trying to do is to take a little bit of the trial and error out of that," says Linda Porter, director of the NIH Office of Pain Policy and Planning. "Instead of 'why don't you try a little bit of yoga' or 'why don't you try a little bit of acupuncture,' this will help individualize that with a good assessment and a clearer path toward treatment."

This is especially important when you consider the complexity of chronic pain. Medications that work for one kind of pain might exacerbate another. Pain may appear for no obvious reason, then mysteriously disappear. And when pain arrives and then refuses to leave, it might be conflated with any number of other conditions.

It's no exaggeration to say that the initial mystery of pain and the dogged pursuit of a solution presents anew with every patient who walks through the door, no matter how similar to other patients they may seem. And yet, ironically, the solution for any given individual might come through compressing reams of data from many other pain sufferers to produce patterns of pain that can inform how we help that person.

High-tech data analysis is already aiding in this process. The NIH is sharing its growing database, and some other institutions have made theirs available to help create promising matches between pain patients and treatment options.

Even as providers look forward to the advances in pain assessments that technology is expected to provide, a couple of issues are uniquely ours to address. One is the value of human connection. A consistent theme in pain research is how vital the connection is between patients and doctors and between people living with pain and their families and friends. Pain can be all encompassing, invading every aspect of your life. Yet at the same time, it can be an intensely private experience. Finding people you trust—including your doctors—and having honest conversations go a long way toward healing. In my practice, I have found that many of my patients have been particularly grateful for my care simply because I listened, even if I didn't provide any new therapies for them. As I was reminded when my own mom was suffering, simply holding one's hand can be healing.

Second, one of the most humbling aspects of the quest for diagnostic clues is the realization that the brain and body are already on the case, aware of everything we need to know and with healing capacities we've barely begun to tap or even identify. In other words, our efforts to diagnose and treat pain are really efforts to learn what the body already knows. The most updated pain science reminds us that the brain, in constant dialogue with the body, is always calling the shots. We need to make sure we are listening.

CHAPTER 3

Mastermind: The Brain as Pain Maker

I remember the first time I felt intense pain. Just after my twelfth birthday, I set out to jump over a fence that had spikes all along the top. Running toward it, I put one hand on the smooth part, then tried to vault my legs over at the same time. I didn't make it. I landed directly on one of the spikes, which pierced completely through the right side of my torso, from back to front. I had impaled myself on the fence.

This could have been disastrous, but thankfully the spike pierced through soft tissue rather than my organs. It hurt, but more concerning was the fact that the spike was holding me in place. I panicked, worried that I wouldn't be able to get down, even that I might die there and never be found. After that initial instant of trauma, though, something fascinating happened: the wound stopped hurting so much.

Rather than crescendoing toward a peak, my pain came in waves. Even stranger, the stabbing, stinging sensation I expected from being impaled on a spike wasn't really there. Instead, it felt like I had been punched or slapped. In fact, I had to keep looking down at the side of my body, tracing the spike with my finger to where it entered and touching where it poked out, to be certain of what had just happened to me.

We tend to have preconceived notions of not only how painful an injury might be but also the nature of what it will feel like. Very often, those notions are wrong. For some people, the body's natural defense mechanisms respond so vigorously that feelings of pain are quickly replaced with near euphoria. Others may suffer more, or longer, because those same mechanisms act as part of the pain-generating process that uses inflammation to trigger the release of healing agents.

As I've learned over the years, the amount of pain you might suffer with exactly the same injury can differ from day to day or even hour to hour, depending on seemingly unrelated things like how much sleep you had or whether the weather was nice or stormy. It has been well established that mood, emotions, mind-set, and many other psychological factors can make us more or less sensitive to pain.

On the day I got impaled, I had been having a wonderful morning under a beautiful summer sky with hardly a care in the world. I was in a great mood, well fed, and was active and exhilarated. I had confidence bordering on delusional invincibility, which is what led to the questionable decision to try this jump. In terms of the body's natural painkillers, meaning the endorphins and other endogenous opioids released during exercise, I was experiencing something like a runner's high—right up to the moment the spike pierced my body, and those endogenous opioids unquestionably helped buffer me from a fairly traumatic experience.

The next thing I remember, I saw my mom running toward me. It wasn't until I saw the horrified look on her face that I started to cry. "How bad is it?" I asked, but I don't remember her reply. That's when I started to feel hot and lightheaded. Then I threw up.

Because my legs were dangling, I couldn't get any leverage to hoist myself off the spike. A neighbor of ours ran to get a tool to cut the spike off the fence with me still on it, but I got impatient, partly because I was embarrassed at my predicament. When my mom provided a step for me to push off, while at the same time supporting my torso, I was finally able to lift myself off the spike. I grabbed my side, though I felt more relief than pain at that moment, and my mom and I made a mad scramble for the emergency room. After a few stitches and assurances that this was only a soft tissue injury, I was discharged—but only after the pediatric ER doctor had me share the story (and my wound) with as many staff members as he could find. I can't blame him, because even today I still enjoy telling friends the story and showing them the scars.

As traumatic and humiliating as the experience was, this also marked the first time I became deeply interested in the most mysterious of human sensations: pain. What are these receptors that warn you of an injury yet are diverse and nuanced enough to signal a cut versus a burn, or hot versus cold? How do pain signals travel through the spinal cord, racing through microscopic paths to the brain where they're processed and deciphered? Learning how that process worked became an early obsession for me, fueling an interest in the central nervous system and eventually a career as a neurosurgeon.

In my case, I was "lucky" enough to have been impaled on a part of my body that was less reactive than others. The skin and underlying tissue along your back, forearms, and calves is the least sensitive in the body. The most sensitive are the fingertips, lips, and tongue. Each fingertip has thousands of touch receptors, including many that detect subtle changes in pressure. This is why humans can use the tactile braille system. Your entire torso, however, has fewer receptors than just one of your hands. That's why a paper cut on your fingertip can bring you to tears, and a finger-stick prick from a small lancet can cause longer-lasting pain than a larger needle poke in your arm. Because it's your fingertip, people think it will hurt less—but for most people, the opposite is true.

How Touchy Are You?:

The DIY Two-Point Acuity Touch Test

The two-point acuity test is a tool scientists use to understand the fascinating ways the body and brain are hard-wired to sense, differentiate, and manage touch. While not perfect, this test offers a DIY experiment you can try on your own body. Take two sharp objects—a geometry compass, for example, or even just your thumbnail and a second fingernail—and hold them close together while pressing down on your skin (firmly enough to feel but not enough to hurt). Even though they're two separate points, you will still likely feel only a single point of pressure.

Now, gradually move the objects farther from each other until you start to feel them as two distinct points. The farther apart the points are when you start to feel them separately, the less sensitive or reactive that area of skin is. On the wrist, one of the most sensitive parts of the body, the distance should be about an inch. On the back, which is where the spike entered my skin, the distance is much greater because there are fewer sensors—and fewer sensors typically translates to less pain.

Many Pains, Many Mechanisms, One Master

Clifford Woolf, PhD, a neurobiologist, professor, and director of the F. M. Kirby Neurobiology Center at Boston Children's Hospital, has devoted his career to better understanding the mechanisms of pain, with the hope of targeting better therapies. When he tells me that we've "just got to accept that pain is complex," he says it with excitement, not resignation. Complexity offers tremendous opportunity to find new targets and mechanisms for pain treatments.

"We use a single word to describe cancer, but everyone knows there's leukemia, lymphoma, breast cancer, bowel cancer, and all of those are very different and require different treatments," he says. "The fact that we use a single word—*pain*—to describe unpleasant sensation doesn't mean that it's a single entity. It's not at all." The consensus is "there's not going to be a single magic bullet that hits the pain target." Rather, he says, "there are going to be lots of different magic bullets." Even the three classifications of pain that I described in chapter 2—nociceptive pain (tissue damage or potential harm), neuropathic (nerve) pain, and neuroplastic pain (no discernible physical cause)—don't capture the full complexity of how differently they intersect or overlap in common pain conditions.

In our neurosurgery clinic, we often debate which human conditions are the most painful. Any ranking is subjective, of course, as we have no way of objectively measuring pain—though I was amused to learn some of the ways people have tried. For example, childbirth tops the worst-pain list for many. And now there's a "labor simulator" experience for nonpregnant partners, so they can feel what it's like to be in labor. In a supervised setting (please don't try this at home!), technicians connect a transcutaneous electrical nerve stimulation unit known as a TENS machine to electrodes placed on strategic abdominal points to try to replicate typical labor pain. The machine can be cranked up to mimic the intensity and discomfort of labor contractions. I'm not sure it ever truly feels like labor, but the empathetic effort counts for something.

Kidney stones, a condition in which rough, calcified crystals move through the slender, tender channels of the urinary tract, ranked high on the list as well. As someone who's suffered them myself, I can attest to how excruciating the pain is. Shingles, a blistering rash caused by the herpes zoster virus, always makes the list, as does the one condition that any neurosurgeon, anesthesiologist, neurologist, or pain doctor will always put at the top: trigeminal neuralgia (TN), a chronic pain condition characterized by sudden, severe facial pain so brutal that it's also called "the suicide disease."

"A lightning bolt of pain," is how a friend of mine described her condition when she called me early one Saturday morning. She was sitting in a parking lot at a grocery store, scared to drive home because a sudden attack might cause her to lose control and crash. As soon as she described her symptoms and the trail of episodes that had brought her to this frightening moment, I was fairly certain of her diagnosis.

The first time she'd suffered this type of pain was shortly after arriving home from the hospital with her new baby, about three years earlier. At that time, it had come on suddenly, radiating from her ear to her nostril. She thought it might be an ear infection, but a prescription for antibiotics brought her no relief. The pain sometimes worsened when she brushed her teeth, so her dentist recommended replacing a few of her fillings on the right side of her mouth. For a while, she thought that was the solution. But within a few weeks the pain had returned.

A CT scan and MRI appeared normal, and high-powered pain meds made her sleepy without alleviating the pain. Afraid to chew food on the right side of her mouth, she began to lose weight. She hardly ever went out anymore and was having a hard time caring for her toddler. For anyone familiar with trigeminal neuralgia, her symptoms were absolutely textbook. And yet for nearly three years she had been dealing with one of the most painful conditions a human can endure, with no idea why.

Based on her history, I told her that even though there was probably no obvious abnormality in her brain, she might need brain surgery to fix this problem once and for all. I'll explain why that surgery is done—and how—in chapter 9.

Others on the most-fearsome pain list include a fractured femur or humerus; osteoarthritis in the hips, knees, or shoulders, as well as orthopedic postoperative pain; back injuries or severe chronic back pain; and migraines and cluster headaches and other chronic headaches. Endometriosis, abnormal growth of tissue similar to uterine tissue outside the uterus, causes painful adhesions and bleeding. Sickle cell disease, in children as well as adults, causes overwhelming pain and swelling.

Complex regional pain syndrome (CRPS), first described in the mid-sixteenth century, makes today's list with intense and abnormally long-lasting pain and inflammation, often in the hands, feet, and limbs following a traumatic injury, surgery, stroke, or heart attack. Burning, throbbing pain, swelling, or inflamed skin along with changes in skin temperature or color can erupt suddenly and with no apparent trigger. Considered a rare disease because it affects only about 200,000 Americans annually, CRPS nonetheless stands out for its intense, often debilitating pain, as we'll see in one man's story later in this book. Fibromyalgia, chronic and often intense musculoskeletal pain throughout the body, affects an estimated ten million people in the United States (75 to 90 percent of them women) and frequently makes the list.

The mechanisms driving these horrific types of pain vary widely depending on the extent of nociceptive, neuropathic, and neuroplastic components involved; any co-occurring health issues the sufferers may have; their unique genetic, environmental, and social and emotional factors; and any underlying trauma from adverse events that occurred earlier in life.

Top-Down, Bottom-Up: All Pain Pathways Lead to the Brain

One simple model we use to talk about types of pain, and thus potential approaches to treatment, differentiates between top-down and bottom-up pain.

Simply put, top-down starts in the brain, involving the processing that draws from expectations, previous experience, and thoughts about pain—in other words, neuroplastic pain. This generates a signal that travels "down" the rest of the nervous system, creating the perception of physical pain even where there's no apparent physical cause.

Top-down pain originates in the brain's pain-processing circuitry, not in the body. When the brain associates certain movements or circumstances with a past painful experience, it eventually may learn to trigger a pain sensation absent injury or risk of harm. Some examples of pain conditions believed to be neuroplastic when no structural causes can be found include chronic low back pain, IBD, and fibromyalgia.

Bottom-up pain has an identifiable physical (somatic) cause, a structural source triggering the nociceptors to signal the brain for attention to an injury, damage, or threat. That might be a cut or broken bone; tissue, nerve, or joint damage; chronic inflammation; or a disease that triggers nociceptive signaling "up" through the network of peripheral nerves and the spinal cord and on to the brain. The signaling system that alerts you to pull your hand from the flame is also focused inward, constantly monitoring our internal organs, blood vessels and blood chemistry, bones, and connective tissue. In that territory, chronic inflammation is like a constant fire. When it reaches a certain level, you'll feel the pain—alarming pain. Appendicitis is one example: a dangerously inflamed appendix is typically accompanied by sudden and extreme pain.

Surgery, however successful, can be another source of bottom-up pain, at least in those first post-op recovery hours, with pain diminishing as recovery continues. Even the best-planned and -executed surgery is an imposition on the body. Preoperative pain management practices can help lessen some surgical pain, and pain medications taken directly after surgery and through recovery work directly on the pain system to blunt pain. Newer studies suggest that a certain level of the initial inflammation response may be needed to trigger healing responses, so today, postoperative pain management aims to balance the protective pain response with pain relief.

In a practical sense, pain often involves both top-down and bottom-up signaling. Even when there is a clear physical reason for acute pain, how your brain processes it through your individual history of experience and emotional memory will be a top-down factor you can work with to manage pain or prevent it. Getting a shot or having blood drawn is a simple example. Perhaps you remind yourself that the quick prick of the needle is done in a blink, that it's important to get it done, and that you can look away and distract yourself. Most of all, you know it's just what it is: not an injury or a danger.

What Exactly Is Pain?

One of the most significant and surprising developments emerging in pain treatment is the recognition that the brain is at the center of any pain experience. Simply put, if your brain doesn't interpret your discomfort as pain, it won't hurt. This is why, when I was impaled on that spike, my pain intensified when I saw how worried my mom was.

For centuries, science defined pain simply as an unpleasant sensory experience, your body's reaction to a noxious stimulus with potential for harm, such as injury, disease, damage from extreme heat or cold, or chemical irritation. Though different cultures described pain differently, the pain process through the academic lens was believed to be fairly straightforward. Sensory neurons, later named nociceptors, sent the pain signal along defined nerve pathways to the spinal cord and on to the brain. Even well into the twentieth century, scientific theories of pain focused on physiological mechanisms—the biological nuts and bolts, pathways, and processes responsible for generating and modulating pain.

But this mechanistic view of pain, and the definition of pain as strictly an unpleasant sensory experience, didn't explain why the same physical insult can be experienced so differently or not even as pain at all.

In 1979, the International Association for the Study of Pain (IASP) addressed these differences by rewriting the definition of pain to include emotional experience as a dimension of the pain system. The revised definition declared that pain is "an unpleasant sensory *and emotional* [emphasis mine] experience associated with actual or potential tissue damage." This simple acknowledgment transformed the conversation about pain, taking it past the centuries-old dualistic notion of mind and body as separate, where pain is purely a physical malady and the mind, on an abstract mental plane, is removed from the messy mechanics of it.

This new, more accurate understanding, which is now encoded in the definition that guides research and clinical treatment, is that the brain, mind, and body are a fully integrated operating system. Nerves, tissue, bones, blood, fears, thoughts, beliefs, what you eat and how you sleep, your gender, your culture, and even your relationships form a full array of biological, neurological, psychological, social, and emotional components that shape your pain experience. In this hybrid nervous system model, nothing is off the grid. From felt pain to our thoughts about it and the physiological changes that trigger reactions systemwide, everything matters.

No matter how the medical establishment may attempt to compartmentalize causes of pain by physical, psychological, or other factors, that's a moot point to the brain, which doesn't differentiate between the psychological and biological components. Mind and body are one.

There's an old joke that goes: Ask ten neurologists "What is pain?" and you'll get eleven different answers. And yet there's little doubt that you know what pain means for you. Whether it's the ache, the twinge, the stab, the throb, or the hurt, you don't need a scientist to tell you what your body knows.

But there's one thing scientists tell us that may surprise you: pain sufferers generally fare better when they're given a basic understanding of the neuroscience of pain—meaning what is actually happening in their bodies and brains when they feel that stab, twinge, or throb. For too many people, this process is mysterious, and the worry and anxiety that uncertainty creates only add to the severity of the symptoms.

The more you understand about what's happening in your body and brain, the better equipped you are to control your pain, recognize how different treatment options are designed to work, and commit to doing what you can yourself to manage pain.

For example, not so long ago, many scientists believed that a designated region of the brain was the hub or "pain center" responsible for pain processing. Not so. Using brain imaging and other sophisticated technology, scientists have been able to observe different areas of the brain that are activated when you feel pain.

In an fMRI image, for instance, increased blood flow or electrical activity "lights up" in areas where neural activity levels are high. When a person experiences pain, many surprising areas light up, indicating that the incoming signals are traveling through interconnected networks in multiple regions of the brain rather than a central pain hub. While the brain is evaluating those signals, those separate regions are also processing the new input for learning, memory, body awareness, and emotions, all of which ultimately create or color your pain experience. It has even been observed that acute pain and chronic pain light up different regions of the brain, even though the sufferer might describe them as similar experiences.

The point is, your brain is not the Wizard of Oz, dictating in isolation how much pain you may or may not feel, relying on static assessments and old information. In fact, the opposite is true: Your brain is constantly scanning fresh input from throughout the body while accessing memory to predict and anticipate possible sources of pain. And because each one of the pathways, processes, and mechanisms in the pain system can completely change your pain experience, each one can become a potential target for intervention.

The Body Electric: From Metaphor to Mechanisms

Sean Mackey, pain physician, scientist, professor, and director of the Systems Neuroscience and Pain Lab at Stanford University, likes to note that because he got his PhD in electrical engineering, "I tend to think in circuits and in amplifiers." This is how he talks about pain circuitry. When asked how he reconciles the fact that pain is both a physical and psychological phenomenon, he answers as an engineer would. "We've got cognitive amplifiers, such as attention and distraction. We have contextual ones, like your beliefs. Expectation—if you expect to have more pain, it turns up an amplifier in your brain and you have more pain. Your mood—if you're depressed or you're anxious, it amplifies things. And then your individual differences, some of which we can't control—the genes that your parents handed down to you—will determine your sensitivity and your vulnerability to pain. All of that shapes your pain experience."

Think of it like this: In addition to the nerves in your body that provide basic senses and allow you to move, breathe, and digest your food, there are also highly specialized nerves that detect changes in temperature, chemical exposure, and pressure and pinch. When the changes are extreme or sudden, these danger detectors, called nociceptors, relay the information to the brain at speeds up to 270 miles per hour—faster than the blink of an eye. The signals from nociceptors are often described as "pain impulses" relayed to the brain. But that's not the whole story. We now know that those electrical impulses aren't technically pain signals at all. They're more like a warning sign on your car dashboard, a signal that grabs your attention.

After the nerve fibers relay those warning signs through the spinal cord and on to the brain, they're analyzed instantly for memory, emotional links, physiological and survival implications, and other factors based on history to predict their salience—their significance and urgency. Keep in mind that the brain is also constantly looking for efficiency shortcuts, so referring quickly to past experience and outcomes saves the cognitive energy required to evaluate every signal from scratch. Once it has processed the incoming signal, the brain sends out its own response—an instruction to trigger a reaction by your muscle or the release of hormones or neurotransmitters. That signal races back down through the spinal cord and the rest of the nervous system.

You might feel the pang of pain, then instantly feel your muscles clench or your breathing constrict. What you feel depends on what your brain concluded and how it processed those signals in that fraction of a second. It's part of an unconscious process called neuroception—an evolutionary gift of a built-in surveillance system that continuously scans the environment for external and internal or visceral cues of danger or safety.

Neuroception is driven mostly by the vagus nerve. The tenth and longest cranial nerve, the vagus nerve runs in two paths: one along the left side of your body, the other on the right, from your brain to your large intestine and affecting the neck, chest, heart, lungs, and abdomen. You might recognize neuroception in the "gut feeling" you get when something makes you feel uneasy or when that same vague awareness gives you goose bumps or makes the back of your neck tingle. It's also why an unconscious memory related to a past trauma can trigger anxiety or a fear response in you today, beneath your conscious awareness.

Neuroception has become increasingly relevant as scientists delve more deeply into the neurocircuitry of neuroplastic pain, persistent pain for which no physical cause can be found. Many pain experts believe heightened neuroception plays a role—and in some cases is the single cause—in chronic pain conditions such as fibromyalgia, IBS, and some chronic lower back pain and headaches. When that's the case, the brain is receiving a cascade of warning signals, despite the fact there is no actual threat. These types of pain sensations could be described as the brain's overreaction to a minor physical slight. Or it could be that the brain associates the sensation with a memory of something worse that triggered the alarm in the past.

Your neuroception is a necessary, highly sensitive surveillance system that is constantly distinguishing between safe, dangerous, and life-threatening input. Often, though, it may also over- or underreact, depending on outside factors.

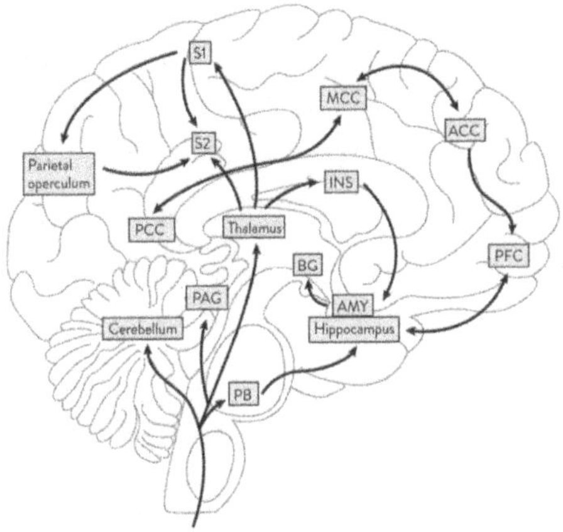

The brain's pain-processing circuitry involves multiple networks, pathways, and processes.

If you were to use imaging technologies to examine the brain closely in the middle of a pain flare-up, you would see many pathways activated, instead of one or two primary pain centers, as was long believed to be the case (see corresponding image above). From the thalamus to the periaqueductal gray, these regions integrate cognitive, emotional, and sensory stimuli affecting memory processes, emotional regulation, motivation, decision making, motor control, and other aspects of human experience. It helps explain the complexity and beauty of pain.

New incoming signals are, in effect, processed through memories of prior pain; sensory input (what you see, hear, taste, or feel in that moment); and your cognitive input, meaning your thoughts about the pain ("I can't stand this," "This happens every time," "This is hopeless"). The network can activate with or without new nociceptive input, and injury or damage may activate it. By the same token, a mere thought—a triggering scent or sound or even an unconscious memory—can flip the on-switch.

The Cloistered King of Pain

Why the Brain Itself Feels No Pain: An Evolutionary Theory

Here's a remarkable fact: Even though the brain has billions of neurons responsible for all our sensations and it commands the processes that create and recognize pain throughout the body, the brain itself doesn't experience pain. It's a cloistered king—one removed from consequences. It is the maestro of pain that is unable to feel pain. What an evolutionary oddity!

One explanation for this, evolutionarily speaking, could be that the brain aims to conserve energy whenever possible, not wasting it on inefficiencies. Protected by the skull, the brain isn't normally exposed to the elements—so from an evolutionary point of view, nociceptors weren't needed for protection.

"Pain can help to stop or avoid damage to skin, so the skin has many pain receptors," explains Randolph Nesse, an evolutionary psychiatrist, scientist, and author considered a founder in the field of evolutionary medicine. "But damage to the brain was generally fatal in ancestral environments, so there would be no benefit to pain receptors." In other words, a blow to the body could trigger pain's protective mechanisms, with a chance of providing effective protective action. But historically, a blow to the skull meant game over.

While that's often still the case, evolution didn't anticipate the sophisticated surgical tools and techniques we now have to enter the brain's protective sanctum. Today, I can perform brain surgery on a patient who's wide awake, their brain oblivious to pain. We can chat as I work on their most crucial organ, just like you might chat with your neighborhood auto mechanic as they work under the hood.

While there are several areas of the brain responsible for pain processing, the periaqueductal gray, in the midbrain of the brain stem, is the chief switchboard operator. It plays a major role not just in perceiving pain, but in deciding how much attention it warrants. Imaging studies show that when these brain regions are activated, pain increases. So if you simply believe something is going to hurt, even with little or no stimulus, it will likely hurt, a self-fulfilling prophecy. When these neural networks are activated repeatedly, the brain remembers and efficiently predicts—and constructs—pain.

Sometimes pain persists even when the nerve that transmitted the signal has been ablated or cut. So where's that pain coming from, if not from the nerve? In those situations, the pain is being created solely in the brain—an astonishing fact, if you really consider it.

The famous "rubber hand illusion" shows how easily and quickly the brain can be fooled. In this staged illusion, a person sits at a table with one arm hidden from view behind a partition and a fake limb positioned in front of them. The experimenter strokes the fake hand and the participant's real hand simultaneously to trick the brain into thinking the fake hand is real. After a few touches, the experimenter slams a hammer into the fake hand. The participant typically recoils in "pain," despite the fact that the hammer never actually touched them. Again, it's an impressive trick that effectively demonstrates just how easily our brains can be deceived, especially when it comes to pain.

In clinical practice, this deception can be used as a healing tool for phantom limb pain. If you hold a mirror next to an amputee's remaining limb, the reflection of the existing limb gives the impression that the missing one is present and healthy. As the person moves the existing limb, the mirror makes it look as though the phantom limb is also moving, without pain. This simple trick helps the brain to resolve the visual spatial disconnect that appears to be at the root of phantom pain. Best of all, it doesn't require any medications or fancy new procedures—just a mirror.

The message for all of us is that our brains have the extraordinary capacity not only to create a sensory reality for us but also to change it, as we'll see next. And the exciting part is that we can tap into that process by choice.

Neuroplasticity, from Promise to Pathology

When I think about all the ways our nervous systems deploy pain as an alert, I feel a sense of wonder and awe at the marvelous interplay between brain and body. That interplay gives me confidence that with continuing advances in basic pain science, surgical techniques, and other treatment options, we'll soon be able to relieve suffering in ways that are less invasive, more direct, and more effective. The brain's capacity for learning and changing how it processes pain—its neuroplasticity—may be our most valuable tool in fighting pain. Yet neuroplasticity is highly flexible, which means the results can be either fantastic or fraught, moment to moment.

Neuroplasticity is the brain's capacity to learn, grow, and change in response to experience. It's one of the brain's superpowers, making it possible to reconfigure existing neural networks, teach old neurons new tricks, and even grow altogether new brain cells at any age. When we're young, neuroplasticity drives essential brain growth and development. Throughout life, it enables us to adapt to new circumstances, learn new habits, and unlearn bad ones. And as we age, it helps keep our brain sharp.

But you might not know that neuroplasticity is also nature's evolutionary master tool for maintaining certain mechanisms essential for our basic survival. Neuroplasticity is critical to the brain's ability to maintain and regulate activity including synaptic transmission (chemical instant messaging between neurons), exciting and calming neurons, and synchronizing networks that connect, well, everything. Including pain.

Ordinarily we think about repetition as the key to learning, based on the idea that "neurons that fire together wire together," a concept that Canadian psychologist Donald O. Hebb described in 1949 to explain neurophysiological changes underlying learning and memory formation. That repetition also saves energy—a critical evolutionary strategy, as it strengthens neural pathways for thoughts and behaviors, eventually turning them into neural shortcuts that the brain uses automatically to respond to stimuli.

Our thoughts and behaviors train the brain, and the resulting shortcuts act as a closed loop to then reinforce those thoughts and behaviors. So when we intentionally study or practice to learn, we're using neuroplasticity to train our brain. And when we develop beliefs or habits of thought and behaviors that repeat connections, those connections become stronger. But here's the catch: that experiential brain training can include pain-related thoughts and behaviors that make pain worse. If the brain learns pain associations from prior experience, then wires them together for a shortcut that creates a new perception of pain with no nociceptive signal at all, that's trouble.

"Because the brain is plastic, when pain grows, it can encode stronger and stronger pain sensations over time, despite the physical injury appearing to be healed," explains Michael Merzenich, professor emeritus at the University of California at San Francisco and a member of the National Academy of Sciences. Merzenich, considered by some to be the "father of neuroplasticity," describes the plastic brain not as hardwired, but more aptly "soft-wired" and open to change.

Call it the dark side of neuroplasticity, but it's nonetheless quite a feat for the brain to create pain with no nociceptive input. When pain occurs without an injury, as it often does in conditions such as fibromyalgia, chronic low back pain, or mixed-pain conditions, the role of neuroplasticity becomes paramount. It's not only the most direct way to change the learned brain-pain patterns; it also explains why some aspects of pain won't respond meaningfully to conventional therapies like anti-inflammatory drugs, surgery, or injections—because the pain is actually due to brain pain-processing issues.

Memory as Mechanism: How the Brain Encodes Pain

Creating a memory starts with your sensory perception of an experience.

Take, for example, the memory of meeting someone you fell in love with. In that first meeting, your eyes, ears, nose, and perhaps even your sense of touch took note of the person's features: the sound of their voice, their scent, their physical presence. Each of these separate sensations then traveled to the hippocampus, the brain's memory center, which integrated these perceptions into a single experience—in this case, the experience of the individual. It is something you are not likely to ever forget. When it comes to pain and neuroplasticity, however, the brain may take a routine acute pain experience and prolong it into chronic pain, an experience that keeps getting played and replayed in your body. For reasons not yet fully understood, the brain "remembers" the pain long after physical damage has healed. And what the brain cannot forget, the body remembers.

All of this analyzing and filtering of your perception occur using the brain's language of electric and chemical messengers. Nerve cells connect with other cells at a point called the synapse, where electrical pulses carrying messages jump across gaps between cells, in turn triggering the release of chemical messengers named neurotransmitters.

Common neurotransmitters are dopamine, norepinephrine, and epinephrine. When they diffuse across the spaces between cells, they attach themselves to neighboring cells. Each brain cell can form thousands of links like this, generating trillions of synapses in a typical brain. The parts of the brain cells that receive these electric impulses are called dendrites—which literally means "treelike"—for the fact that they're short, branched extensions of a nerve cell that has reached out to neighboring brain cells.

All of these connections between brain cells are incredibly dynamic in nature, meaning they can change in an instant. Brain cells work together in a network, organizing themselves into groups that specialize in different kinds of information processing. As one brain cell sends signals to another, the synapse between the two gets stronger, and the more signals sent between them, the stronger that connection grows. So every time you experience something new, your brain slightly rewires to accommodate that new experience—and how you use your brain actually helps determine how your brain is organized. Every experience you have in the real world causes a change in your brain. Next time you learn a lesson or lick an ice cream cone, imagine a beautiful green shrub, full of dendrites and synapses, slowly filling, creating stronger connections from one neuron to adjacent neurons. This process is happening constantly, and goes in both directions. If you have fewer real-world experiences or lessons learned, those shrubs start to wither away as well, weakening the connections inside your brain.

As you take in new information, the brain builds intricate circuits of knowledge and memory. This is how we learn and how we retain what we learn. On a good day, this works in your favor as you learn things that are important to you such as how to read and write, tie your shoes, play a musical instrument, or master a skill.

Many factors affect how well or weakly a memory sticks, but across scientific literature, one stands out: attention. Memory researchers agree on a fundamental point. Memory starts with attention. For many people when they think they have forgotten something, the truth is they never properly remembered it in the first place. For example, you come home and mindlessly place your car keys down and can't find them later. It is not that you forgot where you put your keys down, it is that you weren't paying attention when you did. Many memory problems can be addressed by taking the extra step to pay attention. How you pay attention to information may be the most important factor not only in how much you actually remember but also the way in which you remember it—the sensory and emotional coloration in your mind. This becomes paramount as we consider how the brain remembers pain and processes new incoming signals. Simply focusing your attention toward or away from pain is critically important for changing how you experience it.

Pain Encodes Pain for Future Reference

Our memories work on two different levels: short term and long term. But even before an experience can become part of our short-term memory, there's a brief sensory stage—just a fraction of a second. During this initial stage, your brain logs your perception of an experience as it registers incoming information—what you see, feel, and hear. Sensory memory allows that perception to remain after the stimulation is over, though only momentarily. Then the sensation moves into short-term memory.

Most people can hold only about seven items of information—such as a list of seven grocery items or a seven-digit phone number—in short-term memory for about twenty to thirty seconds. If you take longer than that to dial the number, you may have to keep looking it up again. This happens to me all the time. If you say the numbers out loud, however, that can help reset the short-term memory clock, and if you do this enough, eventually you will create a longer-term memory.

Ordinarily, long-term memory serves us well. It helps keep you sharp as you age. Think of it as your own life narrative, allowing you to recall a lunch last week with a friend or winning a big game as a child. Short-term memories disappear quickly, while long-term memories act more like an unlimited cloud, full of space for more and more of your life experiences that you can access throughout your whole life. When you want to remember something, you retrieve the information on an unconscious level, bringing it into your conscious mind at will. But aside from whatever pain lessons we need or want to remember—meaning those that serve a protective purpose—other memories of pain that replay and reignite the brain's pain circuitry are not helpful.

"It's as if you'd just tangled up a bunch of telephone wires and reconnected them," says Linda Porter at NIH. "How do you take them apart and put them back where they really belong to be non-painful and effective?"

Diverse Cultural Concepts of Pain and Health Focus on Flow and Balance

How people understand and talk about pain, what makes pain, and what relieves it differs across many cultures. Many healing traditions, including those of Indigenous cultures, Chinese medicine, Ayurveda, in practices such as acupuncture, yoga, tai chi, or qi gong, personal spirituality, and others, highlight the flow of energy as a life force. The mind-body-spirit connection tends to be central to preventing and treating pain. These traditions often reflect an alignment with forces of nature—water, wind, heat, cold—and the need for balance and harmony among them for health and healing. There's often a strong therapeutic focus on connecting with nature, a caring community, a higher spirit, or just the practice of mindfulness.

For many people, these ideas can support mind-body practices for pain. As Western pain science inches forward with research that explains the mechanisms involved, the body of literature continues to grow, though it's still far short of the lived experience of those who find relief and optimism through these personal or culture-based practices.

Human Vulnerability and Media: Determinants of Health—and Pain

In a hospital setting, my patients find themselves wheeled into the calm, controlled, sterile environment of the operating room. Once there, my team meticulously calibrates every aspect of pain management, mitigating the patients' experiences of what could have been, if not for anesthesia, some of the most painful few hours of their lives. Most of the pain we experience, however, happens outside such controlled settings, in the wilds of everyday life.

As a medical journalist reporting from the front lines, I have traveled to war zones where many soldiers and civilians are experiencing the most terrifying time of their lives. On several occasions, with a soldier's life hanging in the balance, I've been tapped for neurosurgical duty. It would be logical to assume that for survivors of violence, their physical injuries would have the most dramatic impact. But what I've learned over the years is that for many, it is the psychological trauma that leaves the most lasting scars. As we know now from the science of neuroplastic pain and from decades of research on post-traumatic stress, each person's experience can become encoded in memory.

Far from traditional wartime battlefields, people's brains have created similar neural networks while suffering adverse conditions that were long overlooked or minimized: injustice, inequities, and discrimination. Societal shrapnel inflicts its own wounds—and, yes, pain. Where you live and, in many cases, how much you are exposed to toxic psychological conditions absolutely influence the way pain affects your life.

With all that in mind, I close this chapter on an encouraging note. For all the complexity of the brain and its pain-processing circuitry, it's surprisingly accessible and responsive once you know how to approach it. You might assume that making structural changes to the brain to alleviate pain would require a neurosurgeon's skills or, at the very least, drugs or devices that act on pain through other mechanisms. But the truth is, you can train your own brain to change pain circuitry. This is a tool that all of us can use—no scalpel needed.

As you'll see in part 2, I named the first of my seven strategies *mind your brain.* There's a reason for that. And now that you understand the basics about how the brain creates pain, you can see why the brain itself is one of the most powerful tools for changing your experience of pain. This is especially relevant as we look next at what scientists now suggest we can do to keep acute pain from progressing to chronic pain.

Inflammation: First Responder or Chronic Culprit?

Inflammation is the immune system's response to a variety of factors, including injury, infection, cell and tissue damage, radiation, and toxic substances. Once thought a villain to vanquish at every turn, inflammation has more recently been recognized as essential for health and healing as it marshals a range of responses to minimize infection and begin to repair injuries.

However, continued demands can overwhelm the system and create chronic inflammation that becomes a smoldering source of ongoing pain rather than of relief and repair. The initial redness, swelling, and tenderness that accompany an injury are protective; they're a sign that the cascade of natural cellular and chemical inflammatory mediators is at work. But these inflammatory mediators are a double-edged sword. They can also damage the tissue they came to protect.

A host of physiological processes throughout the body involving specialized cells and biochemical brews can amplify or reduce pain, particularly through inflammation. For example, painful injuries activate glial cells and immune cells, along with cell-signaling molecules such as cytokines, neuropeptides, growth factors, and neurotransmitters to stoke inflammation sufficient to trigger other healing processes. Kept in check, these pro-inflammatory mediators activate just enough to get the attention of other systems that set about to repair, rebuild, and restore tissue and vital functions.

To be clear, inflammation of this kind is part of the healing process: it's the flare that alerts the others. But when these mediators get overexcited and go beyond what's needed—when for whatever reason the "stop memo" doesn't reach them—the continuing inflammation can sensitize nociceptors and that can lead to chronic pain, as we'll see in the next chapter.

In routine procedures, I can effectively quiet amped-up "danger detectors" using a few milliliters of lidocaine, allowing me to perform surgery on your hand without you so much as flinching. If you already have inflammation, however, your nociceptors are on especially high alert and even a slight touch may cause you to scream out in pain. More recently, scientists have observed that "excited" neurons not only amplify a signal but also excite neighboring cells to activate as well. They're now searching for ways to heighten or dampen that excitability. Some have even suggested that inflammation and the inflammatory response could be considered "a unifying law of pain."

New research shows that once again, the body-brain circuit—and the brain stem specifically—has a larger role in regulating inflammation than was previously thought. A study published in *Nature* in May 2024 reported that certain chemicals communicate to warn the brain of an emerging inflammatory response. When researchers silenced this circuit, they reported "unregulated and out-of-control inflammatory responses." By contrast, activating this circuit provided "exceptional neural control of immune responses."

This "dial in the brain" thus controls the immune system, with the cells there acting as "master regulators of the body's inflammatory response," writes Swiss science journalist Giorgia Guglielmi, PhD, in a piece accompanying the study. "The results suggest that the brain maintains a delicate balance between the molecular signals that promote inflammation and those that dampen it," she says. This offers new hope and avenues for research to find treatments for autoimmune diseases and other conditions caused by an excessive immune response.

CHAPTER 4

Hot-Wired: What Trips the Switch for Chronic Pain?

I once performed an operation called a lumbar discectomy on two women on the same day. They were just a few years apart in age, and strangely they both had the same first name, Joanna. They were physiologically almost interchangeable in terms of their blood work, weight, and lifestyle.

The operations, intended to remove the pressure on a nerve from a herniated disc, were performed under general anesthesia on the lower back through a small vertical incision. Both women had the same symptoms, and in both, I operated on the disc between the fourth and fifth lumbar vertebrae, right around the belt line. The operations took around the same amount of time, and there was negligible blood loss in both patients.

In short, I performed two nearly identical operations on two nearly identical women, just hours apart. I fully expected both to do well and go home the next day.

The next morning, I walked into Joanna #1's room. She was sitting upright and greeted me with a smile. She had straightened her bedside table, opened her drapes, applied lipstick, and looked like she was ready to meet a friend for lunch. Having already walked the halls, she was anxiously awaiting discharge. This is almost always a good sign in terms of how someone is likely to progress and heal.

Then I went to see Joanna #2. The room was still dark when I walked in and quietly called her name. She was slumped over in bed with a grimace on her face, her hair a tangled mess. I noticed a morphine pain pump sitting next to her bed. One of the doctors had authorized it overnight, I was told, because she had been in total agony. This Joanna hadn't even been up to use the bathroom, much less walk the halls.

It was the tale of two patients undergoing the same operation with completely opposite recoveries.

As a surgeon, the first thing I thought was, *Did I miss something?* Had I overlooked anything in Joanna #2's initial evaluation, or did something slip my notice during the operation? Once I ruled that out by reviewing the medical chart again and talking to others who were in the operating room, I was confronted with this stark reality: no matter how much we measure, prepare, collect evidence, and use our judgment, pain can defy all of the tools we have.

Such contrasts in recovery weren't uncommon then, nearly twenty-five years ago, and they aren't now. But today, scientists are focusing on them with a new urgency. They want to learn why some people recover quickly, their pain subsiding within the expected healing period, while others continue to suffer for days, months, or even years.

This type of persistent pain presents a particularly perplexing puzzle because the specific physiological mechanisms that drive it are still poorly understood.

In chronic pain, something seems to go amiss. It's possible that tissue damage that seemed to be healed continues to surreptitiously activate pain receptors in the peripheral nervous system. Or perhaps there's some ongoing but undetected nerve damage or other disruption of the nervous system. Or maybe it's the result of neuroinflammation, which has put the central nervous system on a hair trigger and keeps tripping it.

Another fascinating theory now percolating among scientists, however, is the possibility that chronic pain is essentially a learned behavior in which the brain encodes an initial acute pain experience, then plays it over and over again even when no physical threat exists. As those neurons fire together and wire together, the brain learns and remembers that pain pattern, then puts it on a continuous loop. That encoding might be influenced by factors seemingly unrelated to an existing medical issue—in the case of the Joannas, a herniated lumbar disc. A previous history of depression, for example, might be a factor in the outcome, as we'll see in a moment.

I'm reminded of Linda Porter's "tangled up bunch of telephone wires" metaphor when mixed-up neurocircuitry causes the brain to replay a pain memory beyond its usefulness as a cautionary lesson. Now imagine that tangle includes a mass of additional lines—neural networks and symptoms for other coexisting conditions, all impossible to distinguish from each other.

"The hypersensitivity of all these interactions and of all these parts of the circuitry make it really difficult to undo those now fixed," Porter explains. In other words, once a pain experience becomes lodged in long-term memory and the track has been set down through a pain-processing error or circuitry quirk, that's trouble. Accurate diagnosis and treatment become infinitely more complex and challenging.

One of the most pivotal shifts in thinking over the past several years is the recognition that not all chronic pain begins with an acute pain episode; as we've seen, many people develop chronic pain with no clear physical cause at all. And if pain does occur in the wake of an injury, it can persist well after the expected healing time, or even reappear months or years later for no apparent reason. In either case, the aim is to stop that initial progression, called chronification—and, most important, to identify how medical or self-care steps might intervene to minimize or even eliminate it.

Anxiety and Depression Are Dominant in the Mix

Chronic anxiety and depression both appear to have a strong connection to chronic pain. If you have chronic pain, you are nearly five times more likely to have these symptoms. Looked at from the other direction, people living with chronic pain make up more than half of the US adults who suffer from chronic anxiety or depression.

A recent study found that people who had mental health symptoms and chronic pain occurring at the same time were significantly more affected than dealing with either of those conditions by themselves, a destructive synergistic effect.

Researchers are also finding biological connections between chronic pain, anxiety, and depression, often arising from the molecular and chemical mechanisms and brain regions we discussed in the previous chapter. Since the brain shares functions among many regions and neural pathways, it's not surprising that some of the regions associated with pain processing overlap with those active in anxiety and depression.

Neuroinflammation is also associated with both, as it has been shown to lead to pain after surgery, sleep disturbances, and cognitive impairment—all issues connected to anxiety and depression. And the combination of chronic pain, anxiety, and depression is an independent risk factor for new or increased substance misuse, social isolation, and suicide.

When these conditions coexist, they're more difficult to treat, and outcomes are worse than when a person has one condition without the others. So although countless health conditions can co-occur with chronic pain, the particular pairing of chronic pain plus anxiety and depression makes that condition especially challenging.

Are Past Events a Prologue to Chronic Pain?

As chronic pain continues, the challenges associated with it worsen. Treatment failures add to the pain sufferer's emotional burden and low morale, which, unrelieved, can contribute further to pain.

Brain imaging evidence suggests that early in the chronification process, some kind of neural rewiring takes place between brain regions and circuits in the spinal cord and peripheral nerves. Understandably then, much research on the progression from acute to chronic pain has been focused on that initial window of time—the first three months following an acute pain event such as surgery or a serious injury. But recently, researchers have focused on an intriguing new possibility: What if the true cause lies years, or even decades, earlier?

Current research shows that adverse childhood experiences (ACEs) are associated with chronic pain later in life. Physical or emotional trauma in adult life is as well, even more so when they occur together, as with post-traumatic stress (PTS) associated with violent or physically threatening events. And as we've seen, these aren't limited to battlefield trauma. Traumatic brain injury from partner violence or sports injuries is also linked to chronic pain.

Chronic pain's emotional connectors may also have more routine origins. "Sometimes, it's just an injury that led to pain, that led to fear, that led to a spurious medical diagnosis, that created a vicious cycle of pain," says Howard Schubiner, a physician, pain researcher, author, and professor at Michigan State University's College of Human Medicine. "Sometimes, it's simply a fearful life situation, such as a difficult boss or partner. Sometimes, it's fear or guilt. . . . There are lots of roads to pain that come from the brain."

I often think about "the trauma of everyday life"—a phrase that author Mark Epstein, a psychiatrist, used as the title for a book on this subject. Illness, loss, divorce, and other changes can reshape our lives in ways that make us more susceptible to pain.

So, what to do about it?

LIVING IT

Courtney Putnam, expressive arts therapist

I was a gymnast and a track and field athlete—a high jumper. I did a lot of bounding and jumping and was very flexible. Starting in about my twenties, my body started to share with me that, *Hey, those activities don't feel good anymore.* I started to get more chronic neck pain, chronic back pain, and around that time started to get pretty regular headaches—migraines.

A lot of my pain experiences have been kind of elusive, and my doctors diagnosed me with chronic low back pain, chronic neck pain. One wondered if there was fibromyalgia, but I didn't meet the markers for that. When I was in my thirties, suddenly my quadricep tendons and knees hurt, and I didn't know why all this continued to be a problem for me. I've seen several physical therapists who all have different kinds of views about what's going on.

It's quite challenging because it's a vulnerable place to go, to seek help, and I want to trust the process I'm experiencing. It also makes me realize that there *are* so many vantage points, and they all could be valid and maybe they're *all* contributing to the issue. For instance, one physical therapist said the high arches of my feet are contributing to my getting a lot of pressure on my knees. Somebody else said that it's really about not activating my hips and glutes when I walk. I've gotten different perspectives, and I've pieced it together. I still do some of the physical therapy exercises that I've gleaned along the way and use them intuitively. I've always been very in tune with my body and my body's sensations, and that helps with intuition. I think a lot of people who have pain and chronic pain probably have that ability as well—to feel the nuances of their experience.

The Brain That Changes Itself: A Setup or a Solution for Chronic Pain?

A. Vania Apkarian, PhD, one of the world's foremost pain scientists and a poet in his native Armenia, has described chronic pain as "a memory that cannot be extinguished."

"We can talk about it in some fancy jargon and all of that, but it's very simple, and in many ways even Plato and Aristotle understood these things," says Apkarian, a professor of physiology, anesthesiology, and physical medicine and rehabilitation at Northwestern University's Feinberg School of Medicine. "Our brain is in a continuous struggle between our emotional response to our environment and our more cognitive response to the environment, and the battle between the two of them is essentially the (neural) networks fighting each other. In a very simple way, in chronic pain we are losing that battle to the emotional circuit."

In pioneering work using brain imaging, Apkarian's aptly named Pain and Passions Lab has identified brain regions that are activated differently by acute pain and chronic pain, reflecting different neuroplastic changes. With the networked emotional circuits entangled with chronic pain, the brain learns and remembers chronic pain in ways that are "continuously reinforced and thus cannot be extinguished."

The corticolimbic system, which integrates cognition and emotion, is also highly involved in a person's pain experience. So even though the last thing you consciously want is for unhelpful pain memories to stick, the brain processes them through a system that does exactly that. The shared circuits of pain, emotion, and cognition, as well as the brain's habit of learning through repetition, can drive the progression to chronic pain.

I always feel a sense of wonder when I see patients recover after a brain injury. It's as if the brain is teeming with little construction crews laying down new roads to bypass the damaged ones. And seeing a healthy part of the brain take over for an injured part is like watching a new city being constructed for the displaced residents of the old one. That's neuroplasticity in action.

But there's one crucial catch. Neuroplasticity is fundamentally a neutral process, not an inherently benevolent one. So any cue—physical or emotional, a sound or smell—can prompt the brain to tap a neural shortcut and pick up on remembered pain (or fear or joy), in the same way it perks up at the first notes of your favorite song or the sight of a loved one.

Nature's Tipping Point: Inflammation and the Goldilocks Principle

I wrote earlier about the positive role that inflammation plays in activating the immune system to fight traumatic injury. The Goldilocks principle that aims for "just right" applies: too much inflammation can do us harm and leave us vulnerable. Too little offers us no help. We need just enough inflammation to fight infection and promote healing.

A recent study of genetic variables in the progression from acute to chronic pain revealed one surprising facet of inflammation: the timing of when it appears may determine whether it hurts or helps. Specifically, a robust inflammatory response in patients with acute back pain, observable in very active immune cells in the blood, was associated with a more active healing process, helping to resolve acute pain within the predictable time. But in patients whose pain continued past the three-month mark, that initial cellular activity was markedly absent.

This particular study compared patients' blood samples from the time they developed acute lower back or jaw pain to three months later. The goal was to determine what transcriptional (protein-driven mechanism that turns a gene "on" or "off") activity might be associated with patients who healed as expected versus those who still had pain after three months. McGill University geneticist Luda Diatchenko MD, PhD, and her colleagues were surprised when a pattern related to inflammation—which they hadn't even been looking for—showed up unexpectedly in the blood analyses. Among those with chronic pain, "there was absolutely nothing happening in their blood in terms of cellular activation early on, including inflammation," Diatchenko said. It was as if the active cellular processes had been in "a kind of frozen state."

This finding, published in the journal *Science Translational Medicine*, upended prevailing assumptions about inflammation. Before, it was seen as driving the progression from acute to chronic pain, which led to the standard practice of tamping down inflammation quickly after injury or surgery. Now, the research was showing that impairment of inflammatory responses *increased* the risk of chronic pain. So giving anti-inflammatory pain meds too early might be as problematic as giving too many of them. As you will learn later, this is one of the primary reasons that movement and exercise may be a better immediate option than rest and ice for many injuries.

These findings were considered startling, even radical, in the scientific community, and no one was more surprised than Diatchenko herself. In the context of postsurgery pain, she said, "We all think about inflammation as a bad thing, because we know that in chronic pain patients there is this kind of low-grade inflammation. That's why we always think we need to inhibit, inhibit, inhibit this very low grade of inflammation." Now we know otherwise.

Bedside-to-Bench: A New Push for Life Lessons to Lead Chronic Pain Research

Over a hundred years ago, William Osler, the Canadian physician and founding influence on modern medicine and medical education, is said to have instructed his students to "listen to the patient. Quite often he is telling you the diagnosis."

Today, the urgent search for meaningful insights into chronic pain has given that idea a new relevance, with impressive results. Health care providers now encourage patients to engage as partners in the treatment process. Research programs now routinely include people with lived experience—patients, family members, caregivers—as members of committees that advise and direct pain studies.

Pain scientists are calling for a dramatic change that puts greater emphasis on the studies that draw first from people's real-life pain experience, then follows up with lab-based research to develop targeted solutions for effective pain management. This reverse translational research flips the classic bench-to-bedside process that starts in a laboratory and ends with a clinical trial.

Reverse translational research begins with the patient's real-world experience and then tries to decipher the mechanisms through brain imaging and blood tests, correlated with the patient's symptoms and self-reports. Instead of the bench to the bedside, which was taught when I was in medical school, this is bedside to the bench research. The bench scientists then work with the findings to learn more about the basic mechanisms.

Prasad Shirvalkar, a pain physician, neuroscientist, and the director of the Shirvalkar Lab at the University of California at San Francisco, used such a hybrid approach a couple of years ago to find the unicorn in pain science: *objective biomarkers of a subjective experience.* He started by implanting electrodes in the brains of patients, to measure brain signals. He then followed the trial participants home and, with the use of continuous surveys and digital monitoring, tracked their pain through everyday life and correlated those results with direct readings from the brain. The combination of lab-based and home-based monitoring led to a groundbreaking series of clinical trials that made headlines around the world. In 2023, his team was able to directly map signals of chronic pain for the first time in history. In more recent trials, the team used electrodes implanted in the brain to map the unique neural signature of each participant's pain experience over thousands of hours. The result was the ability, for the first time, to create an objective measure of an individual patient's subjective pain experiences.

The AI Assist: Flagging Those at Higher Risk for Pain to Start Preventive Measures Sooner

To be effective, artificial intelligence (AI), its machine-learning subset, and advanced deep learning by computer algorithms require large amounts of standardized and accurate data. While immense quantities of patient and treatment data are now being collected and stored, access to those data, comprehension of how they might be used, and creation of software and methods of analysis all require time, rigorous testing, and extensive clinical trials to validate. The process is exceedingly complex, intensive in computational time, and costly.

Substantial efforts are nonetheless underway to bring AI's potential to pain detection, assessment, treatment, and long-term management. In addition to the NIH's A2CPS study, which focused on identifying factors that lead to chronic pain, other efforts have been organized to detect whether facial expressions, muscle tension, sweating, body movements, or skin conduction can be used as reliable and actionable indicators of pain.

For example, in July 2022, the *European Journal of Pain* published a study of a deep-learning system trained to identify facial expressions indicative of pain. The system was trained to identify and classify 2,810 facial expressions from 1,189 patients, using expressions captured before and after surgery. It was then tested to evaluate postoperative pain on a rating scale of 0 to 10, with the AI pain ratings compared with the ratings supplied by thirty-three nurses. Evaluating 120 face images, the AI system accurately interpreted pain intensity 53 percent of the time. It correctly detected pain rated 4 or greater 89.7 percent of the time, and pain rated 7 or greater 77.5 percent of the time. By comparison, the nurses estimated the right pain intensity 4 or greater 44.9 percent of the time and 7 or greater 17 percent of the time. "The findings represent a major step in the development of a fully automated, rapid, standardized, and objective method based on facial expression analysis to measure pain and detect severe pain," the researchers concluded.

In another study, this one by anesthesiologists at the Leiden University Medical Center in the Netherlands and the Shaare Zedek Medical Center in Jerusalem, researchers employed something known as a nociception, or pain monitor, during surgery to guide later opioid use even as the procedure was still underway. Among patients who received opioids as directed by the monitor, the number who experienced severe postsurgical pain was 70 percent lower than those who received opioids using a standardized manual procedure.

The monitor, attached to the patient's middle finger, has four sensors: a PPG (photoplethysmogram) to measure cardiovascular attributes, one to measure galvanic skin response, an accelerometer, and a thermistor. Collectively, these sensors respectively record variables such as heart rate, heart rate variability, vasoconstriction, and sweating. A trained AI system then generates a score that indicates how much postsurgical pain was expected and the appropriate amount of opioids to blunt it. Over time, researchers expect that advanced systems employing AI will be able to provide reliable information to guide the diagnosis and treatment of pain in a wide variety of clinical settings.

In a more recent and ongoing trial, the maps and electrodes were used to predict a pain burst, which was followed by the delivery of a carefully calibrated electrical impulse—deep brain stimulation (DBS) to interrupt the pain, reducing or even eliminating it altogether. Predicting when pain might occur, objectively measuring its severity, and then quickly inhibiting it is in many ways the ultimate achievement.

The following story is about someone using this remarkable treatment approach, but first a caveat. It's not currently available, or even feasible, for general use, so it can't deliver on the dream of a cure for chronic pain. But it *does* deliver evidence that pain circuitry in the brain is measurable and malleable. It can be targeted and treated, and we'll likely see the emergence of a range of approaches that can do so without brain surgery.

"Lightning Bolt Razor Snakes"

By the time Ed Mowery stepped to the podium to brief the US Congress about his experience on the front lines of pain research in 2024, the audience had already met him—or, at least, had met his brain. And his pain.

Mowery, the fifty-three-year-old founder, vocalist, and bassist of a metal band from New Mexico, had been a chronic pain sufferer for more than thirty years when he signed on to participate in the Shirvalkar Lab's clinical trial of deep brain stimulation to intercept pain in the brain. Now, Shirvalkar and the burly, bald, bearded musician had come to share the results with policymakers on Capitol Hill. They included an elaborate slide presentation of data taken from Mowery's brain by implanted electrodes.

Mowery had been diagnosed with complex regional pain syndrome (CRPS), the long-lasting pain that can follow an injury or medical trauma. CRPS can occur anywhere in the body, but it usually affects a person's arm, leg, hand, or foot. Mowery described his pain as "lightning bolt razor snakes" that would strike in his big toes and wreak havoc all up and down his legs and into his low back. "I would literally reach down to see if I was cut and bleeding when the snakes came out in my legs."

By this point, he understood that his pain was manufactured in his brain. "No cuts, no bruises, nothing at all to see," he said, "with the exception of how I reacted to it."

As Mowery struggled with his escalating pain, a thousand miles west, in a neuroscience lab at the University of California, San Francisco (UCSF), Shirvalkar and a team of scientists were working to find a solution for it. Their tools were implantable gadgetry, a phalanx of high-tech equipment, AI, and one revolutionary idea: if they could track a person's pain as it happened—moving beyond traditional lab assessment experiments—then perhaps they could devise a way to interrupt the pain and dial it down, or even make it stop.

The UCSF team first needed to find biomarkers, consistent biological signals linked to the very subjective experience of pain. Their hope was that these biomarkers would not only create a living map of his pain-related brain waves but also predict when those waves might come, just as a surfer can predict the arrival of the next big swell. The team aimed to use that technology to deliver a dose of electrical stimulation at the precise moment needed to interrupt the pain wave, thus reducing or even stopping its arrival.

I remember the first time Shirvalkar explained this to me on the phone. At first it sounded fantastical, but as he passionately described the science, it sounded more and more possible.

His team had taken the most basic and timeless questions necessary for treating pain—*Where does it hurt?* and *How much does it hurt?*—and found the answer in the brain itself. The implanted electrodes made it possible to at first simply listen to the mind's internal universe. There are nearly as many brain cells inside your skull as there are stars in the galaxy, so the task was daunting. It was as if the researchers were pointing their sensory equipment up at the sky and then waiting to hear what sounds and signals they could pick up. This required a lot of patience, and it was just the beginning.

Next, the researchers hoped to decode all those signals, allowing them to create the real-time circuitry map of the brain as pain was happening. To help verify the strength and veracity of that map, they used patients' time-stamped reports of pain, then correlated those to corresponding brain wave patterns using advanced machine learning tools. Finally, they used a small burst of electricity to target those networks in real time to interrupt, turn down, or turn off the pain.

The goal, Shirvalkar explains, was to determine which brain regions actively generate signals for pain, because they would be the ideal targets to stimulate. Next, the researchers also needed to get the precise timing of the stimulation right. When surfers catch waves too early or too late, they might move hardly at all—or they might be pounded into the ocean floor. The same thing could happen here: the patient may have no reaction to the stimulation, or too much reaction, which might lead to more pain. Finally, the researchers wanted to determine the best pattern of stimulation.

It was a gamble for Shirvalkar, and even more so for the patient. "For better or worse, it's brain stimulation and it's invasive brain surgery, so it's often considered a therapy of last resort," he says. "The folks we recruit often have tried at least two drugs or drug classes, usually four or five injections or other kind of nerve blocks. Many of them have tried nerve stimulators or even spinal cord stimulators. So basically, they're the most severe of the chronic pain population. They have been failed by these therapies."

Mowery fell into this category. He had tried more than twenty medications, steroid injections, a spinal cord stimulator, and physical therapy. He'd had discs replaced and others fused. And still he was disabled, tormented by pain. His pain centered in his limbs, but it had worsened over time and was now a sharp, stabbing, burning over his whole body. Even so, he hesitated to join the trial, which would require a brain operation to implant the electrodes that would constantly monitor his brain's pain signals for the next two years, and hopefully deliver well-timed electrical stimulation to interrupt the pain signals. It sounded like a wonderful technological dream, but he knew there was no guarantee that any of it would work.

"It scared the hell out of me," he said later. "I waited a year and a half to sign on. I was deathly afraid of brain surgery. But the pain got so bad and so brutal that I didn't care what they did to me. I just wanted it to stop. I felt I had no other choice but to go through with the trial."

Target Risk Factors You Can Change with Preventive Steps and Strategies

Risk factors for chronic pain are a mirror on contemporary life:

- Chronic stress
- Inflammation
- Sedentary lifestyle and obesity
- Depression, anxiety, and mental health challenges
- Other chronic diseases
- Social isolation and loneliness
- Social and economic inequities that undermine health care
- Longevity

Some factors, such as our age, genetic predispositions, history of trauma, and social conditions, aren't things we can directly affect in everyday ways. But other factors are modifiable, from our choices of medical treatment and self-management of pain to lifestyle choices that help build physical and emotional resilience.

To reduce your risks and boost resilience, the International Association for the Study of Pain offers these general health guidelines:

- Maintain a healthy diet and weight.
- Exercise regularly.
- Eliminate unhealthy practices such as excessive alcohol use and smoking.

- Work and rest in a variety of healthy postures.
- Manage stress with everything from breathing to having fun.
- Seek counseling or psychological/behavioral therapy whenever needed.

Off the Grid No More: Mapping the Coordinates of Chronic Pain

Pain, suffering, and desperation, but sprinkled with a dose of hope like Mowery had, were considered prerequisites for participants in this pair of biomarker studies, the first of which made international headlines. "First-in-Human Prediction of Chronic Pain State Using Intracranial Neural Biomarkers" was published in *Nature Neuroscience* in June 2023. The senior coauthors of the study, which was funded by the NIH BRAIN Initiative, HEAL Initiative, and DARPA (Defense Advanced Research Projects Agency), included Shirvalkar and a who's who of pain science heavy hitters.

The main takeaway from earlier studies of deep brain stimulation had been that whatever DBS benefits work in the short term seem to fade, so Shirvalkar focused on building a closed-loop (automated) deep brain stimulation (DBS) solution. "Specifically, can we try to engineer a system that looks like a thermostat, and acts like a thermostat," he says. "Could it turn on and off in response to the measurements of the ambient heat?"—by which he meant ambient pain.

In the initial mapping phase, researchers "listened" to the brain, monitoring the brain waves in the anterior cingulate cortex and orbitofrontal cortex, two brain regions that scientists believe are central to pain processing.

Rx: Reframe, Replace, Reset

Rewrite the Script of Unhelpful Thoughts about Your Pain

Pain is designed to get our attention, so it's only natural that your thoughts about it in the moment can feel automatic. But thinking about pain can make you more sensitive to it and even make the pain feel worse. As it worsens, your thoughts may grow more negative, continuing the cycle. Negative thinking can also depress your mood, lead you to avoid activities that could be helpful, and result in isolation that can make pain feel worse and cut you off from sources of pleasure and more positive experiences and thoughts.

Your initial thoughts about your pain may arise uninvited, but you can use them as cues to refocus your attention, identify unhelpful thoughts, and rewrite the script. The US Department of Veterans Affairs suggests this self-assessment and everyday practice.

Common Pain Thoughts	
Catastrophizing: Believing that something is the worst it could possibly be.	
Example of Unhelpful Thoughts	When my pain is bad, I can't do anything.
Example of Helpful Thoughts	**Even when my pain is bad, there are still some things I can do.**
"Should" Statements: Thinking in terms of how things should or ought to be.	
Example of Unhelpful Thoughts	My doctor should be able to cure my pain.
Example of Helpful Thoughts	**There is no cure for chronic pain, but I can use skills to cope with my pain.**
All or None Thinking: Seeing things as "either or" or "right or wrong" instead of in terms of degrees.	
Example of Unhelpful Thoughts	I can only be happy if I am pain free.
Example of Helpful Thoughts	**Even if I am in pain, I can still be happy. There is always something that I can do to have a better quality of life.**

Common Pain Thoughts	
Overgeneralization: Viewing one or two bad events as an endless pattern of defeat.	
Example of Unhelpful Thoughts	I tried doing exercises for my back pain before and it didn't help. So it isn't going to help now.
Example of Helpful Thoughts	Although physical therapy didn't help much before, maybe this time it will help. I might as well try.
Jumping to Conclusions: Making negative conclusions of events that are not based on fact.	
Example of Unhelpful Thoughts	When I move my back hurts, so it must be bad for me to move.
Example of Helpful Thoughts	Hurt does not equal harm.
Emotional Reasoning: Believing how you feel reflects how things really are.	
Example of Unhelpful Thoughts	I feel useless, so I am useless.
Example of Helpful Thoughts	Even though I can't do all the things I used to do, it doesn't mean I can't do anything.
Disqualifying the Positive: Focusing on only the bad and discounting the good.	
Example of Unhelpful Thoughts	So what if I am doing more, I am still in pain.
Example of Helpful Thoughts	Doing more is important for me to live the life I want to live.

Source: US Department of Veterans Affairs.

Note: For more health information materials, visit the US Department of Veterans Affairs website at https://www.va.gov.

After the DBS devices were inserted, including electrodes 1.3 mm in diameter and 400 mm in length, the participants returned home, where the brain monitoring continued. Several times a day, they were asked to log their pain level, answer survey questions, and press the button on the device that started recording their brain signals for thirty seconds. One survey asked participants to rate how accurately a descriptive word for pain—such as *stabbing, crushing,* or *burning*—resonated for what they were feeling.

Participants were asked to do check-ins multiple times a day for up to six months, and these data—the same questions but with real-time variations in responses—plotted their pain fluctuation over time. The data were live-streamed to the San Francisco lab, where the researchers then created an AI model to analyze and correlate each person's daily data, enabling them to predict when and where the participant's brain activity would reflect their pain in real time and at what level.

Every two months, the participants would fly to San Francisco for three days of what Shirvalkar called "mild torture" at the Weill Institute for Neurosciences on the UCSF Mission Bay campus. After a good night's sleep in a comfortable hotel, they'd arrive each day at 8:00 a.m. and settle into a private room in the third-floor testing suite, where the lab team would brief them on the pain test itinerary for the day. Typically, this included a battery of sensory, physical, emotional, and cognitive tests, breaking only occasionally as needed and for lunch. Clock-out was at dinnertime.

In one test, a participant would sit at a table with arm outstretched, palm up, while a researcher placed a temperature probe about the size of a box of Tic-Tacs on the forearm. Temperatures for the testing ranged from about 90°F to 122°F. As researchers controlled the temperature, intensity, and duration of the stimulus, they asked participants to rate their pain and identify where in their bodies they felt it.

In another test, researchers placed the temperature probe on an area of the body adjacent to where the participant normally felt chronic pain. They would then run fifty to sixty trials in which the temperature was slowly ramped up to a target temperature from 107°F to 152°F, with the goal of surpassing the background chronic pain. For context, 115° is about normal pain threshold, Shirvalkar explains. "If you're holding a hot cup of coffee, it's the temperature at which it goes from really warm to just painful. And [122°] is like you've picked up a hot plate from the microwave and it's so hot you want to drop it."

As the battery of tests progressed, the researchers calibrated settings to match each person's subjective pain ratings. From those data, they were able to measure the participant's pain based on the standard 0 to 10 subjective scale, while also adding the objective measure of corresponding brain activity. So, for instance, the person might rate 107°F as 3 out of 10 on the pain scale, 115°F as a 6 out of 10, and 118°F as a 9 out of 10. Correlating all of this together allowed the researchers to create a crude biomarker for each person's pain experience.

Along with a continuous recording of the temperature applied to the subject's skin and their pain scores, researchers also monitored their hearts with EKG and pulse oximetry, which allowed them to track their cardiac rhythm, heart rate, and oxygenation, meaning they could see pain-related patterns happening outside the brain.

The next clinical trial—the one that brought Ed Mowery and others aboard—went an exciting step further. Its focus was not just on *finding* the signals but also on *using* the signals to create direct personalized pain management. Two of the participants had extreme poststroke pain. One had a spinal cord injury. And then there was Mowery, with his raging CRPS.

In this part of the clinical trial, researchers identified the best region of the brain to stimulate in order to produce relief. If the patients felt 50 percent or more relief, the researchers would implant the permanent brain device and follow them for two years. During that time, they continued to collect data from listening, assessing, decoding, and stimulating the brain regions to help create a hyperpersonalized approach to treating pain. Nothing like this had ever been done anywhere.

Along the way, researchers captured stunning amounts of data, including how pain reacts to different sets of medications (like most other pain patients, the participants were taking many) and what really happens in the brain when you experience the sudden onset of pain. Ultimately the system was able to predict and short-circuit the pain signal, significantly calming the pain circuitry for all but one of the participants. The lucky ones now "essentially have a pain thermostat in their brain that's fine-tuned, personalized to their brain," says Shirvalkar, adding that the longest participant is four years out and reports still getting good relief. Shirvalkar is the first to point out that this study illuminates just one facet of the brain/pain story and that one of its acknowledged limitations was that the study group was small. Still, we now have proof that it's possible to "see" someone's pain in their brain, measure it, and then use those data to tailor treatment.

For Ed Mowery, it worked. These stunning therapies chased away the lightning bolt razor snakes. He has been able to return to work and his music, and on the medical front, he has started the careful process of weaning off the multiple pain meds (including morphine) that he used for so long. Mowery still feels pain sometimes, but nothing like before, he says. He's now able to manage it with the DBS thermostat, regular exercise, some daily mindfulness meditation, and other relaxation practices tailored for pain management. And there's his music—his passion, his work, and his joy, all good medicine, as he describes it.

"It's been tough getting better. It takes a lot of work and determination," he says. But his only regret about the clinical trial? "That I didn't sign on sooner!"

Upstream Interventions Beat Downstream Rescue Operations

Most of us don't have access to sophisticated technology such as deep brain stimulation to treat our pain, and even as a neurosurgeon, I don't think invasive brain surgery will be the ultimate answer. Yet Prasad Shrivalkar's work has shown us what is possible: that chronic pain can be predicted and prevented at the source. If you've ever had a seemingly trivial event in your life suddenly spiral out of control, you know why it makes a lot more sense to prevent an issue rather than wait for it to blow up to a bigger, messier problem.

Scientists are discovering new mechanisms in pain and pain processing that suggest we can intervene earlier and more effectively than ever before. With chronic pain, in particular, neuroscience is showing that some symptoms that were once inexplicable have a basis in the brain and are potentially treatable and even preventable through psychological and behavioral approaches. These approaches, along with others that engage our body's physiological processes in new ways, are ready for us to use. We're so much better off if we use them to address known causes of chronic pain upstream to prevent them, rather than ignoring the causes and continually struggling downstream to rescue people once the problems are entrenched.

CHAPTER 5

My Pain, My Self: A Hostile Takeover

Of the many different ways pain impacts our lives, perhaps the most influential aspect, regardless of the diagnosis, is how it can come to define who we are—not only in how we are perceived by others but also in how we perceive ourselves.

Back when I was an intern in surgery, I had an experience with a patient that changed how I thought about pain and the impact that it can have far beyond physical symptoms. I was on the vascular surgery service, where many of the patients had diabetes and suffered tissue loss as a result of poor blood flow to their feet. Some developed gangrene, which caused their skin to turn red, purple, and eventually black. Often there would be tremendous swelling. Ultimately, the tissue would die, after which the patient would feel no pain or sensation whatsoever. Prior to that, however, the pain could be stabbing, severe, and relentless.

The biggest concern was that so-called dry gangrene could turn into wet gangrene, which meant bacteria had invaded the tissue. This can cause sepsis throughout the body, which makes the patient very sick and often leads to death. When all other treatment options have been exhausted, the only one remaining is the most dramatic: amputation. It isn't an easy choice to make, but the patients generally understood that it was necessary. This story is about a man in his late fifties in that exact situation.

He was a lifelong smoker and had diabetes for nearly thirty years. A handsome man with a big personality and quick sense of humor, he was always making the nurses and doctors laugh with wry jokes, often about his own predicament. He was well read and happy to chat about nearly anything going on in the world. But there was one thing he didn't like talking about: his gangrenous right leg.

Despite antibiotics and regular dressing changes, his leg had started to deteriorate below the knee. He had undergone several rounds of debridement, a grisly and painful process that removes dead or infected tissue in the hope that healthy tissue can better grow and heal the wound. Unfortunately, his gangrene continued to progress, and I was there when the chief of service told him he would need an amputation to prevent worse, possibly even fatal, complications.

The patient indicated that he understood the need for the procedure, known as a BKA (below-knee-amputation), and he willingly signed the consent form. But on the day of his scheduled operation, I was surprised to receive a message from the nurse on the floor informing me that the man had refused transport to the operating room. Because he and I had developed a good relationship, I was the doctor dispatched to go speak to him. What followed was one of the most memorable conversations I've had with a patient in my thirty-year career.

When I walked into the room, my typically talkative patient was stoic, refusing even to look at me. "What's going on?" I asked gently. He didn't answer, so I walked to his bed, sat down next to him, and waited silently for a few minutes while he stared quietly at the ceiling. Eventually, he leaned over to his bedside table, opened the drawer, and pulled out a piece of paper. He handed it to me.

It was an old, yellowed photograph of a young, Hollywood-handsome man wearing swimming trunks and flexing his biceps. Grinning at the camera, he looked like the very picture of health—shirtless, tanned, with tautly muscled arms and legs. At first, I wasn't sure who the man was, but as I looked closer, I realized it was my patient. I handed the photo back to him, and he sat for a few moments letting his gaze linger on it, momentarily transported back to that younger, happier time in his life. He touched the photograph, tracing the outline of his body, including his right leg.

As I sat with him, I realized that my patient was facing not just the loss of his leg today but the loss of his very self. Despite the tremendous pain he was undoubtedly experiencing, he was willing to deal with that agonizing stabbing sensation in order to hang on to a vision of himself that he simply could not let go.

With tears in his eyes, he looked pleadingly at me and said, "It doesn't really hurt anymore." It was heartbreaking, because I knew it wasn't true. Taking the medically necessary step that would save his life and alleviate his pain would also take away a critical component of who he was. My patient's leg wasn't just a part of him. It represented the essence of who he had always been as a person.

So often the consequences of a serious medical condition throw our reality into disarray. Pain, and our response to it, may become the most defining feature. Sometimes we need time to process that evolving experience. For many of us, and especially those with chronic pain that corrodes the quality of life, nurturing and strengthening a sense of self is an ongoing challenge. As I looked at my patient's tear-filled eyes, I realized I was watching that difficult, agonizing, very personal negotiation unfold in real time.

He and I sat quietly together for a few moments, and eventually he simply nodded. I unlocked the wheels on his bed, rolled him to the door, and began pushing him down the long hallway to the operating room.

Who Am I?

The idea that something sinister can invade your body and take over your mind, take over your very world, is terrifying. The insidious nature of it. The feeling of helplessness against it. The memories of a life "before" and the dawning awareness that this thing has hijacked not only your attention but also your here-and-now life—absolutely everything, including how those around you see and treat you and whatever vision you may have had of your future.

For Elsa S., seeing a few odd blisters on her face one morning marked the day her normal "before" life took the hellish turn that would become her "after." An educator with a long record of professional success, Elsa, fifty-five, had served eighteen years in a variety of high-level, demanding administrative roles in public schools. Over the previous eight years, she had worked with parents of children with special needs to develop individualized educational programs to support their learning, as well as their social and emotional development. A single mother with three children, she was devoted to her family, and she was proud of having managed to stay present for them. "I had a great job that I loved, was doing really well at work, and my kids were doing well, too," she says. "I felt really good about that."

Then, COVID-19 struck. The pandemic threw her school into turmoil, with sudden closures, partial reopenings, rolling quarantines, and high absenteeism. Children with special needs were especially hard hit, as their essential support system was so profoundly disrupted. Elsa loved these kids and their families, and to witness their suffering through all of this was gut-wrenching. And then those painful blisters erupted on her face.

She arranged a telehealth consult, but at first her doctor wasn't sure what was causing them. Seven days later, the telltale rash was identifiable as shingles. But now she was told it was too late for the standard shingles treatment, which should start within seventy-two hours of symptom onset to be most effective.

Within a week, Elsa's life was completely upended. Even though she had previously been fairly healthy, albeit stressed, a cascade of pain emerged worse than any she'd ever experienced—first in her head and neck, then her back, then her hips. Her deteriorating physical condition made her more anxious and depressed. She felt physically and emotionally devastated, not only by the pain and physical impairment but also by a new and concerning brain fog. The idea that she was literally losing her mind was terrifying.

She began losing her train of thought, fumbling with tasks she'd done a million times. Although her initial pain had been localized to a specific part of her body, it now began to erupt elsewhere, adding to her confusion and baffling her doctors. She was slowly becoming unmoored from the only life she knew.

Eventually, unable to return to work when her leave ended, Elsa lost her job as well as her sense of self as the strong, resilient, capable person she had always been.

"I used to get up at five and run five miles a day, then go to work and run a school, you know? And take care of three kids of my own at the same time," she says. "I'd always thought of myself as strong physically and emotionally—resilient. I'd always been able to handle a lot of life events." Soon, those life events narrowed to experiencing pain and accessing treatment for it, which mostly either failed or offered only temporary relief. She was living a nightmare. It was as if she'd taken a wrong turn off the highway and found herself hopelessly lost in an unfamiliar and very scary place.

When I spoke with Elsa a year and a half into this frightening detour, her pain was continuing to gain momentum, as if it had a life of its own. A shift in meds or a nerve block, an injection of medication around a nerve to temporarily "turn off" the signaling, occasionally provided brief relief. However, the block might work on one pain but not another, and either way, its effects eventually wore off.

The discouraging diagnoses piled up. Following shingles came postherpetic neuralgia, a long-term nerve damage that affects around 10 to 18 percent of people with shingles. People over age fifty, like Elsa, are at greater risk, especially for more severe, lasting distress. Her emerging mix of symptoms now included extensive body pain, headaches, and a flare-up of a connective tissue disorder that causes joint hypermobility.

This debilitating pain kept taking her further and further from the life and self she knew. It's a story I heard over and over again in conversations with chronic pain sufferers: there is a zero-sum equation when it comes to pain. It robs you of your sense of self; the more pain gains, the more you lose.

The Science of Self: Chronic Pain Remasters Neural Networks for Identity

I once heard a psychologist describe the selflessness of parenthood using the Jungian concept of "ego death," which is characterized by a sweeping loss of self and a profound reset of one's identity. As a humbled parent, I can confirm this experience. But in the context of parenting, ego death is considered a good thing; it's nature's way of creating the parenting brain through a system update with enhanced neurocircuitry for selflessness (among other things). I never really thought about the neuroscience behind this transformation until I heard a passing reference to ego death as a "merciless destruction of all previous reference points in the life of the individual." That's when it struck me: this is exactly how people with chronic pain described their lives to me.

Sometimes "various aspects of a person's life may become entangled with their pain experience, and a widening variety of activities that could promote recovery and wellbeing become threatening and are avoided," as Marianne Reddan, PhD, and Tor Wager, PhD, wrote in "Brain Systems at the Intersection of Chronic Pain and Self-Regulation" in *Neuroscience Letters*. Through this "pathological interweaving of pain and self," they say, "chronic pain, unlike acute pain, is conceived as something inseparable from one's sense of *self*."

In the brain, our sense of self is more than just a mental selfie of how we see ourselves and think others see us. It's a neurological construct buried in the circuitry of conscious self-awareness known as the default mode network (DMN), often described as the brain's daydreaming or mind-wandering channel. It gets activated when we reflect, engage in introspection, think about our future or past events, and consolidate experience, processing input from the outside world while at the same time processing conscious and unconscious input from our inner world. As pain takes over, the brain consolidates all the ways we think about ourself into a single identity defined by pain.

"There's a very neurologic component to this," says Timothy Furnish,

MD, clinical professor of anesthesiology and pain medicine at the University of California, San Diego Health, where he serves as chief of pain medicine. "All pain is experienced in the brain and just the way our brain thinks about the world has an impact on how bad the pain feels . . . The mind's ability to modulate pain is pretty dramatic." Furnish is known for his work as part of the University of California San Diego's Center for Psychedelic Research (CPR), where he's done groundbreaking research on the therapeutic potential of psychedelics for pain patients (a topic explored later in the book). He studies how psychoactive compounds act at the intersection of pain, identity, and memory in the brain. According to Furnish, brain scans of people with chronic pain in these interwoven areas of identity and reality differ from scans of people who are free of that pain. The imaging makes it possible to see pain-caused dysfunction and may lead to new ways to treat it.

Studies of chronic pain highlight the dark side of neuroplasticity I've mentioned before. As pain repeatedly interferes with other neurocircuitry, particularly the DMN and our sense of self, the brain changes in response to the constant pain messaging.

When Vania Apkarian and his colleagues used resting-state fMRI to examine functional changes in patients suffering from chronic back pain, complex regional pain syndrome, and knee osteoarthritis, they found that various types of chronic pain conditions are associated with functional connectivity and reorganizational changes within the DMN during that resting state. And the intensity of the pain and length of time someone had chronic pain made a difference in the extent of that neural reorganization, with some of these changes occurring mainly after more than a decade living with chronic pain.

The point is this: it's no surprise that pain alters everyday life, but it does much more than that. Pain can fundamentally alter our perception of ourselves in the deepest way, affecting things that once brought us joy, sense of purpose, and even our outlook on the world, which are forced to adapt to an emerging altered reality.

You Really Are Not Your Pain . . . But It Can Feel That Way

"You are not your pain" is a familiar line heard repeatedly while working on this book. It is meant to remind you that while you may *have* pain, you are more than that. Pain need not define you. We know this is true, and the stories in this chapter attest to it. But they also point to a distinct experience in which people struggled with the fact that in a very real sense pain had hijacked their "self" circuitry (or at least threatened to), and they knew that. Pain had commandeered the driver's seat, and the people felt like hapless passengers. It was like waking up in a highway nightmare just as the car careens toward a cliff's edge: if you don't grab control of the steering wheel, you're flying into the abyss. Your sense of self is that steering wheel. But the struggle to regain control of it is fierce because pain does not want to yield.

Heather Voorhees, associate professor of communication studies at the University of Montana, extensively studied how chronic conditions, including pain, create an "illness identity" which encroaches on the "you" that you once knew yourself to be.

Maybe you knew yourself as cheerful, resourceful, focused, creative, reliable, or disciplined—or spiritual, giving, or community minded. The problem is that with pain at the wheel, just when you most need to draw on those inner qualities, values, and strengths, you're least able to access them.

Pain redirects your thinking. This narrowed vision focuses on the problem—physical pain—but stops short of focusing on what you might do about it. Let's say you hit a particularly discouraging period, feeling stuck in a valley of anger, fear, or hopelessness. Your options for positive action that can pull you to higher ground can suddenly feel distant. Instead, you might curl up, start avoiding social contact, eating poorly, or spending too much time doom scrolling when you can't sleep. This sense of identity paralysis can happen to anyone when a major life change—whether that's illness or the loss of a relationship or a job, for example—upends their world.

"You're entitled to the feelings this causes, and you may need to spend some time in the valley to work through them. But you don't want to live in the valley," Voorhees says. "At some point you're going to have to make a plan for getting out of it."

Acute pain works differently, she notes, because the off-ramp to "normal" is well lit and you can see your destination on the horizon. "When you break your leg, which I've done before, things hurt," Voorhees says, "and you need to modify for a while. People support you, and then eventually you're going to get better. There's always this end goal, this sense that this isn't going to be forever. But chronic pain takes all that away. You don't know if this is going to be forever. You don't know what you're going to feel like from day to day, week to week. So how do you incorporate this into your life? How do you work with this, knowing that there isn't really a set end goal? Or maybe there is, but you don't know what that looks like yet."

Voorhees describes interviewing participants in her studies—adults who had dealt with chronic pain for varying lengths of time, some for six months to a year, others for seven years or more. Their comparisons of life before and after pain took over were revealing in descriptions of feeling like "a ghost" or "a shell" of their former selves.

"I was literally just not myself," said one. "I was painted in color . . . and those colors are fading away," said another. Her description of how it felt to lose herself this way reminded me of the art therapist's earlier point about the different languages for expressing pain.

Voorhees believes you should examine how your life has changed. She suggests starting simply. For example, you might observe: *Maybe I can't be that person I was five years ago. Maybe that person is different, but everyone changes over five years. Exactly what has changed? What do I miss? Is there a way that I can start to get part of that back?*

Some additional questions can open up your thinking: *Who do I think I am as a person, and how does pain change that? How do I fit that into my life? How does this change the way I think about myself and about my relationships? How do I work to incorporate that into my sense of self? And how does that influence how I view the world?*

There are no right or wrong answers to these questions. It's the process of diving into each one for an honest assessment that makes them valuable.

Joe Arcidiacono: Problem Solving with New Purpose

Joe Arcidiacono's view of his world changed in a split second.

A week before his forty-fifth birthday, he was in a motorcycle accident that left him paralyzed, with no sensation from the middle of his chest down. A few months later, his symptoms worsened after he developed a spinal syrinx, a fluid-filled cyst in his spinal cord. The cyst caused diminished sensation down his left arm and inhibited his ability to distinguish hot from cold or sharp from dull. Over the years, he had three back operations, including removal of his T3 vertebra, a fusion, and a spinal cord pump, which infused a steady stream of baclofen to help address spasms. He had survived a horrible accident, but his sense of self, physically and mentally, was forever altered.

"From day one after the accident, I was in pain," Arcidiacono says. "I was stuck in bed most of the time and they had me on some pretty powerful painkillers. Opiates really frightened me from all of the horror stories I have heard. I would find myself not taking them, even if I was in pain, due to my fear of getting addicted." When he was finally able to get into a wheelchair and do a workout, his pain level dropped significantly. "It's still weird to me that lying in bed doing nothing can cause me so much pain, and the cure is to get up and move," he says. "The more I saw the reduction in my pain levels, the more I worked out. I increased my stamina dramatically during those first few years."

Arcidiacono told me that he drew from strengths he had honed during his more than twenty-five-year career in the US Navy, where he developed problem-solving skills, the ability to find the positive in any situation, and a bedrock belief that failure is not an option.

"From day one, I asked the doctors what they needed me to do to improve my life, and I did what they told me to do every time," he says. "They were always amazed at my progress and the fact that I never got down on myself or showed any signs of quitting. I was constantly problem solving and figuring out how to complete the tasks I wanted to do in my new life." While his goals were now wildly different from those he envisioned when he left the navy, he still had goals that challenged him and renewed his sense of purpose while helping him retain his sense of self.

This isn't to suggest that the road is easy. Arcidiacono, now fifty-eight, is candid about the fact that he deals with spasticity, pain, and lots of frustration. Yet it's clear that the active, challenge-seeking lifestyle he had enjoyed before the accident, combined with his military training, helped him find himself once again.

This is a valuable lesson for anyone dealing with chronic pain. The inner qualities and values that defined you to yourself may be obscured by pain, but they remain part of who you are and are strengths you can draw on—albeit differently than you did before. Remember, neuroscience has established the existence of pain-self circuitry in the brain. Pain will push to take over that circuitry with its imposing presence, but you can effectively push back with the very essence of who you are.

Who Am I Really?

It's a scary question for any of us, but Voorhees has some ideas to help answer it.

In a 2022 study of how chronic pain can deeply change the way we define ourselves, the team used the communication theory identity model developed by researcher Michael L. Hecht, to construct the "four frames of identity"—personal, relational, enacted, communal—that you can try yourself.

Think of the four frames as concentric circles, with the personal identity frame as the bull's-eye and the others expanding outward in widening spheres of engagement, overlapping and merging, all part of your identity. Voorhees asks participants how their pain changed the way they feel about

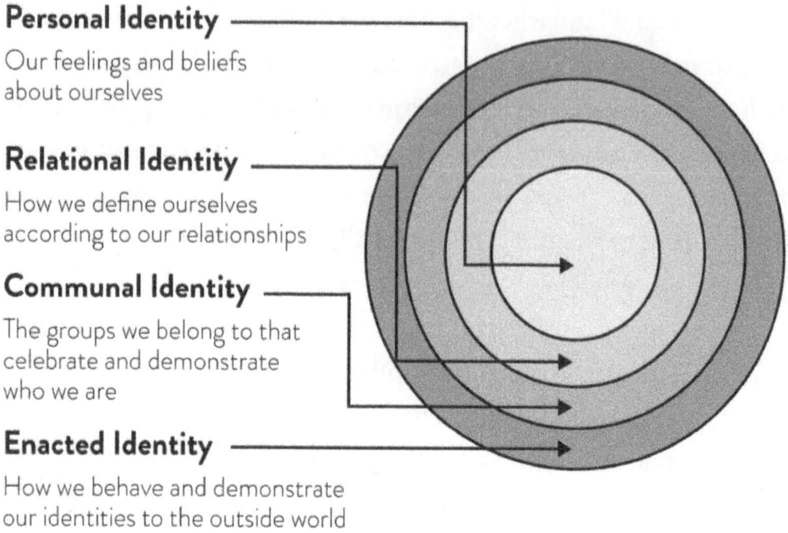
Personal Identity
Our feelings and beliefs about ourselves
Relational Identity
How we define ourselves according to our relationships
Communal Identity
The groups we belong to that celebrate and demonstrate who we are
Enacted Identity
How we behave and demonstrate our identities to the outside world

The Four Frames of Identity

themselves and their relationships with others, within the context defined by each of those frames—starting from their life before pain to their life since the pain began.

The frames serve as a tool for self-review and a prompt for reflection on strengths, vulnerabilities, obstacles, and opportunities. You consider what's working well and what you'd like to change or build on. Voorhees describes each frame of identity and some prompts to help you recognize them in yourself.

Personal identity. "This is what you think about yourself. Maybe you think you're smart, or you think that you're funny. What do you value? What do you believe to be true about the world? Are you a religious person? Do you value curiosity? What is your personality? This is your personal identity. No one can take this from you. This is who you believe you are."

Relational identity. "This is the idea that we exist in relation to other people, and those relationships help shape who we are. So, I'm a wife. I'm a daughter. I'm a sister. Those relationships help determine who I am. But another part of that layer is the idea that you are who other people say you are. Maybe you don't think you're particularly funny, but your friends say, 'Oh my God, you're so funny. I love when you show up!' You're thinking, 'I am? Me?' That starts to influence your overall sense of self. What people say about you is not the be-all, end-all, but it's part of how you move through the world. We don't exist in a bubble. There's a relational aspect to who we are; those relationships create a piece of who we are."

Enacted identity. "The clothes you wear, your hairstyle, the objects that you place in your room, these are all indications of your preferences, your values, your personality. They help show the world 'This is what I am, this is what I believe.' " In the study, Voorhees says, participants reported ways that, because of continuing pain, they'd changed how they physically moved through the world and the things they would show in the world. Some described modifications, such as using a heating pad at work or using a shopping scooter in the grocery store. "Whereas before they were 'not that kind of person'—they would want to hide their pain, basically put on an act for other people—now they were much more open to demonstrating 'I am now in pain.' "

This calls for balance, which isn't always easy to achieve. Too little and you're making yourself invisible; too much and pain becomes the defining self you convey to others and to yourself as well. As someone who's suffered from migraine headaches most of my adult life, I often kept my symptoms quiet. I was worried people would think less of me or as someone incapable of completing a task, especially while caring for patients in the hospital. This was a part of my enacted identity that I'm now striving to change after reading Voorhees's research. While I'm still careful not to let the migraines become part of my central identity, I am more willing to tell people when I am having a headache rather than simply letting them think I'm otherwise cranky or disinterested in the conversation.

Communal identity. "The communal frame of identity consists of the groups you align with. Are you a Detroit Lions fan? If you go to the games, or watch the games at a local bar, or wear their jerseys, that's a community that you are part of and it says something about who you are. Are you a cancer survivor and you go to awareness-raising walks, wear one of the various awareness ribbons, and identify as part of that group? The communities that you join reflect your identity. They communicate who you are, and who others think you are."

In practical terms, the four frames are a way to focus on the spheres in which we can understand how pain is changing our engagement with other people and our own interests, and then shape that with intention. "If you understand more about who you are, and you understand more about your relationships and how you show up in the world and how other people affect you, understanding that is half the battle," Voorhees says. "You can only change something that you understand."

As we think in particular about the central role of relationships in our sense of self, there's plenty of evidence to back up the fact we need social connection to thrive and that social isolation takes a significant toll on those with chronic pain. We'll turn to that more fully in chapter 16. While working on a previous book, *Keep Sharp*, I traveled around the world observing some of the happiest and healthiest cultures. One thing I noticed repeatedly was that societies with robust social practices were heavily protected against the harmful effects of stress on the brain and the increased likelihood of chronic pain.

Be choosy about the company you keep. Focus on people and communities that acknowledge the challenge of your pain, but also see you as more than the pain and respect your choices to be health oriented in the way you live. For instance, community and online support groups can be a valuable source of affirmation and sometimes practical advice. But when the conversation stays centered on pain complaints, your brain absorbs the steady drumbeat of fear and anger, and the ambient sounds of "unsafe" can stoke hypervigilance. Or when they stray too far with anecdotal "cures" or promoting products, it can undermine your confidence or leave you confused and anxious.

Hypervigilance and its anxious twin, catastrophizing, can increase pain intensity and the risk of postoperative pain. They can affect sleep quality, increase negative thinking and expectations, increase avoidance behaviors, narrow cognitive focus to threat-related cues, and add to overall emotional distress. So aim for online and other communities that offer optimism and that share encouraging stories that can be useful or inspiring to you.

When something you've tried gives you a win or gives you hope, a supportive community cheers you on. Remember to celebrate the victories with the same energy you displayed during the grind of the struggle. Conversely, it can also be helpful to take breaks as needed from those social media environments, to focus energy and attention elsewhere to stay grounded in the larger world, or that of family and friends.

The four frames exercise is a great place to start answering the sometimes scary question: Who am I really? And at the very least, you've stepped away mentally for a few minutes, reflecting on things that matter to you rather than focusing solely on pain itself. While you're reflecting, you can look for ways that even small adjustments might begin to reshape your relationship with pain, loosen its grip, and rewrite your view of possibilities.

Also, remember: it's not just the number of social connections you have. The type, quality, and purpose of your relationships matter. Aim for those that carry the energy and message that you need. Your brain is listening.

LIVING IT

Amy Tomasulo, "Laugh Your Face Off!"

Twenty-two-year-old Amy Tomasulo had recently graduated from college and was home with her family when she woke up one morning with searing, stabbing facial pain. "I woke up and I felt like a different person," she says, the memory still vivid twenty-five years later. "I didn't know what was going on—it was so sudden. There was nothing to indicate that this was going to happen to me the day before. It was *extremely* sudden. And quite shocking."

Tomasulo had played Division I softball in college, then had stayed on as a student coach when an injury ended her collegiate career early. "Before the pain I was a very athletic person," she says. "That was always kind of the centerpiece of my life." But now she was living an unsettled life in the grip of chronic pain.

Two years of treatments for trigeminal neuralgia didn't really help. Then she undertook a rehabilitation program focused on working with pain while still living her life in meaningful ways. That shift in focus helped her immensely. Tomasulo and her husband, Pat, a Chicago broadcast sports anchor and host, as well as a comedian, eventually found they could parlay their joint skills into fundraising for facial pain research. Inspired by another local fundraising event they had attended, they decided to do more to support research and add to the movement in their own way.

"I was feeling a little lost," she says. "It's not easy having essentially zero control over how you feel most days. And then it was like, *Great! Finally someone's doing something. We have to be a part of this.*"

Laugh Your Face Off! was born, an annual stand-up comedy show in Chicago sponsored by Northwestern Medicine and more than a hundred other cosponsors, from comedians to corporations, with all proceeds going to the Facial Pain Research Foundation.

In its first year, the event, launched on a Thursday night in a local comedy club, raised about $185,000. As it grew, the Tomasulos shifted the event to a theater venue, which sells out every year. The 2023 fundraiser had topped previous years, raising $640,000; then the tenth-anniversary event in 2024 raised more than $825,000, bringing the ten-year total to $4.6 million. When Tomasulo shared that number in an email, she added, "Just writing that sentence really captures what this event does for my sense of self. To see what we've created blows my mind sometimes."

"Who I was before pain—I was always laughing. I was always the one making people laugh, just always looking to have fun," she went on. "That carries through to who I am today. I still really like to laugh, even though laughing, ironically, is one of the biggest triggers for my pain. Sometimes it is excruciating. But to me it is worth it. Unfortunately, I can't be as big in the action part of the show because I simply can't. But I do what I can when I can, and that's kind of the story of my life."

In addition to raising money for research, the Tomasulos want to raise hope. "There is not a lot of hope when you have a rare disease. And hope is *necessary*, you know?" she says.

As a young athlete, Tomasulo had developed a disciplined practice mind-set she thought would carry her on to a career in professional sports. Today her practice ethos helps her live strategically with pain that can be unpredictable.

"I wake up around the same time every day. I get up. I feed my dog," she says. Wind against her face triggers the trigeminal neuralgia pain, so a good day is a windless one. "If there's no wind, I get to walk my dog. . . . That alone makes my day." Afternoons and nights are harder for her, so on the days when she's able to keep moving after her morning walk, she feels especially grateful. "If I get to be up and not need to lie down after I've done those activities, and I get to continue doing things during the day—walk the dog *twice*—and have dinner with my husband, that's an amazing day," she says.

"When you get trigeminal neuralgia, your life will never be the same. That's an incredibly difficult thing to accept," she goes on. "And there are days where I still fight that. But I've learned that while I can't escape this disease, it doesn't necessarily have to define me. And that is what keeps me going every day."

One Small Thing: The Power of Incremental Progress

Psychologists and health coaches often focus on the power of doing "one small thing," however small or incremental it may seem. A simple example: at any given time, a deep, deliberate breath can help reduce stress and engage the parasympathetic nervous system to calm your nerves. And there are many more such actions within reach, whatever your capabilities: Add a few steps or repetitions to an exercise practice. Take short breaks from sedentary periods, then make the breaks a little more frequent and a little longer. (See the sidebars in part 2 for more information.)

To make a small change stick, pick any metaphor—a pebble sending ripples across a pond, the butterfly effect of a small movement leading to larger change, an athlete practicing a move over and over—and visualize that as you do the one small thing that sets the energy in motion.

Elsa: Pacing, Patience, and Permission to "Just Go with It"

Since her bout with shingles, Elsa continues to suffer from chronic pain. Though it remains a part of her life, she found an exit from that freeway nightmare of pain when she turned deliberate attention to focusing on incremental things she is able to do.

She makes an effort to engage with her family and friends and in activities that give her pleasure. She accepts that her pain fluctuates and with it the types of activities she is able to pursue. Lately her walks have grown longer, and she varies the pace to meet different goals. Sometimes she takes a pleasure walk to focus on the smells or colors of the season; other times she steps up her speed for a few blocks, depending on what feels like a reasonable stretch. She was able to resume swimming at the local community center, which makes her ecstatic. She's bicycling again. She meditates and has found working with a therapist helpful at times. Sometimes the mix of meds, other treatments, and her own practices deliver a good stretch of hours or even days not dominated by pain. She takes advantage of those, but doesn't take pain spikes as a sign of failure.

"There are good days and then there's harder days," she says. "I'm trying to learn to just go with it and when I'm having a harder day, just accept it and try to do the things I can. It's about being okay with going slow and giving myself permission to rest when it's really hard."

She has become a student of gratitude, engaging it not so much with rose-colored glasses as with a magnifying lens and a very specific practice of noticing even small, positive things and giving the feeling a moment to sink in. "Some days that's harder than others," she told me one day in a call she took in her garden. "But when I came out just now to put the chairs out, a little butterfly came on the chair, and I thought. 'Oh, that's so beautiful.' That made me so happy."

Pain, Loss, and a Joyful Life Recovered

A few months after my patient had his amputation, I saw him in the clinic. Actually, I heard him before I saw him—that booming voice, joking and flirting with people as he walked down the hall. He was back to his usual gregarious self.

In the examination room, he sat on the table in a polo shirt and a pair of shorts, not trying to hide the prosthetic leg now extending below his right knee. "Hey Doc, you helped me lose about ten pounds by cutting this off," he cracked. "And take a look at this," he added, as he turned to his somewhat embarrassed daughter, who'd accompanied him that day. He took her hand, twirled her around, and then they embraced sweetly in the tiny exam room. "I can even dance now," he said with a wide grin.

His pain was gone, and I made a notation that he hadn't refilled his pain prescription since being discharged from the hospital. It was also clear that his grief over losing that part of himself had dissipated. While I'd known we could get rid of his pain, I had worried that the cost of doing so would be too high—that while he might report a pain score of zero, he might also report a quality-of-life score as zero. And yet here he was cracking jokes and doing a jig.

As I remembered that yellowed photograph of the muscular young man in swim trunks, I thought to myself, *He's still in there.* He didn't lose himself. Although the prospect of losing his leg had shaken him deeply that morning before the surgery, eventually he had found the strength of self that he needed to recover his life.

As I've listened to these and other stories that people have shared, the range of their experiences and the depth of the impact on their lives have only underscored just how complex and diverse pain is. How unique it is to each person. But one thing has been constant, and that's the power of conversation. Whether that's the conversation with our doctor or therapist, our loved ones, friends, colleagues, or the clerk at the grocery store. And most of all, our conversation with ourself—respecting our experience, cultivating resilience, and believing in our capacity for growth and change in any circumstance.

CHAPTER 6

From Hope to Healing: An Argument for Optimism

What excites me the most about researching and writing books like this is the opportunity to celebrate the scientists, doctors, patients, and advocates who are accomplishing extraordinary things. These are the people who steadily advance our knowledge and understanding of complicated human conditions such as chronic pain, yet they rarely receive appropriate recognition for their work. They're unwilling to accept the status quo, believing that through their efforts, people's lives can and will be improved. And while they are, for the most part, practitioners of science, they're also social justice warriors, fighting on behalf of the suffering and forgotten. I find this deeply inspiring.

These unsung heroes were on my mind recently when I delivered the commencement address at the Georgetown University School of Medicine. "The old adage is, *if it ain't broke, don't fix it*," I reminded the new graduates. But then I told them that after thirty years of practicing medicine, I now had a different take. "Keep fixing, keep tinkering," I told them. " 'Not broken' somehow implies that you've made it perfect. It's not perfect. Nothing is." This is certainly the case when it comes to pain. We've overtreated it, undertreated it, and for too long failed to explore the body's own natural pain-fighting capabilities.

The scientists and others I've introduced in this book never stop tinkering and fixing, and in the process they're changing the narrative around pain. There's a message for all of us in that as well: We can all keep trying new things. While there's no single solution for everyone, there are solutions out there for anyone if we look for them with a fresh eye, an open mind, and a sense of possibility.

Even when progress is chaotic and messy, it's still progress. From quieting the mind to nurturing the myofascia, I'm more confident than ever before that the mechanisms that can prevent or relieve pain are within reach for all of us. They may look different and even work a little differently for each of us, but that's the point: we get to choose. We know our own unique needs if we pay attention to our bodies; we know what matters most to us. Now that we understand the dimensions of pain in the body and the brain, let's figure out what we can do about it.

An Argument for Optimism from the Front Line of the Opioid Crisis: A Systems Case Story

You may never have found yourself in a hospital emergency department in pain or had any personal stake in the conversation about opioid use. But I want to take you behind the scenes just briefly to share one of the most inspiring stories unfolding in pain science and medicine. It's not about the drugs so much as it is a human story—one about passion, purpose, and the power to bring about great change, starting with a simple shift in the conversation.

It was just a few years ago that the vision of an opioid-free emergency department was making headlines, suggesting the promise of reversing the utter devastation the opioid epidemic had caused. The idea wasn't so much a throwback to some idealized time before the opioid crisis, but a new vision to tame pain through nonaddictive drugs.

The ER seemed a practical place to start, as well as an apt metaphorical one. The ER represents everything we fear and hope about pain: fear that pain might blindside and then engulf us, through an accident, an injury, or some odd symptom that sends us there in the middle of an ordinary day or night. And hope that somebody there can do something to make it stop—and fast.

As a physician, I realize that we must recognize the value of opioid medications while also being appropriately critical of them. Talk to any pain doctor about this, and you're not likely to get the impression they either totally condone or condemn the drugs. Many describe them as the most valuable medications known to humans. At the same time, they'll tell you that for too long, opioids became too much of a good thing, with horrific consequences.

During the worst years of the crisis, doctors routinely used morphine (a type of opioid) for any kind of pain that appeared in ER patients, from dislocated hips to toothaches. The use of morphine and other opioids was so prevalent that some doctors worried that *not* prescribing them would result in angry patients and lower satisfaction scores.

Scott Weiner, the McGraw Distinguished Chair in Emergency Medicine at Brigham and Women's Hospital in Boston, recalls an ER patient who screamed at him and accused him of violating the Hippocratic Oath because he didn't prescribe opioids for shoulder pain. "It was yelling, calling the security guard, the whole thing," Dr. Weiner told me, voicing a rising concern over the staff's personal safety. This was one of the first times he realized that something was very wrong with the overall approach to pain management.

During his training, Weiner mostly learned acute pain management by simply watching how experienced attending physicians handled it. At the time, however, there were few guidelines in place, and as a result, pain management could vary widely from state to state, from hospital to hospital, and even within the same hospital.

For example, when the Mayo Clinic medical staff reviewed the twenty-five most common elective operative procedures performed at their institution, they found a huge variation in pain management for the seventy-five hundred patients operated on over a specific time period. They found almost no uniformity in opioid use between doctors or procedures. Dr. Halena Gazelka, professor of anesthesiology and pain medicine, decided with her team to set some parameters, with the hope of creating more consistent and predictable opioid prescribing practices.

They started by categorizing what were reported to be the least painful procedures, such as carpal tunnel surgery in which a tight ligament in the wrist is cut to relieve pressure on a nerve, to the most painful procedures, such as a knee replacement. What they found was surprising. Regardless of the procedure type, patients were still highly satisfied even if they left with a prescription for ten oxycodone pills instead of two hundred (an amount often prescribed). Contrary to popular belief, they wrote in Mayo Clinic's Experience Notes, "People typically just use what they need." In fact, follow-up surveys showed that most patients were actually taking less than half of what they'd been dispensed. So as worried as physicians were about not being able to satisfy patients, the Mayo Clinic's findings showed that this wasn't a legitimate issue.

This insight partly reshaped the debate over the prescription of opioids. In the 1990s, opioids were promoted as wonder drugs, and the number of opioid prescriptions written by physicians in the United States continued to rise until around 2011. But even before the decade was out, that pharmaceutical marketing mirage was shattered with the rising toll of deaths, overdoses, and addictions. "There was finally a real recognition that things had gotten out of control, and that we were causing too much harm," Dr. Weiner recalls.

Dr. James Dwyer, then chairman of emergency medicine at Northern Westchester Hospital in Mount Kisco, New York, recalls the time when doctors began changing their behavior. "At that time, there was a lot of heat and criticism of physicians for overprescribing opioids. But since then, we have spent a lot of time and education about appropriate opioid prescribing," Dwyer said. And in a number of places, emergency physicians and emergency departments led the movement from always-opioids to hardly ever using opioids. In one notable early experiment, the emergency department of Maimonides Medical Center in Brooklyn decided to do something fairly revolutionary: they launched what became known as the "opioid-free shift." To start, they developed a plan to avoid opioid use by substituting other safe and effective pain-reduction medications. Here is an example of what that might look like.

Opioid–Free Shift

Neuropathic Pain

1. PO Ibuprofen-400-800 mg
2. PO Gabapentin-100-300 mg
3. PO Prednisone-25-50 mg
4. PO Clonidine 0.1-0.2 mg
5. IV Ketamine-0.3 mg/kg over 10 min, + IV drip at 0.15 mg/kg/hr
6. IV Lidocaine-1.5-2.5 mg/kg/hr drip x2-4 h (2% cardiac Lidocaine)
7. IV Dexemedetomidine-0.2-0.3 mcg/kg/hr drip
8. IV Clonidine-0.3-2 mcg/kg/hr drip

Post-Operative Pain

1. IV Acetaminophen-1g over 10-15 min
2. IV Ketamine-0.3 mg/kg over 10 min, + IV drip at 0.15 mg/kg/hr
3. IV Dexemedetomidine-0.2-0.7 mcg/kg/hr drip

Dental Pain

1. Dental Blocks
2. PO Ibuprofen-400-800 mg
3. PO Acetaminophen-500-1000 mg

Burns

1. PO Ibuprofen-400-800 mg
2. PO Acetaminophen-500-1000 mg
3. PO Naproxen-375 mg
4. IV Acetaminophen-1 g over 15 min
5. IV Ketamine-0.3 mg/kg over 10 min, + IV drip at 0.15 mg/kg/hr
6. IV Lidocaine-1.5-2.5 mg/kg/hr drip x2-4 h (2% cardiac Lidocaine)
7. IV Dexemedetomidine-0.2-0.7 mcg/kg/hr drip
8. IV Clonidine-0.3-2 mcg/kg/hr drip

Sickle Cell Painful Crisis

1. PO Ibuprofen-800 mg
2. PO Hydroxyurea-100 mg
3. IN Ketamine 1 mg/kg (no more than 1 ml per nostril)
4. IV Ketamine-0.3 mg/kg over 10 min, + IV drip at 0.15 mg/kg/hr
5. IV Lidocaine-1.5-2.5 mg/kg/hr drip x2-4 h (2% cardiac Lidocaine)
6. IV Dexemedetomidine-0.2-0.3 mcg/kg/hr drip

AM J Health Syst Pharm 2015;72(23):2080-6

(FYI Other Options)

For that eight-hour shift, standard painkillers such as morphine, hydromorphone, and oxycodone were out, in favor of alternative drugs such as steroids, lidocaine, acetaminophen (or Tylenol), and in some cases the dissociative drug ketamine. All adults arriving at the emergency department with a complaint of pain were first treated with the alternatives. Opioids were used only in the most extreme cases of pain instead of as a first-line therapy.

Among patients suffering acute pain who arrived during the first eight-hour window of the experiment, five reported musculoskeletal pain, four had abdominal pain, and three had kidney stones. Patients who arrived complaining of chronic pain included one with joint pain, three with neuromuscular pain, and one with long-standing abdominal pain. Doctors assessed the patients' pain by using a standard scale at baseline, at thirty minutes, and again at sixty minutes, after giving the patient the alternative medication. What they found was that these alternatives worked. In fact, only one patient required "rescue" opioid therapy and, crucially, nearly all the patients were satisfied with their pain relief.

When the trial was published in the *American Journal of Health-System Pharmacy*, it shared details of the protocol, including a list of the substituted non-opioid drugs and an extensive discussion of the training and other preparation needed to carry out this approach. Over the ensuing several years, the use of these types of approaches to manage pain became standard procedure and training for all medical staff, while also spreading to other community clinicians, first responders, and affiliated medical schools. In this new environment, the use of opioids steadily declined, while new and previously used (but for a time forgotten) pain control techniques became far more commonplace.

Three leaders of this effort—Dr. James Dwyer; Dr. Sandeep Kapoor, who is Northwell's assistant vice president of addiction services and an assistant professor of emergency medicine; and Dr. Eugene Vortsman, an emergency medicine physician at the Long Island Jewish Medical Center in New Hyde Park—described in detail the alternatives patients and providers are now likely to experience in their emergency rooms.

For mild pain, physicians can order commonplace pain relievers such as ibuprofen, acetaminophen, topical analgesics, and naproxen. For patients reporting more severe pain, the newer medication lists might include non-addictive medications such as ketorolac, lidocaine, and steroids. Rising up the pain scale, providers could prescribe medications such as gabapentin, pregabalin, ketamine, and even nitrous oxide. ER physicians and pharmacists began using combinations of these medications to provide fast, safe, and often surprisingly effective pain relief.

Also altered was the tool chest of pain-relieving procedures. Trigger point injections (used to relieve muscle cramps in legs, backs, and necks) and nerve blocks (injections often guided by ultrasound imaging directly into nerve clusters) became part of provider training and moved into the realm of normalized effective pain treatments. "We said, let's try heat packs, let's do lidocaine patches, let's talk about other things we can do," says Dr. Vortsman. "We educated people about trigger point injections and how to treat lower back pain with local needle injections. These are things that historically have never been present in the emergency department."

Sometimes the new approaches are just multiple types of analgesia used together. "Instead of just using Tylenol or a nonsteroidal anti-inflammatory drug, use both of them, and it might be that the patient never needs an opioid," says Dr. Dwyer. "We try to identify the type of pain the patient is having and pick the alternative for that type of pain." A patient suffering from the excruciating pain of a kidney stone might first receive ketorolac, an anti-inflammatory drug, perhaps with Tylenol. There's an option for intravenous lidocaine, which may be a useful adjunct. Only in the most extreme cases will a physician turn to opioids. By 2010, the tide had shifted: fewer opioids and more alternatives were catching on across the country.

"I would never say that we're done. We're still learning," says Dr. Kapoor. "But we have had widespread culture change." As I write this, all eighteen of the emergency departments grouped under Northwell Health in Long Island and the New York metropolitan area have received American College of Emergency Physicians (ACEP) accreditation for opioid-alternative prescribing. The opioids-free culture has also spread to other departments at Northwell hospitals, with specialists in all areas of care now adopting many of the same protocols.

Among those pioneering this movement, Dr. Alexis LaPietra is often credited as the person whose vision and tenacity infused it all. LaPietra, an emergency medicine physician at RWJ Barnabas Health in New Jersey, echoes what other medical providers faced in the early days of the opioid crisis and how it inspired her to action. A habit of "just giving oxycodone had created a culture where people expected it," she says. "'I have a broken bone; I expect to get medicine where I feel quite good. My pain is gone, and I feel pretty good.' We really were at that time giving out oxycodone for almost everything. There wasn't much utilization of alternatives."

At the time, Dr. LaPietra was a young ER doctor at St. Joseph's University Medical Center in Paterson, New Jersey. Many new emergency medicine physicians in training ride with paramedics for several weeks to get a feel for what's called *prehospital medicine.* As a third-year medical resident, Dr. LaPietra rode with the paramedics in a diverse urban area and saw how overdose calls cut across demographics. It was a time when the opioid epidemic had shifted back to heroin, another type of opioid.

During those ride-alongs, she saw people who'd overdosed "with needles in their arms, just dead in a car," she recalls. "ER doctors see naloxone-reverse patients who survive. And that's good. But there were also all these people who were dead on arrival, opioid overdoses that were going on right outside our doors that we weren't seeing. It was really gutting."

Those gut punches were part of what pushed Dr. LaPietra and her colleagues to rise to the challenge. "So we put together evidence and research, a lot of it from other specialties, that could be scalable in emergency medicine, for example, combining different medications for migraines, like neurologists do. So, this was just a period of discovery in emergency medicine where we realized we played a big role, and we could really impact many lives. It was just a matter of getting it together, protocolizing it, and then disseminating it."

"We're Going to Have the Power to Get Answers"

As the novel becomes the norm, not only do those in all medical specialties need to have a voice in the conversation about pain—everyone does, especially those who have suffered with pain, because as we have learned by now everyone's pain experiences will be different. That individual diversity has the potential to drive innovation. We saw Ed Mowery's remarkable outcome when scientists used real-time data to personalize the deep brain stimulation that relieved his pain. And a raft of new technologies is enabling scientists to harvest data like that from Mowery, aggregating those data in such a way that one day soon, data-driven matches between patients and treatments will become as common as a blood test in the emergency room that could help individualize the best strategy to reduce your pain.

Dr. Kim Burchiel, professor of neurological surgery at the Oregon Health & Science University, is particularly excited about the strides we're making in that sort of precision medicine, made possible through massive data analysis enabled by machine-learning models.

"There are many, many examples of pain conditions that were not well understood, but with the power of large data analysis, we can better understand and even individualize the conditions and treatments. When you can do these analyses," he says, pausing with a sense of wonder and excitement, "we have the capability to do things now that you couldn't do five years ago. If you want to look at all the various pain conditions and the associated medical conditions as a spreadsheet, there might be twenty-five million categories. No human could do that. But we have the power now to analyze things and determine best options for specific patients."

Emerging pain science is calling on all of us to broaden our viewpoints. We must re-envision possibility, as the emergency physicians described above have done, collaborating across divides and disciplines—and with patients themselves—to address the scourge of pain once and for all.

PART 2

Taking Charge for a Pain-Smart Life

CHAPTER 7

Reset

As you learned in part 1, the world of pain science is pushing harder than ever to find safe, effective, and accessible treatments for acute and chronic pain. The search for ways to manage pain and stop chronic pain from developing in the first place is beginning to show promise.

A few things have become increasingly clear. First, when it comes to treating chronic pain, a mix of approaches offers the greatest promise of relief. For example, steroids mixed with Tylenol and a trigger-point injection may be a better option than a single monotherapy, especially opioids alone. Second, it's preferable to fail fast—discover what doesn't work as quickly as possible—so you can move on to the next option that may offer relief. Also, remember that you're the most trustworthy judge of what's working and what's not. Stay in contact with your doctor and pay close attention to how you feel in response to an intervention, how long it took to feel relief, and whether you had any side effects. Don't forget that lifestyle changes that improve diet, exercise, sleep, and stress management can also enhance the effectiveness of pain meds and potentially reduce the amount you need.

Finally, finding the right doctors can take time, especially when it comes to pain. After all, you want a team that has not only excellent clinical skills but also the time and patience to listen to your complete story. Pain rarely occurs in isolation, and connecting the pieces of the puzzle is critically important. As daunting as it may be, if your existing team isn't as engaged as necessary, you may need to find a new one. (See "Finding the Right Fit," on page 121.) Most doctors don't mind if you seek out other opinions, and many even encourage it.

Reset: Choose a Different Lens

Doctors are typically focused on pathology—the question of what's wrong with you—so they can find the problem and fix it. That's the conventional medical orientation, because an accurate diagnosis is essential to developing an effective treatment plan. But what's sometimes missing is the focus on what's *right* with you: your natural capacities for healing and health, for growth, change, resilience, and well-being.

This isn't a new idea. But you may be surprised at the many extraordinary mechanisms for pain relief that are woven through every system in our body and brain, working continuously whether we notice them or not. If you find that notion a stretch, there is concrete evidence to make it real for you: the cut that heals on its own, the bone that fuses, the bruise that fades. From scabs and scars to cellular-level repairs and maintenance, the body has an extraordinary capacity to heal itself, without our even thinking about it.

If we had to consciously micromanage all those processes, we'd likely always be in pain. Instead, these systems enable us to address our pain robustly from within. The best news is that decades of rigorous research into these healing mechanisms have produced evidence-based practices that we can easily adopt into our own lives. As I told my mother after she broke her back, think of it as learning to harness the amazing capabilities of your own biology.

Reset: Mind-Set Matters

Cultivate Confidence. Self-Advocate for Your Needs and Take Charge of Your Choices.

Albert Bandura, an eminent social cognitive psychologist who wrote extensively about self-efficacy as "a unifying theory of behavioral change" famously said, "Given that individuals are producers as well as products of their life circumstances, they are partial authors of the past conditions that developed them, as well as the future courses their lives take."

Decades of chronic pain research have borne this out—first, in the suffering that mounts when we feel helpless and hopeless in the misery of pain, and second, in the positive effects of pain education, self-advocacy, and self-management that can reduce pain or at least change our pain experience for the better. We are more likely to do well when we feel like proactive producers rather than passive products of our health circumstances.

Consider these highlights from several recent studies:

- Patients who reported higher self-efficacy levels experienced less functional impairment and severe pain than their cohorts who reported lower self-efficacy levels.
- Physical and mental health can be influenced by a person's beliefs about what's affecting and controlling their health. These beliefs can be internal, when patients see themselves in control, or external, when they feel medical experts, or even luck and fate, are in control.
- Patients who feel more in control of their life despite their chronic pain feel less psychological distress, feel better able to manage their chronic pain, and function better in their daily lives.

The idea that we are the producers as well as the products of our own lives is a powerful reminder that we do have a great deal of control over our pain, and there are new strategies emerging to do just that.

Reset: Prioritize Preventive Health

Preventive Health Steps Are Also Active Agents in Pain Relief

The idea of preventive health has been around since ancient times, passed on in apple-a-day aphorisms and healthy lifestyle advice so ubiquitous that it's easy to tune it out as background noise. The "should do" list becomes something we'll get around to when time allows.

Of course, time never seems to allow for things we consider optional, and mainstream medicine has traditionally treated preventive practices as just that: optional. They're barely mentioned or perhaps recommended in a general sense but left for patients to pursue on their own. Unless you have a chronic illness such as diabetes, where careless attention to diet could land you in a diabetic coma, preventive health might seem removed from your everyday priorities. Historically, doctors didn't have the training, time, or inclination to incorporate pain prevention into medical practice. The conventional wisdom was that some people would get pain in their lives, others wouldn't, and there wasn't much they could do to alter your fate. But all of that is changing.

Now that emerging pain science has established its objective value, preventive medicine has finally begun moving from the background to the forefront. We have learned that lifestyle practices involving diet, exercise, stress management, sleep, mental health, relationships, and social engagement all act on pain in direct ways: lowering inflammation, increasing cell-to-cell communication, and setting in motion a range of physiological, neurological, and psychological processes that can either produce pain or reduce it. Maintaining a healthy lifestyle is the single most effective preventive approach to pain—reducing your risks and boosting resilience.

Exercise is an excellent example. By improving your balance, strength, and flexibility, you're better able to avoid a painful injury. And when you do have pain, physical activity is now a recognized critical part of pain management and rehabilitation. This is about more than building muscle or burning calories. Exercise works so deeply across pain mechanisms, pathways, and systems that it "change[s] the underlying causes of pain itself," says Kathleen Sluka, PT, PhD, a leading researcher in the science of exercise for pain control, and a professor in the Department of Physical Therapy and Rehabilitation Science at the University of Iowa. "Exercise is the most effective multimodal treatment there is."

So, it is time to start thinking about movement for many pain conditions. Too often, we are told to decrease activities and do little more than rest. Simply moving, however, is the better decision in most cases. Besides quickly improving mental health and facilitating deeper sleep, it has now been well established that regular physical activity can reduce pain, improve pain tolerance, and lower the likelihood of developing chronic pain.

Start thinking of preventive health as a classic upstream approach: stopping pain before it begins. So if pain's not in your picture right now? Great—these practices can help keep it that way. And if you're already downstream, dealing with pain, then these approaches address its root causes, bolstering your resources for effective self-management and healing.

The Seven Reset Strategies for Pain-Smart Living

In previous chapters, we've explored at length what makes pain so complex and chronic pain even more so. I've shared some of the science that reveals dimensions of pain processing that interweave and overlap through the brain, mind, and body. We've unpacked the biological, psychological, social, and emotional components of pain. And we've seen the newest evidence that reveals how the brain's pain-processing circuitry is shared among other more generalized brain functions that govern how we think, feel, and behave. Suffice it to say that pain is one of the few human experiences that can cut across every facet of our lives.

To help you prevent that from happening, I've created seven strategies. They're based on the merged best practices recommended by leading pain and preventive health experts, supported by science, and offered up by pain sufferers I've interviewed—enthusiastic and generous contributors with a desire to help others. I've listed each one here with just a brief example of practices, techniques, or specific approaches that support it. Here are the Seven Reset Strategies, and over the next several chapters you'll find practical tips, stories, and more for each one. I will explain what they mean and how to best incorporate them into your life.

1. Mind your brain: Mindfulness, psychotherapy, hypnosis, self-hypnosis
2. Befriend your body: Mind-body practices, myofascial release and other manual therapies, acupuncture
3. Move more: Exercise, movement, yoga, tai chi, dance
4. Sleep well: Relaxation and restorative sleep, developing habits that improve sleep
5. Eat well: The pain-smart pantry, anti-inflammatory eating plans, gluten-free or other dietary considerations as needed
6. Cultivate connection: Personal, social, and community relationships that support and strengthen a sense of connection
7. Savor moments and memories: The power of your focused attention on positive experience

Each of these strategies targets three basic components: active pain management, building resilience, and active prevention. All seven principles dovetail with the others, synergizing benefits. Keep these in mind as you engage the strategies and fine-tune them to work best for you.

Twin Targets: Manage Stress, Build Resilience

In many ways, all seven of the pain-smart strategies function by managing stress and building resilience. This is important because excessive or chronic stress fuels inflammation, which creates a simmering source for pain. Chronic stress also puts you at higher risk for anxiety, depression, digestive problems, and weakened immunity, which all increase your pain reactivity.

This isn't to say that all stress is bad. We need some stress to get us out of bed in the morning, study for an exam, or prepare for an important meeting. The stress we're looking at here is the type that's relentless, churning out inflammation and increasing your pain sensitivity.

Think of resilience as strength training for the mind, brain, body, and spirit, with the added benefit of helping buffer against stress and corresponding pain. Increasing resilience can be accomplished in several ways, but when it comes to pain, these three have the greatest value:

1. Engage in activities that you enjoy and help foster a sense of community. Find your tribes.
2. Focus on optimal recovery from stressful experiences by returning to equilibrium as quickly as possible and processing your experience from a calm state of mind.
3. Seek out a physical or psychological challenge as an opportunity for personal growth.

Resilience is defined as "reflecting overall individual well-being despite the presence of a significant stressor." Through that lens, it's clear that you can build resilience in many ways—by overcoming adversity, or investing time and attention in things you enjoy or find meaningful. It's also helpful to recognize the value of "good stress" and appreciate how your response to it, and navigating challenges or working toward personal goals, can stoke your confidence.

Finding the Right Fit

When to Seek a Second Opinion or Simply Explore Alternatives

Reasons you might seek a second opinion or explore other options for pain care include insurance coverage, concerns about recommended surgical interventions, and, of course, treatment failure. But your gut feeling is important too.

- Do you feel listened to and respected?
- Does your practitioner explain things in terms you can understand—do they decode technical terms as needed and avoid medical jargon?

- Do they show the kind of interest and commitment that make you feel that they genuinely care?
- Do they welcome your questions and make a clear effort to respond helpfully?
- Do they welcome your self-advocacy and the role of someone you may bring with you to appointments as an advocate?
- Do they provide referrals for specialists outside their area of expertise? This could include pain psychologists, physical therapists, and others in pain rehabilitation medicine, including those from outside the mainstream.

The more informed you are about a pain diagnosis, options for treatment, and the risks, benefits, and potential for any treatment's success or failure, the more fully you can partner in the process. Studies show that feeling comfortable with a particular practitioner's approach—which includes intangibles like their communication style and the "vibe" they give off—is a big predictor of a successful outcome.

"With complex pain, it's important to find someone to work with, the right person," advises Jane Ballantyne, a pain physician, professor of anesthesiology and pain medicine at the University of Washington–Seattle, and past secretary of the International Association for the Study of Pain. "It's not going to come easily; you may need to try out a few relationships until you find someone that really is helpful. Don't be afraid of saying 'this isn't working' and moving on to someone else, because there's no point in working with someone who's not helping you. With complex pain, that relationship is key."

A recent study of two hundred adults with chronic neck or back pain found the first visit was crucial. If there was effective patient-physician communication during the initial consultation, it helped patients manage their uncertainties, including their fears and anxieties, strengthened their confidence in their ability to cope with their condition, and helped foster a mutually open and honest relationship. The study, led by University of Illinois Urbana-Champaign communication professor Charee Thompson, PhD, found that patients' feelings of distress were reduced when they and their physician mutually agreed that the other person was effective at seeking and providing medical information, and when the patients felt emotionally supported by their doctors.

Thompson suggests four ways you (and your provider) can foster a positive, productive conversation from the start.

1. Be honest and direct about your priorities for treatment—and specific types of treatment you'd like to consider or which you have reservations about.
2. Ask each other questions to understand different perspectives, show curiosity, and navigate uncertainty. For instance, you might ask, "What do you think is causing my pain, and how do you explain what's happening in my body?" Your provider could ask you the same thing to learn more from your experience and perspective. Talking about pain can be frustrating for both patients and doctors, and statements may come across as accusatory or overly definitive. Questions, on the other hand, keep the conversation open and encourage more dialogue.
3. Discuss clear plans to maintain open communication. Managing chronic pain is an ongoing process, and you need to know you can reach out with concerns. Physicians also benefit from follow-ups and open dialogue, which provide essential insights into a patient's health. You might say: "Open communication is very important to me. How can we be in touch about developments or concerns when they arise?"
4. Finally, always review instructions for the period ahead. You might ask your provider to give you a printout and review those notes together before you leave. Be sure you both agree on what you should do if anything comes up between now and your next appointment.

To find a recommended pain management provider, try the following:

- ask your primary care provider for a referral
- check with your insurance company for in-network pain management specialists

- search online directories for pain specialists and patient advocacy organizations
- ask trusted family, friends, or local support groups with experience with pain management
- check credentialing organizations such as the American Board of Pain Medicine, which assesses a provider's experience and skills

Remember Bess Talbot in Alabama, whose story of decades-long migraine pain opened this book, and the turning point she described when she found Dr. Saper in Michigan. She encourages others struggling through hard times with chronic pain to persevere in the search for a compatible doctor and treatment team. "If you can find the right physician, one who is willing to work with you and listen to you, do know there's hope at the end of the tunnel. You may have to keep searching but I think with pain, until you can find someone who's really willing to work with you, that's your job—to keep searching."

Short Take: A Word about the "Small Voice" of Prevention

We can't really prevent pain in a conventional sense. There's no vaccine against it. But one thing we can do is listen to that little voice in our head that tries to protect us from ourselves.

Whenever I'm called in to consult about a patient's situation in the ER, I often hear some variation of the same story. Someone looked at a box on a high shelf, or a fallen branch blocking a rooftop gutter, or a stack of heavy file boxes that *really* needed to be carried out to the garage, and despite hearing a little voice saying, "Wait . . . don't do that!"—well, you know what happened next. We've all done it: lifted something too heavy, forgot to use our knees rather than our backs, stood on a wobbly chair instead of grabbing a stepladder. The worst case I had was a ninety-three-year-old patient who took his leaf blower up to his roof—and then came tumbling down.

This is how preventable injuries happen, and unfortunately, it's often the genesis of chronic pain and a new, unwelcome way of life. The slip and tumble that dislocates a hip. The careless chopping of vegetables that leads to stitches in your hand (or worse). The sudden lane change on the highway that leads to an accident. Or in my sweet mom's case, the decision to lift a too-heavy suitcase, leading to a fall and a fractured spine.

A brief lapse of judgment can lead to a lifetime of pain. So in the category of low-hanging fruit, I'd like to turn the volume up on that little voice in your head and encourage you to listen to it. Slow down, take care, don't fall. Ask someone to give you a hand or to steady the ladder. Use your judgment and always consider the consequences. Don't paralyze yourself with fear that you might hurt yourself—but *do* anticipate that possibility. And if you don't hear your own voice in these situations, let mine be a stand-in. Here's the shorthand: If you're wondering whether a situation is safe, it's probably not safe enough to attempt.

Believe in Yourself

You can change the conversation, change your brain, and change your pain.

You don't need a placebo; you *are* one. "Engaging in the ritual of healthy living—eating right, exercising, yoga, quality social time, meditating, whatever you choose—probably provides some of the key ingredients of a placebo effect," says Ted Kaptchuk, professor of global health and social medicine at Harvard Medical School. Adopting healthy behavior is generally a good thing, but deliberately doing it as self-care intensifies the positive effects, actively contributing to your physical, mental, and emotional resilience and enhancing your quality of life. Placebo is more than simply positive thinking or belief in a treatment, he says. "It's about creating a stronger connection between the brain and body and how they work together."

I have mentioned Dr. Michael Merzenich, who has contributed so much to our understanding of neuroplasticity. I'll end this chapter with something he said that's so relevant to pain: "Moment by moment, we choose and sculpt how our ever-changing minds will work. We choose who we will be in the next moment in a very real sense, and these choices are left embossed in physical form in our material selves."

It's time to choose who you will be in the next moment, as well as the things you can do, whatever your circumstances, to feel as able, stable, strong, and pain-free as possible. Let's get started.

CHAPTER 8

Pain Relief: What's in Your Toolbox?

When headaches or sore muscles strike us at home, we reach for everyday painkillers. Usually it's something like ibuprofen, aspirin, or naproxen, all analgesics known in the medical world as nonsteroidal anti-inflammatories (NSAIDs). The most common non-NSAID pain reliever is acetaminophen, or Tylenol, which isn't an anti-inflammatory but works well to reduce fever and is typically easier on the stomach. Even before reaching for those over-the-counter meds, we may ice a sore elbow or lower back, or soak in a hot tub to ease achy muscles or joints.

In the clinical setting, we certainly appreciate it when the dentist numbs our mouth with Novocain. We take anesthesia for granted when rolling into surgery (having had an IV sedative first), or receiving an epidural during childbirth—as my wife did for all three of our girls. Then, of course, there are post-op meds—including, when necessary, prescription opioids to manage acute pain through recovery. In all these ways, we've become accustomed to pain relief being an "outside job." But in truth, elaborate biochemical systems, molecular mechanisms, and mind-body networks for pain control and prevention already exist within us, an "inside job" that science is only beginning to unpack.

Mind, body, brain, bones, and blood: every part of us is wired not only for pain but also for pain relief. It's an incredible system that gets little attention, one I first experienced all those years ago while lying impaled on that spiked fence. Even before I went to the ER or received any medications, I could feel my body starting to soothe itself, my own healing mechanisms taking over. The pain didn't disappear, but it came in waves, with periods of real relief in between. And then, simply having my mother arrive provided not just mental and emotional comfort but actual physical comfort too.

Having a caring person in your life can improve your resilience to pain, whereas isolation or loneliness can exacerbate it. I remember the first time one of my children got a shot. I didn't even have to think about what to do: my first instinct was to comfort her with voice and touch. Sometimes when we're sidelined with a painful injury, a call from a friend or even just listening to music can make a difference in how we feel by flooding the brain's pain-processing circuitry with positive feelings and emotions. Training your brain in this way is a crucial piece of the healing mix for pain relief.

Think of this healing mix as an expanded toolbox that goes beyond what most people consider the "real" tools for pain relief. The conventional conversation tends to focus on medications and medical interventions, but I want to bring your attention to other, less appreciated tools. Let's start with your body's built-in painkillers, the endogenous opioid system.

Your Body's Natural Painkillers: Endogenous Opioids, Placebos, and More

By now you know that opiates are some of the world's most powerful painkillers. But what you may not know is that your body is adept at producing the natural form of these same chemicals. They're called endorphins, a term that merges the Greek word *endogenous* (meaning "from within") and *morphine.* Though endorphins are just one of several types of protein molecules with this painkiller quality, the word is often used to refer to them collectively. And as you're about to learn, they can influence your mood as well as your perception of pain. Pump up the endorphins—decrease the pain.

The natural world serves as both an inspiration and a guide as scientists search for ways to tap into or mimic its unique problem-solving genius. A bird in flight, the strength of a spider's web, a gecko's sticky grip—all have served as models for scientific inventions. Bioinspired innovations are all around us, from skyscrapers to syringes.

Many years ago, when drug developers began to search for molecules and mechanisms that could safely reduce pain, they drew inspiration from our own human bodies and their endogenous opioid system. Keep in mind that in addition to reducing pain, the system is involved in emotional regulation and mood, neurogenesis (growth of new neurons in the nervous system), neuroplasticity, learning and memory, and the brain's reward-processing system.

So how does it work? Opioids, whether endogenous or those found in narcotics (called exogenous opioids), bind to opioid receptors located on the outer membrane of nerve cells in the brain, spinal cord, and other organs. Like molecular keys in locks, when opioids bind to these receptors, they trigger a cascade of chemical changes within and between neurons, producing feelings of pleasure as well as pain relief.

The receptors are also present in the brain's reward circuitry, which uses the neurotransmitter dopamine to tag experiences of pleasure. That is why we often want to repeat certain experiences. That's true of all opioids. But endogenous opioids have an insider advantage as a natural part of the body's interwoven system for pain modulation. Like software programs that are part of the same operating system, they mesh seamlessly. Evolution has fine-tuned their actions with meticulous precision, including the way the body metabolizes them so they can constantly turn on or off, as well as micromanaging doses. This prevents some of the complications that arise with outside opioid medications, including constipation, brain fog, slowed breathing, nausea, and drug tolerance and dependence.

Nature even added an emergency survival tool: stress-induced analgesia that temporarily suppresses pain. Under extreme stress, the fight-or-flight hormones aggressively trigger the endogenous opioid system, which greatly reduces the pain. The pain does eventually come back when this emergency hormonal response subsides, but in the meantime, traumatic injuries may not immediately register as painful to a wounded soldier or a kid impaled by a fence. "When you look at the release of norepinephrine and opioids for the flight and fear response—it is one of the most potent analgesic, anti-pain molecules that exists," says Daniela Salvemini, PhD, William Beaumont Professor and director of St. Louis University Institute for Translational Neuroscience. Having devoted her career to understanding the mechanisms that drive neuropathic pain, and the molecules that may relieve it, she remains in awe of "what our bodies have given us as survival kits." For some, it kicks in right away, and for others, it takes considerably longer, but everyone appears to have this naturally occurring plan B for the most dire circumstances.

A variety of stressors, not just physical pain, can trigger the endogenous opioid system. These include psychological, neurological, physiological, even ontological (spiritual or metaphysical) factors, which can activate the system to:

- Disrupt pain.
- Reduce pain intensity.
- Decrease the emotional unpleasantness of pain.
- Calm the nervous system and enhance stress resilience.
- Support robust brain health and even grow brain cells in response to pain.

Because most of these endogenous opioid benefits take place at a subconscious level, these processes have long been assumed to be inaccessible, meaning not something you can control in the same way you can pop a pill. But now we know that simply moving—jogging or going for a brisk walk—can trigger an endorphin release that delivers the rush we call an endorphin high, or "runner's high." Gazing at a sunset or a loved one can help do it as well. You can activate your own endogenous opioid system and experience the surprising power of your neural circuits to disrupt pain *and* amplify pleasure. We now know that just by choosing to focus on something beautiful or positive, a wondrous cascade of events unfolds in our bodies that can change our experience of pain.

Placebo: Phantom Force for Pain Relief

Let's take a closer look at the term *placebo effect,* which many think of as a fake pill or sham treatment used in clinical research to compare effects with the "real" treatment being studied. Researchers typically compare the two, because any health improvements from a new or experimental medication must outperform the placebo by a measurable amount before being deemed worthy of taking forward.

Recognizing a placebo's intrinsic value as something that can improve pain, however, scientists are now investigating the placebo effect on the endogenous opioid system. This makes sense because we know cognitive factors—our thoughts, beliefs, and expectations—can affect our physical and emotional well-being by activating the endogenous opioid system. We also recognize that the effect of any treatment, placebo or "real," may be affected by the meaning we attach to it, in addition to the physical property of the treatment itself.

Two important findings about placebos have become clearer over time. First, there is no single placebo effect; placebo effects are influenced by a multitude of factors at any given time, including expectations (positive or negative) about treatment. Second, these expectations, while intangible, are the product of subjective and physiological experiences that are wired into the brain's pain-processing circuitry and can be modified over time. This means that far from just being a sham treatment, placebo is a legitimate tool in your pain toolbox.

New Knowledge Continually Changes Pain Medicine

Now let's turn to the external tools. Keep in mind that these can change, or how we use them can change, as scientific understanding evolves. Here's a simple example that involves a routine home remedy so common and widely accepted, you'll be surprised to learn that it's been at the center of a simmering debate for nearly fifty years—and counting.

You've probably heard of RICE—rest, ice, compression, and elevation—and may have even used it to treat a sprain, strained muscle, or painful bruise. For as long as I can remember, RICE was the recommended first response for treating acute tissue injury.

The concept of RICE dates back to 1978, when a sports medicine physician named Gabe Mirkin coined the term, which coaches and health care providers quickly adopted. At the time, conventional wisdom was that reducing inflammation, along with resting, would reduce pain and hasten healing. Slightly elevating an injury to decrease blood flow and applying gentle pressure presented no red flags medically, so the RICE treatment grew in popularity.

Whenever I had a mild injury, I used these steps too without ever giving it much thought. Recently, though, amid a flourishing debate, some newer candidates include PEACE (protect, elevate, avoid anti-inflammatories, compress, and educate); LOVE (load, optimism, vascularization, and exercise); and POLICE (protection, optimal loading, ice, compression, and elevation). Without going into all the differences—from vascularization (blood vessel formation) to gauging the proper load for an injured muscle—I'd just point out that the expanding conversation reflects that focus on tweaking health and medical approaches as new scientific findings emerge. What I see as most compelling is a loose but well-reasoned growing consensus that suggests the better option is to replace RICE with MEAT, which stands for movement, exercise, analgesia, and treatment.

Here's why. The downside of RICE is that it tamps down inflammation. As you've read in previous chapters, some level of inflammation is necessary to activate healing processes and reduce the chance of developing chronic pain. While dialing down inflammation may initially ease pain, it also can delay or inhibit long-term tissue healing. The lesson is a critically important one when it comes to pain: let the body take care of itself as naturally as possible. Given what we now know, unless you have a fractured bone or can't bear weight, RICE should no longer be the blanket recommendation for pain management.

Instead, the emphasis is now on these four steps:

Movement: Mild movement or exercise improves blood flow and circulation of healing agents to the injured area. It stimulates muscle, tendons, ligaments, cartilage, and other tissue, whereas stagnation can stall healing and lead to continuing pain.

Exercise: This component is meant to kick in once the pain has lessened. For a muscle injury, this would involve gentle moves designed to slowly restore function and flexibility. For other types of bruised or swollen soft tissue, for example, from surgery or trauma, mild exercise further improves circulation.

Analgesia: Cautious use of pain relievers if necessary, as well as the use of natural options such as turmeric or capsaicin instead of anti-inflammatories, which may inhibit healing for the reasons already described (see box starting on page 137). Also consider topical anesthetics and analgesic patches, or mild transcutaneous neurostimulation such as the TENS device, which applies a low-voltage current to the skin.

Treatment: The final component of MEAT refers to the range of tailored early treatment through various therapeutic approaches. These might include physical therapy, massage, acupuncture or other "dry needling" (solid needles containing no medication), myofascial release (and other techniques using targeted massage to release tension in a specific muscle area), joint mobilization (to improve range of motion), as well as use of ice and heat.

Heat and cold therapy both can help relieve pain, though they work in different ways and are best for different situations.

Cold therapy is best for short-term pain, applied within the first seventy-two hours to counter swelling. Keep in mind that while cold temperature slows blood flow, which can help reduce pain from sprains, strains, and other acute injuries, it may also decrease inflammation, slow healing, and increase the likelihood of chronic pain. Regular cold-water plunges have gained a popular following in recent years, and some studies suggest that regular cold exposure through ice bathing or plunges may ease discomfort after intense workouts and help with stress regulation. These may not be the best options, however, for treating an injury. The practice continues to be the subject of debate because it may also carry risks for some people—in particular those with cardiovascular issues. The concern is something known as a cold shock response, which can lead to an increase in blood pressure and heart rate. Some may also hyperventilate, which can lead to fainting as well.

Heat therapy is best for long-standing muscle pain, stiffness, and chronic pain conditions. Because it boosts blood flow, which can help relax muscles and ease aching joints, heat therapy is often recommended before exercise or stretching or to ease morning stiffness. Applying low-level heat for a longer period, such as with heat wraps you can buy at the drugstore, may reduce stiffness and tension and increase flexibility. Just be sure to follow product directions.

Either way, don't overdo it. When using a hot or cold pack, wrap it in a thin towel to protect your skin and apply it for no more than ten to twenty minutes to avoid skin damage. You can do this several times a day, but be sure to take breaks in between to let your skin and tissue recover. And stop using heat or cold therapy immediately if it worsens your pain or discomfort or if your skin reacts.

Neither MEAT nor RICE is all wrong or always right. But with a basic understanding of these points of difference, you're better equipped to evaluate your options. The bottom line is that a desire for a quick fix may slow your overall healing process; as a general rule, be conservative with initial interventions like these and pay attention to the way your body responds; let the body heal itself and intervene only when necessary.

Renewed Urgency about Extended Use of Aspirin and NSAIDs

Now let's return to your home medicine cabinet and the nonprescription painkillers you probably keep on hand. If your everyday go-to for pain relief is aspirin or another NSAID (nonsteroidal anti-inflammatory drug), it's time to take a fresh look at how you use it. We now have not just new information, but continued findings over time, that have renewed urgency about the serious risks NSAIDs present for some people, as well as the adverse effects of taking too much or taking them for too long.

NSAIDs provide predictable relief for so many routine aches and pains—arthritis flare-ups, headaches, fever, menstrual cramps, colds, flu—that it's easy to lose track of how often you're using them and how much you're taking, and overlook their potential for toxic or other adverse effects. And because these drugs are sold over the counter, it often means you're making a decision about medication without your physician's guidance on how to avoid potential problems based on health conditions you may have or medications you may be taking. Keep in mind that these nonprescription medications were mostly intended for short-term use, so relying on them long term might put you at risk for complications.

Aspirin is a good example. For decades, aspirin has been used for primary prevention of atherosclerotic cardiovascular disease, which is heart disease from plaque buildup in the arteries. In light of recent trial data, however, that practice is now controversial. The risk of bleeding might simply be too high to justify the benefits of preventing heart disease in someone who's otherwise healthy.

That is why in 2022, the US Preventive Services Task Force recommended that people over sixty years old should not take aspirin to prevent primary heart disease. Even for those aged forty to forty-nine who may have a lower bleeding risk, the benefit is still thought to be small. If you've already had heart problems or have a strong family history and no evidence of bleeding problems, your doctor may recommend a daily baby aspirin. But in general, many doctors have moved away from the practice.

Supplements: Considerations, Caution, and Careful Use

People are turning increasingly to dietary supplements, seeking out substances they perceive as natural. Unfortunately, because there are very few good, randomized trials, it's hard to find solid evidence of the benefits of this approach. Additionally, many of these "natural" supplements are unregulated, meaning there's no guarantee that they're safe or consistent. There may also be interactions with prescription medications you're using or other health conditions the supplement could adversely affect. Still, even given the above caveats, I will name a few that are worth considering:

Coenzyme Q10 or C0Q10. There is evidence that this coenzyme can improve mitochondrial function within cells and also act as an anti-inflammatory. Given the way it works, it may be most beneficial when taken after intense activity or with the use of statin drugs—both of which can be associated with muscle aches. It may also effectively lower blood pressure.

Magnesium. Evidence exists that this simple mineral, which is found in all our bones, can help with pain, particularly in the lower back. By blocking calcium from entering cells, magnesium may reduce the excitability of your muscles, allowing them to relax and reduce spasm, especially after exercise.

Turmeric. Growing up in an Indian household, I've been eating turmeric since I was a kid. The active ingredient, curcumin, is thought to be a potent anti-inflammatory, particularly effective for osteoarthritis of the knees. Recently it has been recommended to help reduce the symptoms of irritable bowel syndrome. In recent lab experiments, however, turmeric inhibited some chemotherapy drugs from working against breast cancer cells and also increased the risk of kidney stones, so make sure to check with your doctor if there is a concern. And buy from a reputable source. Turmeric is among spices that have recently been flagged as potentially being contaminated.

Willow bark. The active ingredient in willow bark is salicin, which is very similar to aspirin. It is broken down into salicylic acid, which helps decrease pain and fever, and like aspirin may have side effects such as upset stomach and bleeding problems. If you're sensitive to aspirin, have kidney disease, or you're taking a blood thinner (or planning surgery) check with your doctor.

Nonopioid Analgesic Medications

Acetaminophen (paracetamol)
Brands: Tylenol, FeverAll, Panadol

An analgesic medication that works in the brain to reduce mild to moderate pain by increasing the body's pain threshold and changing the way the body senses pain. It is also your best bet to regulate body temperature and bring down fever.

Best for: Headaches, muscle aches, sore throat, toothaches, backaches, and sprains and strains. Best painkiller for people with gastrointestinal issues

Don't use for: Nerve pain or inflammatory conditions like arthritis

Avoid if: You are a heavy drinker. Take no more than 1,000 mg at a time, and no more than 4,000 mg over a twenty-four-hour period, to avoid liver issues.

Ibuprofen (Advil, Motrin, Midol), Naproxen (Aleve, Naprosyn, Naprelan), Meloxicam (Mobic)

Consult your doctor to determine dosage and frequency of use that is best for you.

What it is/What they are: Nonsteroidal anti-inflammatories (NSAIDs) that reduce fever and block prostaglandins, compounds that cause pain and inflammation

Best for: Headaches, musculoskeletal pain, arthritis, toothaches, backaches, and sunburn. These are safer choices than aspirin for those with bleeding risks but are still associated with gastrointestinal issues.

Don't use for: Nerve pain

Avoid if: You take blood thinners or have uncontrolled high blood pressure, heart failure, or a history of ulcers or liver or kidney disease.

Aspirin

What it is: An NSAID that stops the production of prostaglandins, which cause pain and inflammation. It also reduces fever and blood clotting.

Best for: Headaches, arthritis, toothaches, muscle aches, sprains, strains. It's also the only NSAID that reduces heart attack and stroke risk, though updated guidelines say that adults sixty and older should not start an aspirin regimen to lower their risk of a first heart attack or stroke, due to the risk of gastrointestinal bleeding.

Don't use for: Wounds or bruises (aspirin may promote bleeding) or nerve pain (it just won't touch it)

Avoid if: You take blood thinners or have uncontrolled high blood pressure, kidney disease, ulcers, or bleeding risk.

Topical pain relievers

What it is/What they are: Anesthetics that temporarily relieve pain at the skin's surface. A topical NSAID called diclofenac sodium topical gel 1 percent (Voltaren, and over the counter as a generic drug) can be effective for joint pain.

Best for: Neuropathic pain, nerve pain, and soft-tissue injuries

Don't use for: Wounds or open sores

Avoid if: You are allergic to lidocaine or if you have liver or heart issues.

Final reminder: Always tell your doctor about all the medications you are taking. Even if you buy them over the counter, they might still cause some concerning drug interactions.

As you consider these or any of the many other options for pain relief we're about to explore, keep this in mind: pain relief isn't just about physical relief; it is an integral part of a complex, dynamic healing process that involves every other system in your body.

One reason opiates have proven so destructive, especially when used as ongoing treatment for chronic pain, is that over time they corrupt those natural systems. In exchange for initial pain relief, they slowly disable processes essential for normal functioning and healing, and they can create new complications: constipation, nausea, slowed breathing, dizziness, depression, brain fog, and the obvious—dependence and addiction. All of these compromise healing and health, often prolong pain, and carry even greater health risks.

Drugs Old and New Expand the Toolbox . . . Slowly

We've seen remarkable progress in pain management since the days when opioids and steroids were used to treat most pain maladies. For neuropathic pain, that shooting or burning sensation, we now have drugs such as gabapentin, a prescription medication originally developed as an anticonvulsant, which regulates how pain messages travel from the brain through the spinal cord and reduces the excitability of nerve cells in the brain. "Gaba" (sold under the brand names Horizint, Grayliese, and Neurontin) was approved for treatment of neuropathic pain about twenty years ago, but it is far from a perfect drug. A 2017 review concluded that while around half of those treated had objective pain relief, they also often experienced adverse effects such as dizziness, drowsiness, tiredness, headache, nausea and vomiting, memory loss, weight gain, coordination problems, and eye problems. The drug worked best for postherpetic neuralgia; evidence for other types of neuropathic pain was very limited.

We've also seen an uptick of interest in the use of antidepressants for pain, especially for chronic migraines and long-standing arthritic pain. It's not entirely clear yet why they help relieve pain for some people. The fact that they increase serotonin, which can improve mood, might be one reason. It may also be that they affect the *perception* of pain, reducing the focus the person puts on it and thereby distracting them from it. What is clear is that these medications take a long time to work, sometimes up to several weeks, and even then, the patient may need regular dosage adjustments to minimize side effects. A 2021 systematic meta-review of thirty-three trials showed that serotonin-noradrenaline reuptake inhibitors (SNRIs) reduced back pain with moderate certainty, osteoarthritis pain with low certainty, and sciatica with very low certainty on pain and disability scores.

A 2023 Cochrane network meta-analysis examining antidepressants across all chronic pain conditions concluded that after investigating twenty-five different antidepressants, "the only antidepressant we are certain about for the treatment of chronic pain is duloxetine. Duloxetine was moderately efficacious across all outcomes at standard dose." There is also promising evidence for milnacipran, the study said, but higher-quality research is needed. "Evidence for all other antidepressants was low certainty." Additionally, after randomized controlled trials excluded people with low mood, the review was unable to establish any beneficial effects of antidepressants for people with chronic pain. The review concluded that currently there is "no reliable evidence for the long-term efficacy of any anti-depressant."

In people who suffer chronic pain, there's emerging evidence that their sensory neurons are more excitable than usual and can therefore be more easily triggered. For that reason, there's new interest in the use of sodium channel blockers, an established tool for quieting seizures, which are also caused by overexcited nerve cells in the brain. Novocaine, which dentists inject into the tissue they want to numb for a procedure, is one example of a sodium channel blocker. The goal has been to turn that into a pill that works for chronic pain conditions, and researchers are currently making progress on that front.

Just this year, the FDA approved the first new drug in a new class of non-opioid pain medicines, approved to treat moderate to severe acute pain in adults. The approval of Journavx (suzetrigine) marked the first approval of a new class of non-opioid pain relievers in more than two decades. While opioids primarily work by dulling sensations in the brain, the new drug, in fifty milligram oral tablets, is reported to reduce pain by targeting a pain-signaling pathway involving a specific sodium channel in the peripheral nervous system, before the pain signals reach the brain. The efficacy of Journavx was evaluated in two randomized, double-blind, placebo-controlled trials of acute surgical pain, one following abdominoplasty and the other following bunionectomy. In addition to receiving the randomized treatment, all participants in the trials with inadequate pain control were permitted to use ibuprofen as needed as a "rescue" pain medication. Both trials demonstrated a statistically significant superior reduction in pain with Journavx compared to placebo, the FDA said in announcing the approval.

The discovery of this drug has a fascinating backstory. Nearly twenty-five years ago, researchers learned about a family of fire walkers in Pakistan. They could walk on hot coals without flinching. Importantly, they felt the coals on their feet and even knew they were hot, but it was the specific sensation of pain they weren't feeling. It wasn't that their feet were numb, given that the nerves responsible for heat and touch seemed unaffected. Rather it was just the pain-conducting nerves that were affected. That observation led to a quarter-century investigation, the identification of a gene unique to this family, and ultimately helped inspire the development of the new medication.

Medical Interventions and Medication Management

Following are some of the many available options for pain relief and management:

- Prescription pain medicines, including opioids. These provide stronger pain relief than nonprescriptive options, but because they have potential for abuse and unpleasant and potentially serious side effects, they should be reserved for more severe types of pain.
- Prescription drugs approved for other conditions but repurposed "off-label" for pain. These include antidepressants and anticonvulsants.
- Neuromodulation, including spinal cord stimulation (SCS), an implanted device that sends low levels of electricity directly into the spinal cord to relieve pain; deep brain stimulation (DBS); and local (external) electrical stimulation, applying brief pulses of electricity to nerve endings under the skin to provide pain relief (Scrambler, TENS).
- Injection therapies, including:
  - *Epidural steroid injections*
  - *Nerve blocks*
  - *Joint injections*
  - *Trigger point injections*

- *Dry needling: Usually as part of a larger pain management plan, dry needling is sometimes recommended. The treatment, which can be initially painful, involves placing thin sharp needles through the skin and into what are known as "trigger points," areas of muscle that have become knotted and tender. The needling can decrease tightness, improve blood flow, and reduce pain. It's called "dry" because there are no medications in the needle, as with trigger point injections.*
- *Botox*
- *Gel injections (hyaluronic acid to mimic cushioning fluid in joints): often used for knee pain, especially mild to moderate arthritis*
- *Prolotherapy injections (concentrated sugar water to relieve pain in joints, ligaments, and tendons)*
- *Regenerative medicine (orthobiologics): a newer category including injectables made from your own blood or tissue, or application of dressings using biomaterials (such as placenta), used to restore tissue in skin grafts and other wound or surgical sites.*
- *Platelet-rich plasma injections and cell therapy: PRP injections involve taking the patient's blood, isolating and concentrating the platelets, and injecting billions of them into the joint, ligament, or tendon. Some newer injectables, called cell therapies, collect cells and tissues from bone marrow or fat tissue. The cells are collected, cleansed, and injected into the patient's joint, ligament, or tendon.*

▸ Others, including:

- *Nitrous oxide (laughing gas)*
- *Radiofrequency ablation, which treats spine pain by using radio waves to heat and destroy nerve tissue, preventing the associated pain signals from reaching the brain. There's also pulsed electromagnetic wave therapy, a noninvasive FDA-approved treatment that uses magnetic field pulses to improve blood flow to a localized area of pain, such as that from rheumatoid arthritis.*
- *Transcranial magnetic stimulation (TMS) is performed by placing a coil on the head to send magnetic pulses that can change the brain's*

activity in areas associated with pain. A recent trial showed that the treatment, typically daily sessions for four to six weeks, results in about half of fibromyalgia patients experiencing a meaningful reduction in pain.

- *Extracorporeal shock wave therapy: Think of it as using high-energy sound waves through the skin right on top of the painful area. This type of therapy seems to trigger the body's natural healing mechanisms, break down scar tissue, and stimulate the formation of new blood vessels.*

▸ Surgery. This can effectively relieve some kinds of pain, primarily that caused by structural issues. Most pain is not caused by structural issues, however, and in those cases, an operation not only won't resolve the pain, it may even make things worse.

Neuromodulation Offers Stimulating Options

Remarkable technological advances are being made in the area of pain control and management. The holy grail, as we learned from Prasad Shirvalkar's pain signature work, would be a device that could prevent pain by predicting and interrupting it before it even registers as pain the person would feel.

A deep brain stimulator (DBS) of the kind that Ed Mowery received requires an aggressive operation and thousands of hours of collecting personal brain wave data, which isn't currently possible to achieve outside a research setting. But emerging innovations are making spinal cord stimuator technology accessible for treatment of lower back pain. Inceptiv, an implanted device from Medtronic that was recently approved by the FDA, works by sensing biological signals along the spinal cord and adjusts stimulation in real time.

A number of simpler devices have been developed in recent years that use electricity to influence the flow of pain signals to the brain. The general theory is that by interrupting or overriding pain signals with electrical stimulation, immediate feelings of pain can be reduced or eliminated.

Scrambler therapy uses a machine that conducts, through up to five electrodes placed on the skin, electrical "nonpain" signals of various intensities and forms. By surrounding areas of chronic pain with these nonpain signals, the brain receives scrambled signals with the hope that it can lead to a reset, diminishing the chronic pain. Scrambler therapy is administered in clinical settings, but patient access has so far proved a significant challenge. Few pain practices have invested in the expensive equipment; insurance rarely covers the treatment costs, which puts it out of reach for many.

Transcutaneous electrical nerve stimulation (TENS) uses low-voltage electrical current to try to block pain—or at least the perception of it. Like many other treatments, it has been highly effective for some people and not at all for others. For those who do get relief, it can be used at home.

A vagus nerve stimulator is similar to a cardiac pacemaker, but instead of sending signals to the heart, it sends electrical impulses to the brain to interrupt pain caused by conditions such as cluster headaches. As a primary pain signal transmitter, the vagus nerve is one of the most important of the cranial nerves. Clinicians can use either surgically implanted electrodes or, more recently, external devices to activate it. And although vagus nerve stimulation has been used to treat depression and epilepsy for many years, its use in pain reduction is more recent and requires further study.

As these technologies continue to advance, researchers hope that some might provide effective long-term pain relief.

Psychological Approaches that Can Help Change How Your Brain Creates Pain—and How You Experience It

Pain psychology focuses on developing self-awareness of pain-related thinking and behaviors, as well as on learning skills and techniques to work directly with pain and to manage emotions and stress in productive ways. Clinical hypnosis (with a trained therapist), self-hypnosis, mindfulness-based pain management (MBPM), and other mind-body approaches are among several techniques that have been shown to help some people not only manage pain but also improve sleep, eating habits, exercise choices to support a more active lifestyle, and relationship dynamics. The most frequently applied therapy approaches include:

- Cognitive behavioral therapy–Chronic pain (CBT-CP)
- Acceptance and commitment therapy (ACT)
- Pain reprocessing therapy (PRT)
- Emotional awareness and expression therapy (EAET)

Options for psychological services are growing dramatically as the medical community has awakened to their value for patients and the need to make them more accessible. In addition to one-on-one therapy and group therapy, other options are programs or sessions by telehealth, online, apps, and other digital platforms.

A fuller exploration of approaches is coming up in chapter 10.

Opioids: From Crisis to Question: Where Do They Belong?

As a journalist covering the opioid epidemic, I often felt that the story was difficult to tell, in part because it was in fact hundreds of different stories. The common through line was that too many of these pills were being prescribed, which led to skyrocketing addiction. And then when prescription opioids became harder to access, many who were addicted started using cheaper, more easily available heroin to satisfy their cravings. That same sad story could be told in any number of ways, but the story that didn't get enough attention was about the benefits of these drugs when used properly.

I believe opioids still have a specific, though limited, role in responsible pain management—and I treat many chronic pain patients who depend on them and take them responsibly. For them, these medications are necessary and even lifesaving.

The problem is that opioids are still too liberally prescribed; recently, even my sixteen-year-old daughter received a prescription for them after having her wisdom teeth extracted, despite recent studies showing that young people who receive opioids after dental procedures are nearly three times more likely than older users to still be using them months later. Incidentally, recent findings have shown that a combination of over-the-counter pain relievers can actually be more effective than opioids in managing pain after wisdom tooth extractions.

As a surgeon, I'm always amazed at the diversity of pain pill use among my patients. Some absolutely want the pills after surgery. Others never ask for them, despite having undergone the same operation. That is why I want to briefly highlight the story largely missed starting with the first wave of the epidemic in the late 1990s: too often, people who have been able to use prescription opioids without abusing them have gotten caught in the crossfire of the broader opioid battle. They've been demonized as addicts, or as people likely to become addicts, and denied the medication that helps them. Some have other health conditions that make alternative pain medications riskier or ineffective.

I asked Dr. Carmen Green how the response to the opioid epidemic has affected patients who suffer from chronic pain and get relief from opioids.

"It's been heartbreaking," she told me. "The stories of people who've been on opioids for a long period of time, who lived high-quality lives, were present for their kids, who never abused their medications, never called in early, never 'lost' a prescription, have been caught up into a system in which all of a sudden they may be viewed as drug addicts."

She shared the story of a woman in her seventies who had been a patient at her clinic about twenty years earlier. "We'd recommended her to be on a long-term opioid pain medication. She was doing well after a couple of years, there was never a problem," Green said. "We sent her back to her primary care physician [and] that primary care physician continued the plan. Then the primary care physician retired, and a new person came in and said, 'I'm not writing [a prescription] for this.' "

The patient had no history to suggest she would misuse the opioid, Green said. "So do we just allow her to suffer? I would say that in this country we have."

If someone has a history of opioid misuse, that clearly needs to be taken into account. "But people who don't have those issues, we also need to be thinking about how we take care of the whole person, and opioids may be a solution for them. So, you know, I always think about that woman." The doctors were eventually able to help alleviate her pain, Green says. "But in the meantime, we put worry in a grandmother who didn't deserve to worry."

When patients can't safely use other therapies—for instance, if they're not able to have a nerve block because they're on blood thinners—that narrows their options. Green notes that to deny those patients pain relief when there are effective options—opioids, if necessary—"is just not humane." Yet too often that's what happens.

Opioid-safety initiatives intended to sharply curtail use have caused unintended consequences for some subgroups of patients—among them, cancer patients. A 2024 retrospective study, "Opioid Use in Cancer Patients Compared with Noncancer Pain Patients in a Veteran Population," analyzed the electronic medical records of 89,569 patients at the VA Medical Center in Palo Alto, California, from 2015 to 2021. Researchers found that the 9,073 cancer patients were nearly twice as likely as noncancer patients to have an opioid prescription. When doctors started to limit those prescriptions, the cancer patients suffered higher rates of pain than the noncancer patients, whose reports of pain remained almost unchanged.

"The consequences for cancer patients, who often rely on these medications for severe pain management, may be unintentional and profound," the study concluded. Other recent studies show that since 2016, cancer patients and survivors have had increased difficulty getting prescribed opioid medications. Many primary care doctors and oncologists, fearing heightened scrutiny by regulatory agencies and the risk of legal action, have reduced or even stopped prescribing opioids. Insurance companies have also imposed more stringent measures for obtaining these medications, contributing to the reluctance among health care providers to incorporate opioids into patient care regimens.

The Cannabis Conundrum

Over the past ten years, I've made seven documentaries examining the use of cannabis as medicine. In some treatment areas—including certain types of epilepsy, symptoms of multiple sclerosis, nausea, and opioid use disorder (chronic use of opioids that causes significant distress or impairment)—the benefits of cannabis are clear. When it comes to pain, however, the data are less compelling. And of course cannabis is not legal for use everywhere.

Part of the issue is that for decades, cannabis was regulated as a Schedule 1 substance, meaning it was thought to have a high potential for abuse with no accepted medical use. That made it difficult to study and collect data. At the same time, we do know that inflammation drives many chronic pain conditions, and several studies show the predominant cannabinoids such as THC (delta-9-tetrahydrocannabinol), CBD (cannabidiol), and CBG (cannabigerol) can drive down that inflammation. So, with that in mind and after reviewing several randomized controlled trials, here's how I'd summarize the findings: around a third of people with chronic pain who used cannabis saw their pain decrease. There were other benefits, such as patients needing smaller doses of opiates, suggesting a synergistic effect of cannabis with other pain meds.

I spoke with Dr. Staci Gruber, familiar to some as "the pot doc" but more widely known as an associate professor at Harvard Medical School and director of the Cognitive and Clinical Neuroimaging Core, which studies the relationship between psychiatric disorders and substance use, as well as the Marijuana Investigation for Neuroscientific Discovery program. Gruber has devoted her career to understanding the effects of cannabis on the brain. We talked specifically about its use for pain, and her advice for anyone using it or considering doing so.

"The first thing is: buyer beware," she says. "The average adult over the age of either sixty or sixty-five is on five conventional medications. So first and foremost, we want to be mindful that we are not creating a new drug/drug interaction. That's really important."

Second: " 'Know before you go.' Before you go to a dispensary or buy something online, know what you're looking for before you buy a product," she says. "Whether it's for pain, sleep, maybe it's both. Maybe it's for mood." Chronic pain can involve all three, but it's important to know specifically what you need as you consider options.

Third: "Start low and go slow," Gruber says. "You can always add—you can never take away. Once it's in [your body], it's in. So be mindful. A little can go a long way."

Dr. Gruber also cautions that "biologically, we are not all the same, so don't assume that someone else's experience with a product means it will be the same for you. Someone with a slower metabolism will have a different experience than someone with a more rapid metabolism, and that will affect how soon the effects will be felt and how long they last. You can go from feeling pretty terrific with a little bit of cannabis on board to feeling absolutely terrible in very short order."

Finally, avoid the trap of "stacking." If you're using edibles, you may initially think they're not doing anything, prompting you to take a second dose. A short time later, you may suddenly feel the effects of both doses, which may not be physically dangerous but can cause dysphoria, a very unpleasant feeling that is the opposite of euphoria.

Wherever you come down on the idea of cannabis use for pain (and there's a lot of cherry picking of studies to support different points of view), one overarching theme is that if you're using any of these products, you should talk with your doctor about it. There may be important individual considerations for you regarding medications you're using or other health issues.

Ketamine

Ketamine is not a new drug, even if you've just started hearing about it recently. In the 1960s, it was used as a battlefield anesthetic during the Vietnam War. In recent years, however, there has been research into using ketamine as a possible treatment for depression, post-traumatic stress, and chronic pain.

Philosophically, I tend to be skeptical of new so-called breakthrough therapies. Too often they're accompanied by more hype than hope. As things stand now, it's important to note that ketamine is currently *not* FDA-approved for the treatment of depression or pain, although the nasal spray esketamine is approved for treatment-resistant depression—meaning, for people whose depression hasn't improved with other existing treatments. But, because it is approved as an anesthetic, doctors can prescribe ketamine off-label for pain, and they increasingly do so.

I spoke with Dr. David Feifel, a researcher, psychiatrist, and one of the first clinicians in the country to prescribe ketamine, about its benefits and drawbacks.

"Drugs that have powerful effects on the mind can be powerfully therapeutic, but can also be incredibly damaging when not used the right way," Feifel told me. "The biggest risk is the fact that the ketamine treatment is associated with an altered state of thinking. When we're talking about psychoactive drugs, there's always a possibility that it'll be very unpleasant, could be emotional, which sometimes could be very scary."

In 2018, the American Society of Regional Anesthesia and Pain Medicine, the American Academy of Pain Medicine, and the American Society of Anesthesiologists offered consensus guidelines for the use of ketamine in managing acute and chronic pain:

- Subanesthetic doses of intravenous ketamine should be considered for patients undergoing procedures associated with severe postoperative pain, such as abdominal and thoracic surgery and orthopedic (limb and spine) procedures.
- Ketamine should be considered for opioid-dependent patients as an adjunct therapy to limit the use of opiates when undergoing surgery or in patients with chronic medical conditions such as those with sickle cell crises.
- For chronic regional pain syndromes (CRPS), there is moderate certainty evidence supporting the use of ketamine infusions for analgesia, which has been shown to provide pain relief for up to twelve weeks.
- Follow-up therapy (after intravenous ketamine infusion) with intranasal ketamine for breakthrough pain can be used.

- Ketamine should be avoided in patients with severe or uncontrolled cardiovascular disease, severe liver disease, increased intracranial pressure, elevated intraocular pressure, pregnancy, and underlying psychiatric disease associated with psychosis.

In 2019, researchers published a systematic review of a randomized controlled trial evaluating the effectiveness of intravenous ketamine for those with chronic refractory pain. The conclusion was that while ketamine provides significant short-term analgesic benefit in these patients, larger, multicenter studies with longer follow-ups were needed to better assess its effectiveness for use in managing chronic pain.

Before we finish the toolbox, a quick word about evidentiary data. Whether we're looking at naturopathic options, high-tech ones, or approaches such as acupuncture, yoga, and meditation, it's important to recognize that there's not much in the way of high-quality data about their efficacy. The measuring scale for such data goes from Level 1 (the gold standard of reliable data) to Level 4 (mostly anecdotal, observational studies), and in the case of these options, the levels of evidence are usually 2, 3, and 4. The unfortunate reality is not just that there is little data on these pain treatment options but that we may *never* have great data on them.

Why? For two primary reasons. First, these are hard studies to do, requiring strict control groups and long-term follow-up. And second, if there's not money to be made, these types of trials aren't likely to be funded. As a result, therapies usually involving expensive drugs and procedures are entrenched. This kind of inertia is a jarringly common problem in the evolution of medicine—perhaps most of all when we consider complementary and integrative options. Though many have evolved through generations of practice grounded in ancient healing cultures, the evidence is still limited, even as their popularity has recently surged. It reminds me of a great conversation between close friends Matthieu Ricard, a Buddhist monk trained earlier as a molecular biologist, and Wolf Singer, a neuroscientist, documented in their book, *Beyond the Self.* Their conclusion is that Buddhism "shares with science the task of examining the mind empirically; it has pursued, for two millennia, direct investigation of the mind through penetrating introspection. Neuroscience, on the other hand, relies on third-person knowledge in the form of scientific observation." Both penetrating introspection and scientific observation are important, especially when it comes to something as ephemeral as pain.

Your Personal Targets for Pain Relief Are Top Priority

What Matters Most to You?

As you consider all the various pain relief options in your toolbox, particularly for chronic pain, experts suggest you focus on what matters *to you* rather than what's the matter *with you*. Short of a medical cure for the diagnosed cause of your pain, what matters is how your pain affects your quality of life. What are your most pressing concerns? What are your sources of joy or pleasure?

Taking an inventory of the areas of self-care below can help you identify how they affect your health. All are important targets for action, but look for the ones that affect you the most and let that be your guide for choosing your pain management options. As a preventive tool, think of these as factors in pain resilience, and use the inventory to appreciate what's going well in addition to identifying any items you can target for improvement.

Sample questions:

- Are you getting enough sleep at night to refresh your body and mind?
- Are you eating foods and drinking beverages that nourish and fuel you?

- Are you surrounding yourself with people you love and care about?
- Do you have as much energy and flexibility as you would like?
- Are you finding opportunities to learn and grow?

Courtesy of the US Department of Veterans Affairs
https://www.va.gov/wholehealth/docs/PHI-long-May22-fillable-508.pdf.

Acupuncture, Yoga, Meditation, and More

Complementary and integrative health options round out your toolbox. An analysis conducted by the National Center for Complementary and Integrative Health (NCCIH) reveals a substantial increase between 2002 and 2022 in the overall use of complementary health approaches by American adults. Researchers evaluated changes in the use of seven complementary practices: yoga, meditation, massage therapy, acupuncture, guided imagery/progressive muscle relaxation, chiropractic care, and naturopathy.

The key findings are these:

- The percentage of people who reported using at least one of the seven approaches increased from 19.2 percent in 2002 to 36.7 percent in 2022.
- The use of yoga, meditation, and massage therapy experienced the greatest growth during that period. Use of yoga more than tripled, from 5 percent in 2002 to 15.8 percent in 2022.
- Meditation became the most used approach in 2022, jumping from 7.5 percent in 2002 to 17.3 percent in 2022.
- Acupuncture, increasingly covered by insurance, saw an increase from 1 percent in 2002 to 2.2 percent in 2022.

The report noted that factors contributing to increased patient use included higher-quality research supporting the efficacy of complementary health approaches, the inclusion of these approaches in clinical practice guidelines for pain, and the expanded insurance coverage for approaches such as acupuncture.

These health approaches are not just for pain, though, as we'll see in the chapters ahead. They're used to improve sleep, stress management, general wellness, energy, and immune health—all of which play a role in pain.

Harnessing those benefits as part of a full-spectrum approach is promising. Think of it as engaging the body's own resources, from our naturally occurring endogenous opioids to the brain's learning processes, as well as therapies and practices that engage those processes on command—our personal command. We need to continue to frame pain management and prevention in the context of our own biological and behavioral arsenal, rather than solely on the conventional focus on "pills, patches, needles, and procedures."

The Geography of Pain Relief: Music in the Mix?

It's easy to assume that people around the world manage pain in the same way, especially where modern Western medicine holds sway. So it might surprise you to discover just how different pain and pain management practices can be depending on geography, history, and culture.

Given that our human bodies are wired in similar ways, it would seem logical that anesthesia for common procedures would be the same in most countries. Yet profound cultural differences exist in pain and pain management. For example, in Japan, China, and much of Europe, colonoscopies are routinely performed without any kind of sedation, while in the United States and the United Kingdom, intravenous sedation is standard. This is an example of not just personal differences but societal ones. If the "standard of care" is not to use sedation, then that becomes the common practice, though it's as much custom as it is science. It turns out that social and cultural dimensions of pain and pain relief are as interwoven in our experience as the most basic biological mechanisms.

Harvey Rich, a physician, psychoanalyst, and founder and past president of the American Psychoanalytic Foundation, spent years as an embedded physician in traumatized, war-torn communities around the globe. He engaged in community-based work alongside local healers and witnessed traditional healing practices—rituals, ceremonies, drumming and healing circles—produce spontaneous recoveries unexplainable by Western medical science. The healing agent, he says, "was the presence of the community and the force of the group. I believe that such matters really do deal with pain and mental anguish. We do not have that in our Western culture anymore; we are relegated to pills and practices that are done in isolation."

In 2019, I traveled to Istanbul to visit a remarkable group of Turkish surgeons, talented not only in their medical skills but also as musicians, as I learned. They took me into the operating room, where I watched them perform a coronary artery bypass graft (CABG, pronounced "cabbage"). The procedure, commonly performed for blockages in blood vessels leading to the heart, involves opening the bone of the chest or sternum with a saw, then spreading the ribs. Though the patient is blissfully asleep during the operation, the postoperative period can be miserably painful—as I saw with my own father after he underwent the procedure. Every movement led to a grimace, and God forbid he had a sudden burst of coughing, which felt like "volcanoes going off" in his body, he told me.

In Istanbul, after we left the operating room and went to the recovery area, the surgeons pulled out their instruments—not surgical ones, but musical!—and started performing a different sort of therapy. As they played and sang Turkish folk songs for the now-awake patient, I watched as his heart rate, blood pressure, and respiratory rate numbers improved, all signs that postoperative pain was being successfully addressed. Another patient, still intubated with a breathing tube, even started conducting with an imaginary wand in his hand. The surgeons were playing a reed flute and a stringed baglama, culturally recognizable to the patient, and the music they chose was relaxing, calming, and without any particularly strong rhythms or percussion.

While the surgeons preferred to play the music themselves, they didn't always have the time to do so. In those instances, the music was "administered" through headphones, which was also very effective. In one study of sixty-eight patients (fifty-two men and sixteen women) who went through CABG surgery, pain perception levels were significantly lower in the group that was treated to music, and the amount of analgesics used was lower as well.

It's possible that the music serves as a source of distraction, drawing attention away from all the negative stimuli. Maybe the benefit comes from the introduction of pleasant and encouraging thoughts. The exact mechanism of how music helps alleviate pain is still a mystery. We do know, however, that it's inexpensive, has no side effects, and is effective.

Presence and meaning, caring touch and reassuring words, music as medicine: there are therapeutic agents for pain relief within reach for each of us.

CHAPTER 9

Brain Surgeon, Pain Surgeon

As a neurosurgeon, I usually see patients who are suffering with some sort of pain—headaches, neck and back pain, often radiating down the arm or leg. Often by the time patients get to me, they've already seen their primary care doctors and maybe even a neurologist. Still suffering, they're now at the point where they're wondering if an operation can help them.

I remember a particular day in the clinic when I saw one patient with lower back pain that radiated down the leg into the big toe and another with arm pain extending into the pinky finger. Both patients were scheduled for operations, while a third who arrived with intractable headaches was sent back to his doctor because he had no clear surgical issue, meaning there was no obvious structural problem causing his headaches. When I informed this third patient that he wouldn't need brain surgery, he told me he felt equal parts frustrated and relieved.

Ultimately, he was diagnosed with cluster headaches, and found significant benefit from simply breathing in 100 percent oxygen for fifteen minutes. He did this multiple times a day, usually at the first sign of an attack. At first, he was skeptical, thinking brain surgery was the only answer. But as is the case with at least 70 percent of patients with cluster-type headaches, a face mask connected to an oxygen tank ends up being the far better and less invasive option.

While pain itself can't be measured or seen on a routine imaging scan, many of its causes can. A herniated disc. Bones or vertebrae that have slipped out of place. An infection or a contused scalp with a fractured skull. A pinched nerve, increased pressure inside the skull. These things can, and frequently do, cause pain—more for some than others. I've seen patients with structurally damaged backs still bounding around with little pain. And I've seen patients with minimal changes in the spine in utter agony.

This last scenario is a primary driver of unnecessary operations, when surgeons attempt to provide relief even though there's no abnormality to correct. With some issues in neurosurgery, such as a blood collection on the brain after trauma, a broken spine causing pressure on the spinal cord, and certain types of brain tumors, the need for surgery is clear. (See "When Surgery Makes Sense" on page 163.) These patients have come to the right place, and they need an operation. But more than half our patients fall somewhere in between an obvious need for surgery and no need whatsoever.

In my experience, only one or two patients in ten referred to me for back pain actually needs an operation. And after a quarter century of caring for neurosurgery patients, trying to figure out which patient is which is still one of the most challenging things I do.

For obvious reasons, nobody wants to undergo unnecessary surgery. It's expensive. It generates risks of various kinds, including the likelihood of acute post-op pain and the potential for developing chronic pain. A 2023 review of studies published from 1997 to 2017 on postoperative pain among a broad swath of patients and types of surgery reported that an estimated 80 percent of patients experienced postsurgical pain, with 70 percent reporting it as moderate to severe. That's not surprising, but once the patients were home, anywhere from one-third to a bit more than half continue to suffer moderate to severe pain.

As you learned earlier, one chronic pain theory suggests that the brain encodes an initial acute pain experience, then continues to replay it repeatedly. And surgery could be considered an acute pain experience. Even routine surgical procedures include the surgical wound to the body, the acute pain it imposes, and the corresponding physical and emotional stress. What's more, the brain's encoding of that surgical stress and pain might be influenced by factors unrelated to the medical issue, such as your emotional distress or that of family members. Other possible factors include work or financial concerns, a previous history of depression, or other underlying health conditions.

Epidemiological studies vary widely, but overall, estimates suggest that between 10 and 30 percent of surgical patients will report some degree of persistent pain at one year postoperatively, with higher rates (over 40 percent) after particularly invasive procedures such as major thoracic surgery. For 5 percent of all surgical patients, their pain is reported as severe and disabling one year later.

Putting it all together, we now know that surgery can be one of the leading causes for the development of chronic pain. This is something I'm fully aware of every time I walk into the operating room. So if we're looking for places to make a meaningful difference in pain and chronic pain, the evidence leads right to my own backyard as a good place to start. Because pain prevention should start before you ever have pain, you should carefully consider whether it makes sense to have an operation. The list of questions, considerations, and especially the preventive steps below could save you from ever needing to go under the knife at all.

When assessing the suitability of an operation to relieve pain, most surgeons will start slowly in order to evaluate carefully. As I told my mom when she fractured her spine, I encourage you to think ahead about your answers to the following questions; then share them with your doctor.

Questions to Ask before Opting for Surgery

- Have I done everything I can to try to treat the pain?
- Is surgery the best option? What other possibilities might I consider?
- How much do I believe the surgery will actually improve my quality of life? (Remember that expectations are highly correlated with outcome.)
- What will the recovery be like?
- What will my restrictions be during recovery?
- How long can I expect to be out of work?
- Will I require physical therapy?
- What will the cost be?

Then ask yourself these questions:

- Is the pain uncontrollable with oral pain medications?
- Have I developed worsening symptoms, especially numbness and weakness, which suggest my body is struggling to manage this?
- Am I no longer able to wait to get better?

The answers to all of these questions will be relevant to your decision. Also, keep in mind that although many conditions at first seem to suggest surgical intervention, they might in fact heal themselves.

Surgery Is Far from a Quick Fix

Consider back pain, for example. Eighty percent of people will experience it at some point in their lives. In fact, one of the most common operations we neurosurgeons perform is on the lumbar spine—the lower back. Yet even with so many people suffering back pain, the vast majority will never need surgery. As I mentioned, only about 10–20 percent of the patients I see for a surgical evaluation typically ends up in the operating room. And again remember, these patients are seeing me after they've been evaluated by their own primary care doctors and sometimes neurologists. That means they often arrive with expectations that an operation will be a cure-all, but most of the time that's not the case.

Here's the point: Even though back surgery is highly effective in some cases, it's rarely necessary.

Keep this number in mind: twelve weeks. Most patients with back pain improve on their own, with nonsurgical strategies, within twelve weeks—and typically sooner. One reason so many people opt for operations is that they don't want to wait—or can't afford to wait—the twelve weeks needed to recover on their own.

I get it! If you're in pain, that seems a long time to wait. You just want to get it over with. We're under constant pressure to be active and productive at work, at home, and in our communities. Who has time to babysit their back for a few months? But opting for surgery with the hope that it will provide a quicker fix too often can lead to the opposite: an even longer and potentially more complicated and unsatisfying outcome. Having said that, recent studies have shown that most patients who undergo operations on the spine, for back pain, or knee-replacement procedures say they're satisfied with the result, with only around 10 percent having some degree of regret.

Nonetheless, I'm struck by the conclusions of Christine Goertz, a professor in musculoskeletal research at Duke University's Clinical Research Institute in Durham, North Carolina.

Writing about low back pain in 2023, she raised the growing concern that "many of these medical diagnostic and treatment approaches—early imaging, surgical consults, corticosteroids injections, prescription opioids—may actually increase the number of patients who transition from acute to chronic pain." Low back pain specifically "has been over-medicalized, making a very bad problem worse," she wrote in an editorial on the medical news website *Med Page*.

"The problem is not the lack of evidence. The problem is that we're not following the evidence," she wrote, referring to well-documented guidelines by the American College of Physicians (ACP), the Veterans Administration, and the CDC that all say other options can be effective. These might include specialized exercise programs, multidisciplinary rehabilitation programs, manual physical therapy approaches such as targeted massage, acupuncture and dry needling, psychological and mind-body practices such as yoga, breath work, and mindfulness meditation; heat and cold therapies; topical products; electrical, magnetic, and light noninvasive brain stimulation; nutrition and supplements; and pain education and guidance.

Too often, she said, many clinicians rush to respond to "frightened patients who understandably want a clear explanation for their pain and a quick fix—a pill, an injection, or even surgery."

"By ignoring the evidence, over-medicating this condition, and continuing to tolerate policies that incentivize the wrong treatments," she wrote, "we are causing real harm to those who turn to us to care for them."

When Surgery Makes Sense

One reason our lower back often hurts so much is that the lumbar spine supports all of your upper body weight, which can result in significant mechanical stress and strain. Just think about all the weight of your entire upper body being concentrated on one area of your spine, especially when you're sitting. That wear and tear, especially in backs that aren't well conditioned, can result in sudden flare-ups or near-constant pain. As with any pain intervention you might be contemplating, there are considerations that can tilt the odds in favor of surgery. Here are a few:

Pain that radiates down your leg. Radicular pain is an indication that you have a pinched nerve, often caused when a disc (the cushioning between two bones in your spine) has herniated or pushed out. This condition, typically confirmed by an MRI scan, results in back pain as well as leg pain, commonly referred to as sciatica.

Spinal stenosis. This is the term for when your spinal canal has become narrowed over time, a condition that can make it painful to walk or stand up straight.

Fractured spine. Often the result of a fall, this is of course what happened with my own mother.

If you suffer from any of the above, surgery may be the best option for addressing pain, but even with sciatica, it may still improve on its own.

Clarifying Expectations Improves Satisfaction with Surgeries

Consider these sobering statistics: The number of spine operations is on the rise in the United States, with more than 1.2 million spinal operations performed here annually, according to the National Center for Health Statistics. This compares with approximately 50,000 in the United Kingdom in 2017–2018, and 100,000 in France in 2019. Even accounting for the difference in population sizes, the United States is a clear outlier globally.

Interestingly, studies have found that most patients are still satisfied after spine surgery, with favorable rates up to 90 percent. And unsurprisingly, patient satisfaction appears to be closely related to clinical improvement in pain and disability after surgery. But the flipside is what I'd like to help you avoid. Recent studies have explored why a certain subset of patients were unhappy postoperatively, even if their operations resulted in "clinically relevant improvement."

The data made it clear that people's dissatisfaction was highly correlated to a perceived reduction in their quality of life, including lingering pain and joint stiffness that limited physical and social activity. There was also often a psychological component that left them feeling more pessimistic about their future.

So, patients need a clear sense of expectations. Many of my patients want to know whether they'll be able to resume a favorite sport, work, play with their kids, or go about daily activities without pain. There are no guarantees, and it's important to have realistic projections for individual circumstances.

You've Decided That Surgery Is the Answer. What Now?

Once you've opted for surgery, there are steps you can take to minimize postoperative pain. First, follow your surgical team's advice about preparations. Surgeons and their staff take steps to minimize adverse consequences and pain after an operation. But there are many things you can do *before* the operation that can help. Think of this as "pre-habilitation": improving your physical and mental fitness for everyday activity prior to a surgical procedure so that you're better prepared to withstand postoperative inactivity and any associated decline in function.

The surprising truth is that what you do before your surgery is just as important, and in some ways even more so, as what you do after your operation. So, instead of shying away from normal everyday activities before your procedure, lean into those activities as much as possible, strengthening your resilience ahead of time to prepare yourself for the road to recovery.

The more fit and active you are going into a surgical procedure, the more likely you are to retain a higher level of function after. So it pays to work on any existing functional deficits, meaning difficulty with everyday tasks, before your procedure takes place.

Recent studies have also shown that preoperative patient education, including behavioral approaches to pain management and skills coaching, can significantly improve postoperative pain management and overall patient satisfaction. According to a 2023 article in the *Canadian Journal of Pain,* inadequate preoperative education about postoperative pain increases patients' anxiety and persistent postoperative opioid use. Additionally, a 2025 scoping review calls out the need and benefit of behavioral interventions throughout various time points in the perioperative pathway—the period covering preoperative planning, inpatient, and postoperative periods—to reduce opioid use and decrease risk of persistent postoperative pain.

Cleveland Clinic uses a number of approaches to help its spine surgery patients throughout that extended period, teaching them nonpharmacological strategies to support their recovery. For example, the clinic adopted Empowered Relief for Surgery, a psychologically based pain education and skills development class developed by the Stanford Pain Relief Innovations Lab in Palo Alto. The class has been well received by spine surgery patients, with the majority of participants rating it highly (median of 9 out of 10 on a 1–10 scale) and reporting that they intend to use the skills they learn in class to support their recovery.

"The patients are focused on the surgery, but once they get in the class, they are so grateful because it gives them tools to go into surgery with to enhance their confidence and to quell anxiety," says Dr. Sara Davin, director of the Center for Pain Recovery in the Neurological Institute at the Cleveland Clinic. "We had to do a lot of education with the patients and the surgery team to get their buy-in on a class for surgery that is behavioral in nature."

For starters, the class participants learn about the neuroscience of pain and how it's processed in the central nervous system, more about the surgical procedures, and about the recovery process. That includes timetables around probable recovery times, such as when the patients will be able to play with their kids again and go back to work. Again, managing these sorts of expectations before operations is critically important. I've cared for patients who expected to be back to normal within a day after surgery, then became highly discouraged when it took weeks.

"As a patient, it is essential that you learn as much as you can about the procedure and what your realistic expectations should be for outcomes," says Davin. Intervening early, before the operation, actually may reduce the chances a patient will transition into some sort of persistent, debilitating chronic pain syndrome. I have often wondered if this level of pre-habilitation might have helped Joanna #2, my patient from years ago.

This cultural shift toward pre-habilitation is gaining currency with medical providers, Davin says. She now works collaboratively with spine surgeons who have embraced behavioral approaches to optimize outcomes. "They're really wanting to consider alternative therapies to support their patients," she says.

Dr. Peter Jannetta: A Historic Surgical Cure Passes the Test of Time

Hundreds of years ago, medical caregivers first described a strange electric shock–like facial pain, referred to as *tic douloureux*. Over hundreds of years, the condition has consistently been characterized as episodic, unexplained, and excruciating, with sufferers terrorized as much by the uncertainty of when it might appear as by the problem itself. Imagine being in a constant state of nervous anticipation, and then suddenly, without warning, a zap of pain shoots through your face, eyes, and jaw. It's the stuff of nightmares, a sort of physical and psychological torture.

Dr. Peter Jannetta, a neurosurgeon who was a leading expert on this disorder, called it the "worst pain in the world." Tic douloureux was known in medical circles as prosopalgia or Fothergill's. In less formal settings, however, it was given the tragic moniker "the suicide disease."

When Dr. Jannetta started his neurosurgery residency in the 1960s, not much was known about the disease apart from the fact that it involved the trigeminal nerve. This is the fifth nerve of the brain stem, that part of the brain that connects the cerebrum and the spinal cord and acts as grand central station for messages going back and forth between the two. Many of the cranial nerves responsible for hearing, eye movements, and facial function go through the brain stem, with the trigeminal nerve being one of them.

The trigeminal nerve divides into three branches, each of which provides sensation to the face, from the chin to the forehead. The ophthalmic, or uppermost branch, so named because it covers the eyes and upper eyelids, provides sensation for the upper part of your face and scalp. The maxillary, or middle branch, covers the middle part of the face: lower eyelids, cheeks, nose, upper lips, and gums. Finally, the mandibular branch, named for the lower jaw, covers that part of the face as well as lower lips.

For patients who suffer from tic douloureux, an electric shock of pain can hit any of these three branches or all of them at once. For decades, the only solution was to essentially obliterate the functioning of that nerve, rendering it incapable of transmitting any sensation whatsoever. The nerve could be cut, burned, electrified with a probe, or pickled in alcohol, but the result was the same: a complete loss of feeling on that side of the face. In essence, the patient was replacing profound pain with profound numbness—a significant price to pay. And even after making that devil's bargain, the pain would sometimes return as the nerve still figured out a way to send out an SOS signal.

More than a hundred years ago, when one of the founding fathers of American neurosurgery, Walter Dandy, first speculated that the trigeminal nerve was the culprit, he tested his hypothesis by severing a patient's trigeminal nerve completely. One day nearly forty years later, in the 1960s, Peter Jannetta was staring closely at that same nerve under a high-powered microscope when he made another discovery, one that completely changed our understanding of why some people suffered this awful pain.

Jannetta found that in a patient with tic douloureux, the nerve was compressed, with the pressure appearing to come from a blood vessel draped across the top of it. The blood vessel was tiny, even microscopic, and at first Jannetta wasn't sure whether it was causing damage to the underlying nerve. When he gently lifted the blood vessel off the nerve, however, a visible groove remained, which suggested that the compression was long-standing and severe. Jannetta hypothesized that addressing that microscopic compression could help alleviate one of the worst pains a human being could suffer. And he was right.

The operation to treat trigeminal neuralgia, known as a microvascular decompression, is now commonly performed in most major hospitals around the world, and I've been fortunate enough to be trained to do the procedure as well. Let me give you a visual description of how it works.

Take a moment to feel the bone behind your ear, known as the mastoid. I start with a small, slightly curved incision just behind that bone, on whichever side of the face is suffering the pain. After creating a half-dollar-sized opening in the skull, I can see the outer layer of the brain known as the dura. I then open the dura with a scalpel, revealing the cerebellum, which we gently nudge toward the brain's midline.

At that point, we have one of the most extraordinary views in all of neurosurgery: the brain stem and several of the major cranial nerves of the brain, including the trigeminal nerve.

Using an operating microscope, the compression of the nerve can be addressed by simply placing a piece of nonsticky cloth, known as telfa, between the blood vessel and the nerve. And that's basically it. The professor who taught me to perform this could complete the entire operation in less than an hour, and that's often the case today. With a long-term success rate of about 80 percent at alleviating pain, it's an incredibly gratifying operation for neurosurgeons, and one of the greatest breakthroughs in the surgical management of pain over the last several decades. MVD doesn't work for everyone with a diagnosis of TN. The reasons may range from subtle structural differences in the nerve and surrounding tissue, to inadequate imaging that fails to clearly identify the culprit compression sites. Or the problem may be a misdiagnosis of TN in the first place. With an accurate diagnosis of TN, however, MVD is a promising option to explore and discuss with your doctor.

Is Pre-Hab a Good Idea for You? The Answer Is *Yes.*

Pre-Hab Sets You Up for Success

Rehabilitation is a postsurgery program designed to relieve postoperative pain, improve strength, and restore function. It's typically undertaken with a physical therapist, who can design a program geared specifically to your condition and capabilities. In addition to exercise, postoperative rehab may include manual therapy, ice and heat therapies, ultrasound, and electrical stimulation via patches or other devices. Somatic exercises and other mind-body therapies such as hypnosis are also becoming more common in rehab, and some physical therapists are professionally trained in those approaches and can teach you those skills for self-management.

In contrast, as described above, pre-habilitation is preventive and protective, designed to prepare you for surgery by modifying probable risk factors, bolstering your physiological reserves, and decreasing the adverse stress response. Recent studies have found that doing pre-hab at least a few weeks before any type of operation is just as beneficial as postsurgical care. And yet until now, it has hardly received any widespread attention.

A good pre-hab program will help you in these ways:

- Strengthen key areas of your body that will be affected by the operation or are important in supporting you as you recover movement and strength for the tasks of daily living.
- Learn techniques for simple tasks such as getting out of bed or chairs, going up and down steps, lifting and bending, and other routine physical demands.
- Practice the above mind-body techniques to self-regulate the stress response, manage pain, improve mood, and cultivate a mind-set that promotes healing and good health (more on this below).

Studies on adjustable risk factors point to a number of protective elements that can reduce surgical complications and improve postoperative recovery. These include good physical fitness, functional reserve, and nutrition. The NIH recommends the following before heading into the operating room:

Stop Smoking

Smoking is a known preoperative risk factor that affects up to one-quarter of surgical patients. Its detrimental effects on cardiac, respiratory, and immune function contribute to prolonged recovery, slower wound healing, and increased chances of a heart attack due to the impact of nicotine on blood vessels. Studies show that preoperative abstinence of just four to six weeks results in a significant decline in postoperative complications.

Decrease Drinking

For patients indulging in more than two drinks daily, alcohol appears to aggravate the neuroendocrine response to surgery, which can lead to perioperative complications.

Definitions of what amounts to "a drink" vary internationally, but according to the commonly used definition by US health agencies, a standard drink contains approximately 0.5 fluid ounces (or around 12 grams) of alcohol and corresponds to the following beverage amounts:

12 fluid ounces of regular beer
5 fluid ounces of wine
1.5 fluid ounces of 80-proof distilled spirits

Personally, I believe the most recent data that strongly suggest no amount of alcohol is good for you. In many ways, alcohol acts as a mini-sledgehammer to the brain, never a good idea—and especially not before surgery.

Move More, and More Strategically

As a general rule, keep doing your daily activities before surgery as you normally would. You don't want to lose muscle memory of the most important activities in your life. It's also helpful to use a combined aerobic and resistance exercise program approved by your surgeon or physical therapist. This can include walking, cycling, and swimming, depending on what's best and most convenient for you and taking into consideration your capacity and preference. Developing a personalized program that you enjoy will help you stick with it.

Other muscle-strengthening exercises, using suitable equipment and under the guidance of a physiotherapist or a physical educator, are recommended a minimum of two days a week. This program should aim to reinforce all muscle groups that support daily life activities, including muscles of the chest, abdomen, back, and upper and lower limbs. Yoga can be an ideal way to engage mind and body in moves that both strengthen and relax.

Personalize Your Pre-Hab: Things to Consider

The following checklist is a helpful guide to discuss with your health care provider to tailor your pre-hab plan most effectively.

- Do you have physical limitations, or are you frail? If so, ask for pre-hab recommendations that reflect your age, fitness, and mobility. At least a single visit with a physical therapist in person or using telehealth services like Sword Health may be beneficial. The goal is to optimize your strength and mobility as much as possible before an operation. If you're over sixty-five, ask your surgeon or primary care provider for a referral to a geriatrician.
- Do you have any underlying cardiac disease? If yes, then ask for a preoperative consultation with a cardiologist. Make sure you have plenty of time to make an appointment before surgery, and be aware further testing may be necessary.
- Do you have pulmonary disease? Same as above, but ask for a pulmonologist.
- Are you exercising or physically active? If not, then consider starting a daily walking program that's within your physical capability. If possible and comfortable, try adding a lightly weighted vest.

—From the American College of Surgeons, Prehabilitation Checklist

Breathe In, Breathe Out

Simple breathing exercises help your lungs work more efficiently, supporting not only your pre-hab routine but also your postoperative recovery. Practiced regularly, deep breathing exercises can help rid the lungs of accumulated stale air, increase oxygen levels, and help the diaphragm do its job of helping you breathe, according to the American Lung Association. The association suggests two useful exercises recommended by respiratory therapists: pursed lip breathing and belly breathing exercises. The following instructions are suggested on the association's website:

Pursed Lip Breathing: This exercise is designed to keep your airways open longer. With fewer and deeper breaths, airflow in and out of your lungs is increased, allowing you to stay physically active longer without getting as easily "winded." The key is to breathe out at least twice as long as you breathe in. And best to breathe in through your nose and out through your mouth, with pursed lips.

Belly Breathing, also called Diaphragmatic Breathing: Start by breathing in through your nose, but now visualize your abdomen filling up with air. If that is hard to do, you can put your hands on your belly and directly feel the expansion and contraction. As with pursed lip breathing, the exhalation should be significantly longer than inhalation.

Eat Right

Think of this as nutritional conditioning. At least four weeks before surgery, start to tailor a plan for your specific dietary considerations. Because inflammation is a special concern following surgery, it's best to opt for the inflammation-fighting foods outlined in "Eat Well," chapter 15, tailored to fit your specific needs.

Learn More, Worry Less

Surgery is a stressful event, and preoperative stressors include receiving the diagnosis itself, as well as anticipation of the surgical procedure, anesthesia, pain, and recovery. All of these can cause worry and anxiety that affect your post-surgical recovery. So in addition to physical and mental conditioning ahead of surgery, you might want to examine how pain works, how you've dealt with it in the past, and what you can do to reduce it. Taking these steps can reduce your worry and stress, bolster your confidence, and improve your outlook.

Keep It Slow But Steady

The weeks leading up to surgery are no time for setting aggressive new fitness goals, but they're also not the time to let yourself slide physically, emotionally, or nutritionally. And remember—when you work out, do it with a very specific target of readiness for the challenge of surgery and successful postoperative recovery.

When Surgery Isn't the Recommended Option

I recently cared for a forty-seven-year-old woman I'll call M. A mother of two with chronic back pain, she told me she'd been going regularly to a chiropractor since her college days, nearly thirty years earlier. While the treatment would intermittently bring relief, her back pain persisted, and she soon found herself unable to be active; even chasing after her children became difficult. She gained weight, and her primary doctor kept telling her to exercise to treat her pain, not seeming to comprehend that the pain was what kept her from being active in the first place.

By the time she saw me, she was significantly overweight, had become antisocial, and, perhaps not surprising, was highly suspicious of all doctors. She was depressed and anxious. Despite all that, treating her as an acute pain patient would be the wrong approach to address her back pain—and yet, until recently, that's how chronic pain was often treated, with surgery and high-powered pain medications. Neither of those approaches is likely to work well if pain has been present for years, let alone decades, as was the case for M. As hard as it may be to distinguish, acute pain and chronic pain should be thought of as fundamentally different medical problems with different treatment options. Chronic pain is often entangled with lots of other psychosocial factors, and learning to separate those from the pain is where we started with M. Then we continued with a more directed approach to address her pain using nonoperative options.

The Value of a Second Opinion If You're Considering Surgery

If your doctor has recommended surgery and you'd like a second medical opinion, don't hesitate to get one. The more you know, the more confident you can be in your decision—whatever you choose. A 2017 study looked at 485 patients who were choosing whether to have surgery to treat degenerative spine conditions. Of those who received initial recommendations for surgery, more than half were subsequently advised to have conservative (nonsurgical) treatment and only about one third (33.6 percent) received a final opinion continuing to recommend an operation. Given these numbers, the study's authors unsurprisingly concluded that getting a second opinion can reduce potentially unnecessary operations.

In our department, after advising a patient against surgery, we don't just show them the door. We refer them to other resources, including specialists and support organizations that we feel may be helpful. There are all sorts of different doctors who treat pain, which is part of the beauty of it and the complexity of it. What we often do in such cases is refer patients to the pain clinic, though admittedly it's one of the most challenging appointments to get because there aren't enough of those doctors. But when you talk to pain doctors such as Carmen Green or Joel Saper, you realize that one of the most remarkable aspects of the treatment they provide is *time*. The epidural shots, prescription drugs, and other medical interventions they provide aren't unique to pain clinics. But these doctors spend a lot of time with patients to dive deep into the intricacies of their pain and closely track their progress.

If you're using painkillers or epidural shots, then your pain team tracks your progress with them. Pain clinics try to replicate the kind of close monitoring and responsiveness you receive from an inpatient program in an outpatient setting. This allows the team to be more nimble in, say, changing a medication if it's not working—failing fast—so you can more quickly try a different medication or treatment. Ultimately, I think that's very helpful.

Some Alternatives to Consider

A 2016 NIH evaluation of eleven studies of postoperative pain, covering 682 participants, found that patients treated the day after surgery with conventional acupuncture and related techniques such as transcutaneous electric acupoint stimulation, called TEAS, ended up having less pain and using less opioid pain medicine. Techniques such as acupuncture, yoga, breath work, and mindfulness-based practices have been used in some cultures for thousands of years, gaining traction in the United States only as evidence-based research has found that they can help improve pain for many people. Even so, as I mentioned earlier, these practices have still been slow to spread.

Why? I've asked that question of pain experts (especially those involved in patient care), as well as people responsible for shaping policies in hospitals, professional organizations, medical schools, and research centers. What I've learned is that recent promising data about these treatments doesn't always reach people—not the patients living with pain, not the doctors treating them, and not the students training for careers in health care. That is why I have taken the time to repeatedly amplify their potential benefits here.

I've always felt strongly about disseminating all the remarkable treatment possibilities for brain health, and I feel the same about pain health. The choices you make around basic approaches to behavioral health, physical and mental wellness, and preventive health are vital to your recovery.

The hard truth is that accidents, injuries, and unexpected health complications are usually not under your control. But your susceptibility to pain and chronic pain can be. It's smart to develop a lifestyle that makes you more resistant to pain and better able to manage it, heal, and get on with your life. That lifestyle prioritizes restorative sleep, physical movement and exercise, an anti-inflammatory diet, social connection, and some kind of mind-body practice that is calming for you. If you haven't got all those pieces in place already, now is the time to start.

Self-Advocate for Access to What You Need after Surgery

After any kind of surgery, access to postoperative rehabilitation and other health care services will have a significant impact on your quality of life. If those services aren't readily accessible due to cost, transportation, or geographical distance issues, then that's as important to discuss with your doctor as any medical details. You should be aware of them, discuss them with your provider, and find the rehabilitation strategies that most closely align with your personal needs and goals.

It's Not "Surgery or Nothing"

Many people believe the choice about surgery is binary: you get an operation, or nothing else will help. Thinking about this reminds me of something Amy Tomasulo, whose story I shared earlier, told me regarding her first appointment with a new pain doctor.

Over a two-year period, she'd had a string of best-guess treatments and an operation that had failed to remedy her severe, constant face and head pain. When she turned to a new doctor, he reviewed her file, then listened intently as she described her everyday experience of pain, as well as the fear and hopelessness she felt when thinking about her future. In addition to truly listening in an empathetic way, this new pain doctor did something else the others hadn't. He referred her to the Mayo Pain Rehabilitation Program, an intensive multiday outpatient program where patients work with a multidisciplinary team and other patients to learn to manage pain.

"I did that, and that was kind of my turning point," she recalls. "There'd been so many failed treatments and medications, and then this came about, and it was the right thing."

So what did this program provide that all her other treatments didn't? It wasn't a magic pill or even a particularly new therapy, but rather a deep connection with other people around a shared experience. "I sat in the room with twelve other people every day for five weeks and went over ways to live with it," she told me. "Just talked about our pain. And it really helped. I hadn't been around anybody else with that same experience." Pain has a shared language that's obvious to sufferers and often opaque to those looking from the outside in.

"It was just comforting to be around other people going through a really hard time and say, you know, we're all in this together. Maybe we can just figure out how we can best deal with this. It wasn't about, 'We're gonna cure this.' It was about, 'How do you live with it?' And that was the turning point." For Tomasulo, the group therapy not only provided relief; it vastly improved her quality of life.

That's the fascinating thing about treating pain. In the space between doing nothing at all and finding an absolute fix, there are many roads to relief. The treatment that finally helped Tomasulo wasn't a quick fix, and it wasn't a traditional cure. But it was good medicine nonetheless.

All of this reminds me of my own "Doctor Dad" reflex. Whenever my kids tell me about something that's bothering them, I immediately go into my Doctor Dad "must fix it!" mode. What I've realized over the years, and particularly as they've grown into teenagers, is that "fixing" the problem isn't necessarily what they want from me. Sometimes they just want validation of their feelings, sprinkled with a good dose of empathy. Learning from my kids to press pause on the fix-it reflex has helped me as a doctor. While I'd like nothing more than to be able to fix a patient's pain with a surgical procedure, I recognize that sometimes that's not the best answer.

CHAPTER 10

A Powerful Pairing Against Pain: Mind and Body

The list of Dan Kruger's wins over his forty-year career as an international motorbike racing champion is impressive—and even more so when you see the list of injuries he's accrued. Even a partial inventory is wince-worthy: a broken back, ribs (four of them twice), hand, wrists, fingers, legs, ankle, toes, jaw, collarbone (both sides), and multiple concussions. Kruger's impressive career comes with a parallel journey through the landscape of the fragile human anatomy.

A professional endurance athlete who adopted the racing life when he was just twelve and went pro around sixteen, Kruger started out as a kid from Canada scrapping to make a life he could call his own. While not a glutton for punishment, he long ago accepted the inevitable risks, injuries, and pain that come with his passion for racing, observing that "it's the nature of the sport and doing extreme sports."

What he didn't bargain for, however, was opioid addiction. But after thirty-five years of injuries, mounting health issues, and an overdose that nearly killed him, he knew he had to quit—not racing, but the drugs. What Kruger didn't expect was that a mindfulness-oriented therapy developed by a psychotherapist-scientist in Utah would provide the off-ramp he needed.

Eric Garland, at that time director of the Center on Mindfulness and Integrative Health Intervention Development at the University of Utah, had been working in that lane for two decades. An opioid addiction researcher and therapist treating pain patients, Garland had found meditation personally helpful. He'd made it the focus of his earlier doctoral studies as a coinvestigator in an early NIH-funded clinical trial of mindfulness for irritable bowel syndrome (IBS), then had continued to pursue his interest in the neuroscience of chronic pain, addiction, and emotional distress.

At a time when mind-body approaches were still largely dismissed in Western science, Garland's path lit up like a neural network. He was awarded a fellowship with the world's premier scientific organization for the study of meditation—the Mind & Life Institute, which was established by His Holiness the Dalai Lama and the Chilean neuroscientist Francisco Varela to help foster dialogue between scientists and Buddhists.

This was a heady environment for the young researcher, who found himself working alongside world-class cognitive neuroscientists, as well as what you might call the Olympian athletes of meditation: Buddhist monks who had lived for years alone in Himalayan caves, meditating. Garland was thrilled when the Mind & Life Institute funded the first research grant for his mindfulness-oriented therapy model to study it as a treatment for addiction.

Twenty years and a lot of serendipity later, Garland, now professor of psychiatry in the School of Medicine at the University of California, San Diego, and endowed professor in health sciences in the Sanford Institute for Empathy and Compassion, has channeled more than $90 million in federal grant funding to study, develop, and test mindfulness-oriented recovery enhancement (MORE) interventions. In a large clinical trial recently published in *JAMA Internal Medicine,* MORE was shown to reduce opioid misuse by 45 percent—more than double the effect of standard therapy.

Dan Kruger came across Garland's work while doing an extensive online search for drug rehab programs. When he reached out for help, the motorbike champion was in a very dark place. Though he was under no illusions of finding a quick cure, he didn't realize just how profound a change he would undergo as his journey moved inward. With Garland's guidance, he learned to work with his mind not only to overcome pain and addiction but also to find greater joy in his life.

MORE draws from long-established principles of cognitive behavioral therapy (CBT), mindfulness- and meditation-based practices, and other treatment models that use mind-body practices as a way to calm the nervous system, relax muscles, focus attention, and engage the brain's reward circuitry to reduce or manage pain. Over time, an extensive body of research has established its benefits, as other psychologically based approaches have also proven to be increasingly valuable components in chronic pain management.

Using Your Head to Get to the Heart of the Matter

At its core, psychotherapy for chronic pain aims to help you manage pain more effectively by working with the way you think and behave in relation to it. By improving your coping strategies and skills, the treatment improves your physical, emotional, social, and everyday functioning. And while the most popular approaches differ in their focus, they often incorporate a mix of talk therapy, relaxation training, stress management, and pain-coping skills training. From therapist-guided sessions to the solitude of mindfulness meditations, a range of techniques use different mechanisms to quiet the central nervous system's sympathetic fight-or-flight energy, engaging instead the parasympathetic nervous system and its calmer rest-and-digest mode.

Cognitive behavioral therapy, often described as the gold standard of therapies, is the most established and well-researched approach. As its name implies, it focuses on working with cognitive processes—how the brain processes information and experience—to change how they contribute to pain, distress, and disability. Cognitive behavioral therapy-chronic pain (CBT-CP) has been further tailored to address chronic pain more specifically. In short, CBT-CP helps individuals identify and manage negative thoughts and behaviors by developing skills to change them.

Another popular option is acceptance and commitment therapy (ACT), which fosters a nonjudgmental approach to distressing thoughts and emotions, encouraging acceptance of them while committing to living a full, engaged life despite the presence of pain. It also cultivates mindfulness and maintaining a balanced view of thoughts and feelings.

Emotional awareness and expression therapy (EAET) focuses on identifying, understanding, and developing skills to effectively communicate and manage emotions. In particular, it targets lifetime levels of psychosocial adversity, trauma, and emotional conflict that confront many people with chronic pain.

Pain reprocessing therapy (PRT) is a newer approach specifically for those whose chronic pain is deemed neuroplastic, meaning it has no discernible physical cause. PRT focuses on retraining the brain to interpret signals associated with the pain as "safe." It explicitly draws from the concept of exposure therapy, helping people confront their fears of pain in a safe environment so they can break the cycle of avoidance and reactivity. In this case, with a therapist, you confront that pain while changing the mental message that goes with it.

After returning from covering the war in Iraq, I underwent a form of graded exposure therapy for concerns about post-traumatic stress. While the technology was relatively new then, I was immersed in a form of imaginal exposure using virtual reality to help place me in situations that had caused me anxiety and increased my heart rate. With the help of a skilled therapist, I was able to overcome my apprehension about going on a big hiking trip to the Grand Canyon, which reminded me of some dangerous treks during my war coverage.

As the therapist described it to me, I had placed "Do Not Enter" signs in certain areas of my brain around things that had frightened me, and this exposure therapy helped tear those down. The difference with chronic pain, however, is that unlike fears of flying, spiders, clowns, or even war zones, the person is in the presence of their feared thing—pain—constantly. And still the evidence is clear that the practice of pain psychology can make a difference, often in ways that defy scientific measure.

Despite the growing evidence for and appreciation of these approaches, they're not always available to patients, providers, and organizations. But recently, innovative methods such as telehealth, Zoom sessions, YouTube talks, webinars, seminars, virtual reality, and animated guides have made remote access to these psychological interventions much easier. Apps exist for everything from brain-calming tones to remote sessions with providers, and wearable technology can ping you to pause for a calming breath or mindful moment when your pain indictors are escalating.

As diverse as the treatment approaches can be, what they have in common is the premise that you can "get your mind working *with* your body rather than against it," as Vidyamala Burch, cofounder of The Breathworks Foundation, likes to say. Burch, a former film editor, speaks and teaches from experience. At age seventeen, she sustained spinal injuries that required multiple surgeries and left her with a complex back condition, chronic pain, and partial paraplegia. Ten years down the road, after a string of unsuccessful operations and treatments, she was angry, hopeless, despondent, and hospitalized yet again. That's when she was taught meditation and realized the potential to train her mind as a tool to help her manage.

"I discovered mindfulness as a way to ease the mental torment associated with the physical pain," Burch says. "Soon I was meditating every day." At some point, she realized the effects went beyond relieving her mental torment; they changed her experience of the pain itself. "The results were truly life changing and transformative," she says. Burch went on to become a mindfulness and compassion teacher, coach, speaker, author, and cofounder of The Breathworks Foundation and the Mindfulness-Based Pain & Illness Management (MBPM) program. In 2022, she was awarded the distinction of OBE (Officer of the Order of the British Empire), one of the United Kingdom's highest honors, for her service to pain management and well-being.

It's remarkable that something as simple as how you breathe or focus your attention are now as much a part of the evidence-based scientific conversation as, say, the molecular mechanisms of inflammation.

And it is all the more important as scientists discover surprising new twists and turns in the intricately interwoven nature of pain. Molecules, cells, or circuitry that were long thought to be bit players in the pain process suddenly appear as elegant, exquisitely precise participants in it all, susceptible to hormones and neurotransmitters triggered by emotions. The idea is that through these mechanisms, your very attention can override pain—think about that! Even if the effect is temporary, the mechanism is there. It's a proof of concept that your mind can objectively change your body.

The basic idea that pain affects our minds isn't new. We all know how a nagging headache or even a little muscle twinge can distract or annoy us. But the idea that we can turn the tables and use our minds to refocus attention and interrupt pain: that's a game changer. These insights, now with growing scientific evidence supporting them, are bringing into focus evidence of the links and mechanisms of the thinking mind, the processing brain, and the body.

Here's how I like to think of it: the top-down power of the mind and brain, coupled with bottom-up input from biological processes, creates a sort of third plane of operations—a healing domain where everything comes together. In addition to rewiring neurocircuitry in the brain, as you engage your mind and body mechanisms, you're activating systemwide endogenous opioids and the mechanisms of the placebo response. And you can accomplish that activation with mindfulness meditation, among other practices, creating the analgesic effect.

One thing the extensive pain science literature has made clear is that techniques that help us tap into our natural capacity for self-regulation—working to upregulate or downregulate the nervous system—can modify our experience of pain. Self-regulation involves multiple domains—biological, cognitive, social, and emotional—that continuously interact through the shared circuitry in the body and brain. We can use our attention, even on something as simple as watching a majestic sunset, to alter how this interconnected neural circuitry focuses on pain, pleasure, or simply positive input that can tip the pain scales in your favor.

This conversation shift in mainstream medicine is long overdue, says Mark Jensen, PhD, a clinical psychologist, professor, and pain researcher at the University of Washington in Seattle. Jensen has researched the efficacy of psychosocial pain treatments and facilitated national and international workshops on these approaches for over three decades. Outdated perceptions about mind-body modalities have been slow to change, placing an unnecessary burden on pain sufferers who've been discouraged from trying new treatments, he says.

"This concept of brain versus body, one bucket or the other, is just wrong," according to Jensen. "Get the body taken care of, healed, but get the mind on board as early as possible. And if pain is chronic then this should be the *first* line of treatment. Not the last line of treatment." Remember, that is where we decided to begin with the patient named M in the previous chapter.

In his work with patients, Jensen combines cognitive-behavioral approaches, clinical- and self-hypnosis, and motivational approaches to help patients better manage chronic pain and its effects on their lives. He describes scenes I've witnessed in my own practice of patients arriving deeply discouraged after repeated medical interventions have failed. Getting over the hurdle of that resignation becomes the first challenge—including helping them deal with the fact that they're coming to see a therapist, still considered by many a stigma or sign of weakness.

People need to understand that seeking therapy doesn't mean they're giving up on finding a physical remedy for their pain, he says. "It means that we're addressing this based on our current scientific understanding of pain, which is that the brain and body work together to give you this experience, and you can learn some skills so that you can hurt less in this process of changing that experience right from the start."

He knows a thing or two about stigma. While clinical hypnosis, Jensen's research and practice focus, is a well-established therapeutic modality, it is often portrayed as gimmicky stage-show "hypnotists" and their tricks. We now know that clinical hypnosis is a therapeutic tool, used to arouse a biological state of deep absorption and focused attention, which the therapist or patient can use deliberately to encourage cognitive, emotional, or physical healing responses. Over the last several years, hypnosis has been studied for many pain conditions, including irritable bowel syndrome, lower back pain, and headaches.

While not found to be equally effective for all these conditions, clinical hypnosis has been found to be remarkably beneficial for some—and that should be our focus of attention, Jensen says. Unlike the pills-patches-and-procedures options, hypnosis presents zero to low risk for most people. That is why many pain physicians now place it in the top tier of the pain management toolbox.

Studies comparing hypnosis with CBT and meditation have shown that all three are about equally effective, Jensen says. However, when significant differences do occur, clinical hypnosis tends to emerge as more effective.

"Although our research indicated that hypnosis is a little better than other treatments, there are people who don't respond as well to traditional clinical hypnosis as they do to cognitive therapy, so we're curious about how we can understand the factors that predict who benefits the most from different treatments, in order to enhance outcomes for everyone."

Jensen's ultimate goal is to create a mix of options for people when they're exploring psychological and behavioral approaches. "If we know that different people respond more to some approaches than others, then that tells us we ought to be offering a variety of treatments. We shouldn't just have one antibiotic. We shouldn't just offer cognitive behavior therapy or only hypnotic approaches. We should offer our patients the options of training in mindfulness meditation, self-hypnosis, cognitive behavioral therapy, emotional awareness and expression therapy, acceptance and commitment therapy—a whole variety of pain treatments," he says.

And, just like those Turkish heart surgeons, Jensen has also been betting on music as a useful tool in the pain treatment mix. Jensen has one study now underway that involves a body tambura, a twenty-four-stringed instrument created for music therapy, which is based on the four-stringed tampura, an instrument of Indian origin. With a sound that resembles an autoharp, therapists use the body tambura to transmit relaxing sounds to a patient's ears and vibrations to the body. The results have not yet been published, but look promising, he says.

As Beth Darnall, the clinical pain psychologist, professor of anesthesiology, and director of the Stanford Pain Relief Innovations Lab, points out, "So often there's a focus on medication, and medication can be incredibly helpful. Medication can make all the difference in the world for some people. But as a psychologist," she advises, "also look beyond the pill bottle to what else you can do."

Sometimes Surprisingly Simple Tactics Can Trick the Brain

In the fascinating "Cognitive and Emotional Control of Pain and Its Disruption in Chronic Pain," published in *Nature Reviews Neuroscience*, Catherine Bushnell, scientist emeritus of the NIH Pain and Integrative Neuroscience Laboratory (PAIN), and her team point out that even simple psychological tactics such as distraction or diversion can activate specific circuitry in the brain, triggering cascading effects quite literally from head to toe. Among those the study identifies:

- Pain experience can be profoundly influenced by emotional states, including how much or little attention someone is paying to their pain.
- Even the expectation of relief activates your endogenous opioid pathways.
- When pain becomes chronic, structural changes are seen in multiple brain regions, including the areas that control emotions and attention.
- There is evidence that chronic pain alters cognitive and emotional processing and can impair decision making and learning tasks.

Dr. Helene Langevin, director of the National Center for Complementary and Integrative Health, sees hope in deepening the connection between conventional medicine and evidence-based mind-body approaches to pain management and prevention.

"When it comes to pain, we know that the mind and body connection runs deep and coping skills can have a profound impact on how—and how much—people experience pain," she says. "Deep breathing, relaxation techniques, techniques to calm down the sympathetic nervous system so that the body can start to rest and eventually have the pain subside. It's very important that we understand how to use these tools. It requires education. It requires patience."

The Power of the Purposeful Pause, Reappraisal, and Savoring the Positive

The three main therapeutic components of the MORE model are mindfulness, reappraisal, and savoring. A fourth is what Garland describes as an expansive feeling of self-transcendence, or a sense of connection with something beyond one's self.

Mindfulness

Mindfulness meditation, as widely practiced, focuses attention and awareness to observe your present moment, thoughts, emotions, and sensations without judging or reacting to them. The aim is to be a witness, an objective observer, intentionally paying attention to the process of your own thinking. This process, called meta-awareness, engages specific neural networks that are important to the therapeutic process. Mindfulness meditation is generally used as a calming practice that helps activate the relaxation response, slowing the heart rate and lowering blood pressure. This not only counteracts stress; it may reduce pain intensity and increase pain tolerance.

Reappraisal

Reappraisal is the process of reframing an adverse or stressful life event to see it as a potential learning opportunity, a means of growing as a person or of finding meaning. It's the practice of "finding the silver lining"—a thought process in which we shift our perspective in a helpful way.

An example might be surviving a heart attack, then deciding to shift to more heart-healthy eating and exercise. One physician I spoke with, who became a paraplegic in an accident and now uses a wheelchair, described how the sudden and nonnegotiable change of pace in his work and life slowed him down in ways that made him a better doctor. He explained that the shared experience of being given a life-changing diagnosis has made him more empathetic and able to forge a quicker and closer bond with his patients. This post-traumatic growth, as it's called, has become what he refers to as his "superpower." Sometimes we naturally recognize positive aspects of otherwise adverse events. But we can also choose to practice this skill and strengthen this quality of mind.

Savoring

Savoring is the process of mindfully focusing your attention on what's pleasant, beautiful, and good in life, then appreciating and absorbing the positive emotions and pleasurable body sensations that emerge, according to Garland. "We focus on the beautiful sights, the pleasant sounds, pleasant smells, the textures, the touch," he says. "We turn our attention to the pleasant senses in the experience, and then as we attend to what's pleasant about the object that we're savoring, it starts to stir up positive emotions in the mind or sensations of pleasure in the body."

We'll discuss this more later in the book, but when I experimented with savoring, I discovered that the feelings extend far beyond gratitude. This isn't about simply being thankful; this is about thoroughly enjoying life. In clinical studies, participants were taught the skills to turn attention inward and to savor the positive inner feeling, absorb it, and, as Garland puts it, "breathe it into the center of their being, deep into the mind and body, like water seeping into the soil."

Self-Transcendence

Self-transcendence, which is the feeling of being part of something greater than yourself, can develop from the practice of the other three techniques, Garland says. Some might call it awe, flow, or a moving spiritual experience. With or without a spiritual aspect, "it's the experience when the normal sense of self starts to quiet down, begins to fade away, and is replaced by a sense of connectedness to the world around you, or potentially even a sense of oneness with the world or the universe. That experience is often coupled with feelings of peace, love, compassion, or even bliss—a powerful, positive emotional state. Those experiences can emerge out of the synergy between mindfulness, reappraisal, and savoring. And I think the synergy of all of them together is pretty important."

MORE therapy has recently been adapted for "just-in-time adaptive intervention," in which wearable technology prompts the user to practice mindfulness on their own when it detects internal cues warning of impending pain. But at this point, MORE is still typically delivered as a group therapy.

In full-length sessions, patients practice their skills of mindfulness, reappraisal, and savoring. The training includes an informational segment about the nature of pain: how it works in the brain, the relationship between emotional responses and physical pain, and how we react to it. Group members also discuss topics oriented around finding a sense of meaning in life. What is your purpose in life? What matters most to you? The aim, Garland says, is to help people use these skills to alleviate symptoms of chronic pain and emotional distress and to reduce reliance on opioids if that's necessary.

This is the program that motorbike champion Dan Kruger discovered worked for him. During regular fifteen-minute guided meditations and his own mindfulness exercises, Kruger found that his physical pain temporarily evaporated. "It's amazing that while meditating to the fifteen-minute guided recording, my chronic pain or migraines disappear during the session," he said. "Typically, the pain comes back after, but not always to the same extent. The meditating is sometimes surreal in terms of how deep I get lost in it."

He compares it to his workouts at the gym, training to stay in shape. "I train every day because it gives me these endorphins that help me get positive, reduce stress, and stay fit. Meditation does much the same thing for me."

Over time, Kruger carefully weaned himself off opioids, even refusing them after injuries and operations that followed. After one particularly gruesome injury and emergency surgery, he says, he was given ketamine instead, which proved sufficient. After a full year of his opioid-free recovery, the combination of brain-training techniques and other conventional and complementary pain management tools continued to deliver uniquely effective relief, he said.

Shorter Skills-Based Program Still Boosts Mind-Body Pain Relief

At Stanford, pain psychologist Beth Darnall is focused on developing novel evidence-based pain treatments that can be delivered via Zoom conferencing with certified instructors and scaled up using technology, making them accessible to the greatest number of people while reducing the burden of time and cost associated with them. At the forefront of these so-called analgesic innovations is Stanford's Empowered Relief program, the one that got high marks from spine surgery patients at Cleveland Clinic. In a single session, the two-hour class incorporates pain management skills for ongoing, long-term pain relief. In addition to learning these skills, participants create a personalized plan for daily skills use. They also receive a free app they can download onto their smartphone or other device for unlimited, ongoing access to the tool.

Four separate randomized controlled trials conducted at Stanford, and another six clinical trials there and elsewhere, have confirmed that patients benefited and were able to manage a range of symptoms for up to three to six months after taking the single-session class. It means that the more accessible, less expensive short course delivered the equivalent benefits of a longer, more costly approach.

Despite such encouraging results, it has still been a challenge to take these pain-relieving techniques mainstream. When Dr. Davin of the Cleveland Clinic originally proposed the program as a pilot project for spine surgery, there was some skepticism from patients and the surgical team, Davin said. And some fear "that patients might think 'Oh, they think I need this class because something is wrong with me psychologically—or maybe they don't think my pain is real.' Some providers worried that the class might deter patients from surgery altogether." She continued to lobby for it, cheerfully calling herself "the brain coach" with patients, and over time the idea became more normalized in the clinic culture.

Pain Reprocessing Therapy: A Closer Look

Training the Brain to Switch Signals from "Threat" to "Safe"

What if the brain could "unlearn" pain by rewiring its response to certain signals that trigger a pain experience? Or what if, through therapy, patients could shift their beliefs about the causes and "threat value" of pain and the fear it generates? What sets pain reprocessing therapy (PRT) apart is the focus on pain as a reversible, brain-generated phenomenon that can be resolved with a mind-body approach to retrain the brain. That means the goal of the technique is not about developing skills to cope with pain or manage it, but rather to eliminate it altogether by retraining the brain.

Developed by Alan Gordon, a licensed clinical social worker (LCSW) and founder of the Pain Psychology Center in Los Angeles, and colleagues, PRT draws from aspects of existing psychological treatment models, including cognitive behavioral, acceptance-based, mindfulness-based, and exposure therapies. But it tailors them to work in a distinct way: to reprogram the pain response, retraining the brain's pain-processing circuitry to respond to a signal as safe rather than threatening.

Gordon was part of the research team that conducted PRT treatments for patients in the first randomized clinical trial of the therapy, published in *JAMA Psychiatry* in 2021. The trial, conducted at the University of Colorado in Boulder, enrolled 151 people whose chronic pain had been assessed as mostly driven by brain sensitization. Participants received one of three treatments: four weeks of PRT, a placebo injection of saline into the back, or a continuation of their usual care.

Participants randomly assigned to receive PRT participated in a telehealth session with a physician, followed by eight psychological treatment sessions over four weeks. The treatment, which used a combination of cognitive and somatic (or body-based) techniques, involved having a PRT therapist guide participants through painful movements while helping them reevaluate, or "reattribute," the sensations as nondangerous brain activity with no physical injury or damage.

The participants were asked to rate their pain before the treatment and four weeks after starting it. They also underwent fMRI scans documenting brain activity before and after treatment. Finally, the team followed up with them a year later.

Four weeks after treatment, thirty-three of fifty participants (66 percent) who received the PRT treatment reported they were pain free or nearly pain free, compared to 20 percent who received the placebo and 10 percent who'd been randomized to usual care. Even more remarkable was that those gains largely remained through the one-year follow-up. When asked about it afterward, the participants mostly attributed the success to their reduced beliefs that pain automatically indicates tissue damage. The study concluded that changing fear beliefs about the causes and threat value of pain may provide substantial, durable relief for people with primary chronic back pain.

Yoni Ashar, PhD, lead author of the study, said the outcome highlighted the untapped potential for working through people's minds and brains to change the pain experience in their bodies. "I think it made a lot of sense for people that if the brain has learned the pain, then the brain can also *unlearn* it, and we found a set of techniques that seem to do that effectively for some people."

Physician Howard Schubiner, clinical professor at the Michigan State University College of Human Medicine, and a coauthor of the study, puts it simply. "The bottom line is that pain is a message," he says. "Our brain is giving us a message and it's up to us to decode that message. The message might be that you fell on your wrist, you have a fracture, and you need a cast. But the message might be something completely different. It is now clear that pain can be generated in the brain in the absence of tissue injury. This is surprising and counterintuitive. The pain is real and your brain is producing this. It's not your fault. You're not crazy. Things in your life have happened to you that caused your brain to turn on these warning symptoms. And we have techniques to help reverse it."

Some in the field are wary about overstating the promise of PRT. They point to the difficulty of determining whose pain is indeed structural versus whose isn't and might benefit from PRT—and the risk of misjudging that. There's also an obvious potential downside of training the brain to ignore pain as a valid warning signal. And there's concern that the high success rate in early studies sends a message that if you try this and it doesn't work, then it's your own fault—a particularly cruel message for people who've been hearing and internalizing that message from doctors for years.

Often unnamed, but undoubtedly a factor, is the specter of Dr. John Sarno, the late maverick rehabilitation physician at New York University Hospital. Starting in the 1980s, Sarno famously promoted an unconventional treatment of chronic pain as a brain-based condition caused by repressed emotions. Turning first to back pain—which was then, as it is now, the most common type of pain driving people to seek medical help—he insisted that any pain not caused by traumatic injury or damage was purely psychosomatic. He expanded the list to include headaches, gastrointestinal disorders, and fibromyalgia, focusing on muscle inflammation that he attributed mostly to repressed anger.

Sarno scoffed at the need for scientific research, saying that his patients' positive outcomes were proof enough. He held that the cure for pain came in learning about brain-pain and mind-body connections, creating a new context for thinking about it, then following through with new responses when it occurred.

Rigorous research published in the most respected journals would later bear out some of Sarno's conclusions, including that evidence of structural abnormalities doesn't always mean they're the cause of pain, and that the brain has a central role in creating and modulating the pain experience. But many of his peers deemed Sarno's unscientific method, promoted heavily through his books, patients' testimonials, word of mouth, and an eager media, an affront to medical science. His 2017 *New York Times* obituary characterized him as "revered by some as a saint and dismissed by others as a quack"—a fair epitaph for his storied career.

Ashar, Gordon, and Schubiner all acknowledge Sarno, if not as a saint, then at least as a prescient pioneer in the brain-based approach to chronic pain. Evidence-based science now shows how deeply intertwined emotions are in the brain's pain processing. Sarno's focus on anger and repressed emotions was "a little off," Schubiner says, "though the emotional component is clearly central." For example, there's now robust research showing that adverse childhood experiences are associated with chronic pain later in life. And even if those adverse events are repressed or forgotten, they may manifest in the strangest ways later in life, including through unexplained pain, as my friend Bessel Van der Kolk wrote in his brilliant book *The Body Keeps the Score.*

PRT has advanced since Sarno's time, mostly by drawing from the current evidence-based support for mindfulness as a useful tool in pain treatment. Schubiner offers a glimpse of how PRT now fundamentally works. First, the exercises require you to focus intently on a specific pain sensation while consciously reframing it as nonthreatening. That alone changes the neurocircuitry driving the pain, which can change the mind-body experience, dialing down the pain response systemwide. "When you change the categorization of the pain or the other sensations from being body damage to being brain derived, it's basically a thought you can approach with curiosity and interest, moving through it," he says.

To determine whether PRT may be beneficial for you, you can participate in a PRT evaluation exercise known as provocative testing. This involves visualizing the activity that typically produces the pain. If simply visualizing it can produce the pain sensation, as it does for some, "that's a really powerful way of demonstrating that the brain is doing this," Schubiner says. "It's a great way to start reversing it, by imagining the activity with joy as opposed to fear. Replacing the brain's mind-set from fear and worry in anticipation of pain to a mind-set of reassurance and joy. That makes a huge difference."

I want to be clear about one thing: a diagnosis of neuroplastic pain—meaning, pain without a discernible physical cause—is essential before considering PRT. If your problem is structural, then it should be treated medically, and in some cases surgically. PRT would not be the initial recommended therapy.

Closing the Gap between Science and Lived Experience

While writing this book, I had a revelation. It may be that pain, which is often thought of as ephemeral and immeasurable, responds to treatments using equally immeasurable methods. In other words, the mystery of pain is often met with the mystery of relief. Just because we don't always understand the mechanisms by which some of these strategies provide relief should not diminish their tremendous potential value to those suffering with chronic pain.

CHAPTER 11

Mind Your Brain

A few years ago, I had the honor of spending some time with the Dalai Lama at the Drepung Monastery in Mundgod, India. When he invited me to meditate with him, I wasn't initially sold on the idea. In fact, I was terrified. Just thinking about meditating with His Holiness gave me performance anxiety, but at the same time, who says no to a chance to meditate with the Dalai Lama? So I agreed to join him early one morning, around 5:00 a.m., at his private residence.

I sat down near him, crossed my legs, closed my eyes, and tried to focus on my breathing—but unfortunately, all of my meditation insecurities kicked in. My back started to slouch, and my shoulders sagged. Random intrusive thoughts going back to my childhood began to invade my brain. I found that the meditation session was actually making me anxious, instead of calming me down. Every now and then I'd sneak a peek at His Holiness, and I remember thinking how envious I was of the total tranquility and peace on his face. After a few minutes, though, I heard his deep, distinctive baritone voice: "Any questions?"

I opened my eyes and looked over to find him smiling, before suddenly breaking into his characteristic head-bobbing laugh.

"This is hard for me," I said, starting to laugh along with him.

"Me, too!" he exclaimed. "Even after doing it daily for sixty years, it is still hard."

I was surprised and reassured to hear him say this. The Dalai Lama,

Buddhist monk and spiritual leader of Tibet, can also have trouble meditating! In a strange way, I felt like that insight offered hope for all of us.

"I think you will like a type of analytical meditation," he told me. Instead of focusing on a chosen object, as in single-point meditation, he suggested I think about a problem I was trying to solve, perhaps a topic I'd read about recently or about one of our recent philosophical discussions. He wanted me to separate the problem or issue from everything else by placing it in a large, clear bubble. With my eyes closed, I thought of something nagging at me, a problem I couldn't quite solve. As I placed the embodied frustration into the bubble, several things started to happen very naturally.

The problem was now directly in front of me, floating weightlessly. In my mind, I could rotate it, spin it, or flip it upside down, staring at it from different directions. It felt like an exercise in developing hyperfocus.

Less intuitively, as the bubble rose, it also disentangled itself from other subjective emotional attachments. I could now visualize the problem isolating itself, coming into clear-eyed view.

Too often, we allow unrelated emotional factors to blur the elegant and practical solutions right in front of us. Through analytical meditation, His Holiness told me, we can use logic and reason to clearly identify the question at hand, separate it from irrelevant considerations, erase doubt, and brightly illuminate the answers. For me, this was a simple and sensible approach to meditation, and, most importantly, it worked. After meditating, my disposition was sunnier than normal, and I felt more patient, less hurried. My restlessness was reduced, and my mind felt lucid. I was also able to look directly at problems in my life and approach them in a more clear-headed way.

As a neuroscientist, I never expected that a Buddhist monk would teach me how to better incorporate deduction and critical thinking into my life, but that's what happened. The experience changed me for the better.

I now practice analytical meditation every day. The first two minutes are still the hardest as I create my thought bubble and let it float above me. After that, I reach what can be described as a quintessential flow state, in which twenty to thirty minutes pass easily. The process also helps me get crucial rest in my day—rest that's different from sleep.

After seeing the Dalai Lama, I relayed his teachings to my family and friends and taught them the basic principles of analytical meditation. This was the gift I most wanted to share with them. And now I share it with you.

After my mom suffered her spinal fracture, she was in agony, even writhing at times. I showed her the MRI of her spine fracture, so she could get a clear visual image in her mind of the crushed bone in her lumbar spine. Then we settled into the most comfortable positions we could—her in a chair, and me on the floor. We started with a few minutes of deep breathing, and then I told her to place the spine fracture in a bubble and allow it to float in front of her, disentangled from her body. Her breathing slowed even further as the spine fracture became an object of curiosity, removed from her body, instead of a nagging source of pain.

My mom told me later that she spun the bubble around, examining the spine fracture from different angles. She was able to imagine the broken bone leaving her body and entering the bubble in front of her. She initially told me that it seemed illogical to focus intently on the source of pain, even staring at it. For those twenty minutes, however, her pain nearly vanished and my no-nonsense, math-minded mom felt relief that had been otherwise desperately hard to obtain.

Analytical meditation became another effective tool in her toolbox, and it worked faster than most of the medications she'd been prescribed. When she finished meditating, she smiled, walked over to me, and gave me a hug. "Thank you," she said. I felt as gratified as if I had done a surgical procedure on her myself.

Mindfulness practices are on the rise, and they share a common theme: being present in the moment and intensely observing what's happening in your life. We often hear anecdotal stories of mindfulness activities decreasing stress, but it's important to know that this is substantiated in medical literature as well. And now these habits are making their way into places where you'd least expect them: military combat zones. In 2014, for instance, a group of US marines who received training in mindfulness-based techniques were subsequently found to have enhanced cardiovascular and pulmonary recovery after exposure to high-stress simulations of military activity.

Whether practiced by highly trained soldiers or an eighty-two-year-old grandmother, mindfulness practices appear to lower levels of the stress hormone cortisol, diminishing the negative impact it can have on our mental and physical health. One of the most comprehensive reviews found mindfulness "could significantly reduce anxiety, depression, and pain."

Another meta-analysis looked at the effects of a different type of mindful practice, transcendental meditation, on 1,295 people across sixteen studies. It too found that the practice led to significant reduction in anxiety, an impact that was even more pronounced in those who started off with high levels of it. And as we saw earlier, mindfulness-oriented recovery enhancement (MORE) is showing success in clinical trials as a treatment for chronic pain.

The point is that researchers are finally acknowledging the measurable benefits of mindfulness therapies and, even better, understanding how these types of practices affect the health and functioning of the brain itself. Much of the current wave of research started in 2005, when researchers at Harvard's Massachusetts General Hospital published an imaging study showing that particular areas of the cerebral cortex were thicker in people who frequently meditated. Following that, numerous studies by that same group and others documented that "thick-brained" people show stronger cognitive skills and memory. This made intuitive sense, as these cortical areas are involved with attention, sensory processing, and judgment. But now, for the first time, there was objective evidence.

Since then, studies have focused not only on the "thickening" phenomenon but also on the thinning of gray matter associated with inadequately managed chronic pain. Among others, the authors of "Brain Gray Matter Decrease in Chronic Pain Is the Consequence and Not the Cause of

Pain" found that the "gray matter abnormalities found in chronic pain do not reflect brain damage but rather are a reversible consequence of chronic nociceptive transmission, which normalizes when the pain is adequately treated." And the opposite is likely also true.

All of this raises the possibility that "thickening" certain areas of the brain may make a person more resilient to pain, and meditation has been shown to accomplish that.

Meditation, however, is not the only way to achieve the relaxation response. Breathing exercises can accomplish the same thing, and so can progressive muscle relaxation and prayer. All of these strategies can trigger a parasympathetic or relaxing nerve response, the opposite of a sympathetic or stressful nerve response. When you perceive stress, the sympathetic nervous system springs into action, resulting in surges of the stress hormones cortisol and adrenaline. The parasympathetic nervous system can trigger a relaxation response—and deep breathing is the quickest way to get these responses to trigger. In a deeply relaxed state, your heartbeat calms down, breathing slows, and blood pressure lowers.

You can do deep breathing anywhere, anytime. If you've never meditated before, a deep breathing practice twice daily can get you started and give you a foundation for trying more advanced techniques. Here's how to do it.

Sit comfortably in a chair or on the floor, close your eyes, and relax your body, releasing any tension in your neck, arms, legs, and back. Inhale deeply through your nose, for as long as you can, feeling your diaphragm and abdomen rise as your stomach moves outward. When your lungs feel full, take in a last little bit of air. Slowly exhale to a count of twenty, pushing every breath of air from your lungs.

Continue this for at least five rounds of deep breaths—but slowly, don't hyperventilate! Too much, too fast can make you lightheaded or have a more intense emotional effect than desired. Calming breath work sounds easy, almost too easy, and that's one reason people may be skeptical. Try it, maybe even right now if you have a few minutes. Like my mom, I think you will become a believer.

PRACTICE

Box Breathing

There are many different types of deep-breathing exercises, but box breathing can be particularly helpful with relaxation. Box breathing is an exercise to help with stress management, whether you do it before, during, and/or after stressful experiences.

It's just four simple steps; try visualizing four equal sides of a box as you "breathe the box."

STEP 1 Breathe in through your nose, counting slowly to four. Pay attention to the air entering your lungs.

STEP 2 Hold your breath for a count of four. No inhaling or exhaling.

STEP 3 Breathe out through your mouth for a count of four.

STEP 4 Hold the out-breath for a count of four. Repeat steps.

You can adjust the length of the hold to match your personal comfort level.

Source: Adapted from "Relaxation Techniques" by Samantha Norelli, Ashley Long, and Jeffrey Krepps in "Stat Pearls," an online educational resource.

PRACTICE

Guided Imagery

Guided imagery is a relaxation exercise in which you visualize a calming environment. Visualization of tranquil settings or pleasing images helps manage stress by distracting from stressful intrusive thoughts.

As we learned in the MORE program, a focus on pleasurable scenes or thoughts registers in your brain as a positive experience, which strengthens the neurocircuitry for pain relief as well as offering broader health benefits.

Guided imagery helps by employing all five senses to create a deeper sense of relaxation as well as distraction from unwanted thoughts. You can practice guided imagery alone, focusing your attention on each of the five senses in turn (see questions below), or with someone who serves as a narrator.

STEP 1 Sit or lie down comfortably, ideally in a space with minimal distractions.

STEP 2 Visualize a relaxing environment, either one from memory or an imagined one. Engage this image with each of your five senses, one at a time, using these prompts:

What do you see? (visual detail such as color, hues, texture)

What do you hear? (the soundscape of the environment, perhaps nature or other relaxing ambient sounds)

What do you smell? (aromas, perhaps of the earth, plants, or sea air)

What do you taste? (or even the absence of taste, e.g., a breath of fresh air)

What do you feel? (gentle breeze, warmth of the sun, rain on your face)

STEP 3 Sustain the visualization as long as needed or comfortable, focusing on taking slow, deep breaths throughout the exercise. Focus on the feelings of calm associated with being in a relaxing environment.

A Tiny Moment of Mindfulness with Eric Garland, PhD, Mindfulness Therapist, Researcher

You can use this technique while standing in line at the checkout, sitting comfortably at home, or whenever you find yourself with a few free moments.

First, pause to become aware of your self and your situation. *What are you thinking about in this moment?*

Now shift your attention to notice the sensation of your feet against the ground. Focus on that feeling. Notice the sensation of the breath moving into your nostrils. *Is your mind wandering? Are you thinking about what you're going to be doing next, or what you're going to have for dinner tonight?*

If you do notice your mind wandering, bring it back to the sensation of your feet against the ground, back to the sensation of the breath moving into your nostrils.

Good work! You've just done one moment of mindfulness, making your mind just a tiny bit stronger. If you were to continue this practice for ten to twenty minutes, you'd increase the sense of clarity, peacefulness, and the calming sense of awareness in your mind.

Doing this mental exercise strengthens the "muscle" of the brain involved with self-control, a self-regulation tool that enables you to manage your response to a stressor. A large body of research shows that mindfulness, by strengthening self-control, alleviates pain, stress, and even craving for drugs.

You now know that mindfulness strategies can be anything from simply taking a calming breath to using an app on your phone to guide you through a fifteen-minute meditation practice. It can also be exploring the Japanese art of forest bathing, or *shinrin-yoku*: being in the presence of trees and surrounding nature. This practice has grown in popularity as a way to lower heart rate and blood pressure and reduce stress hormone production.

Several years ago, I tried it myself, spending time deep in the forests of Japan. As part of a trial, researchers measured my heart rate and cortisol levels through a cheek swab test before and after. Given that I felt so good at the end of my "forest bath," I was not at all surprised to learn that my numbers had dramatically improved. Even better, the effects of forest bathing were durable, meaning they lasted far beyond the time I was actually in the forest.

When you're breathing in the "aroma of the forest," you're absorbing substances known as phytoncides, which protect trees from insects and other stressors. As we've learned over the past few decades, humans also have receptors for these phytoncides, and they can protect us too, by increasing our natural killer immune cells and decreasing cortisol levels. So give it a try! You don't have to go to Japan—any natural green space will do. You can accomplish these same benefits by digging in the dirt of your own garden or visiting a local park. Breathe deeply as you do, and remember that the aroma you're sensing contains something special.

These are not new ideas. There is a wonderful ancient Indian concept called *vanaprastha*, which roughly translates to life as a forest dweller. Starting at age fifty, in your hundred-year life cycle, you need to spend the next twenty-five years living in the forest. While I realize that is not possible for most people, including myself, the message has been clear for a long time. Being surrounded by the real jungle, as opposed to the concrete jungle, is an effective way to regulate stress, improve mental health, and even decrease pain. As a guy in his mid-fifties, I have dreamt about doing just that, so if I suddenly disappear off the grid, you will know where I am.

Some research has found that just walking in nature, as opposed to walking in urban environments, may help people manage stress, calm rumination, and regulate emotion. Even doing your exact same meditation or yoga practice outside versus inside offers up more benefits. For someone like me who spends a lot of time indoors—in windowless operating rooms—I cherish the times I can roam and play outside.

Spending time in green spaces has long been recommended to improve mental well-being, but I've been fascinated to learn that some pioneering pain scientists are also redefining the idea of "greens" and their role in pain relief.

Ordinarily, you probably think of greens as part of a nutritious diet. Many pain scientists, however, also use the term to refer to green spaces, and recently they've even added green light to the mix. In clinical trials of green light therapy using LED light strips, researchers at the University of Arizona Health Sciences made the startling discovery that exposure to green light in a laboratory setting decreased chronic pain, anxiety, and depression, while also improving sleep in people with fibromyalgia and migraine. Other research found that green light taps into the way our eyes communicate with the parts of our brain that control pain and can promote the brain's natural ability to reduce inflammation and pain. Preclinical studies of chronic and postsurgical pain showed that green light acts on a pain center in the brain stem known as the rostral ventromedial medulla (RVM).

"It's more practical—not everyone has the luxury of going to a green place," says the physician-scientist who developed it, Mohab Ibrahim, MD, PhD, director of the University of Arizona Health Sciences Comprehensive Center for Pain & Addiction, director of the Chronic Pain Management Clinic, and professor of anesthesiology at the College of Medicine–Tucson. "Not everyone has a green place available to them within a reasonable distance, so we thought it was a good modality." Dr. Ibrahim is a fan of green spaces himself, which is precisely where he was—meditating, you might say, on a medical mystery—when the idea came to him.

Earlier in the day, his brother had mentioned that when he got headaches, he felt better when he sat in his backyard, with a lot of trees. "I actually made fun of him, calling him a tree hugger," recalls Dr. Ibrahim. But the next time he developed a headache, he decided to try it himself. Instead of reaching for ibuprofen like he normally did, he drove to Reid Park, a rare green area in the desert city of Tucson.

"It's a park. It has grass. It has a lot of trees. It's actually green," Ibrahim says. "So I went over there, and I sat under an olive tree. I can even pinpoint which tree that was. And maybe fifteen, twenty minutes later, my headache went away"—faster than ibuprofen typically took to kick in for him. "I thought, wow, this is interesting! So, instead of going home, I go back to my office—and keep in mind I'm a pharmacologist, so my training is to play with drugs and receptors and intracellular mechanisms. I'm sitting in my office and the first thing that comes to my mind is maybe the trees are releasing some kind of botanical chemicals in the air and I'm just inhaling them and they have analgesic properties. That seemed quite possible because many of the medications that we have, they come from plants, or at least are derived from natural products."

PRACTICE

Zoom In, Zoom Out

A common mindfulness practice used to cope with pain in the moment is to shift your attention and awareness around the pain. Changing focus can change pain perception. Imagine your attention as a camera lens that enables you to focus in for a close-up view to examine the experience of pain; or to broaden out to a "wide-angle" perspective where pain is one of many things.

Drawing on her experience of managing chronic back pain, pain management coach and author Vidyamala Burch, cofounder of The Breathworks Foundation, suggests this step-by-step exploration.

STEP 1 Stabilize

First, stabilize your breathing by settling awareness on the sensations of breathing deep in your body so your mind becomes calmer and quieter, and your attention more focused. Allow your body to settle into the support of gravity.

STEP 2 Zoom In

Now gently and sensitively turn the spotlight of your attention onto the pain itself.

What sensations can you feel in the part of your body that is hurting?

Is there heat? Tightness? Tingling? Is it stabbing, dull or sharp?

Or are there other sensations?

Can you notice how the sensations are changing and how they aren't exactly the same one moment to the next?

Can you soften tensing around the sensations and let them be more fluid?

Look closely to see whether the sensations have edges. Are they defined enough to tell where they are and where they aren't? Or are the edges more fuzzy than sharp?

Do the sensations have a center or are they diffuse?

Look even more closely, to see if you notice spaces where the sensation is and where it is not.

STEP 3 Zoom out

Now pull back to a wide-angle perspective and become aware of your whole body. Notice the flow of sensations that are both painful and pleasant and allow your pain to rest in a much bigger space.

"What people begin to discover is that this thing they perceive as pain that they thought was so solid, this solid, terrible, awful thing that's always there, is actually more of a fluctuating, vibrating, spacious experience," Burch says. "Many people find as they focus deeply in on the pain experience itself, the sensation starts to become more insubstantial, more ephemeral, kind of like a cloud dissipating in the sky and then they can be aware of broad experience where the pain is less dominant."

We have this word, *pain*—but it's just a word, a concept. When you zoom in, you can break down the actual sensations that make up the experience of pain. So rather than focusing on a singular terrible, awful, anguishing experience of pain, mindfulness allows you to zoom into that experience and break it down into individual feelings of heat or tightness or tingling. You can parse the actual sensations, and then, rather than attaching judgments to them, just perceive them as sensations like any others happening in your body. It's a process that shares many similarities with the analytical meditation I practiced with the Dalai Lama.

But tackling this as a research question was admittedly challenging. "To go in an open park and just collect an air sample, where you will have who-knows-how-many chemicals in there? Identify each and every one and then test it? As a scientist, I can tell you this would take more than a lifetime." So he thought again about his brother's house in San Diego and what the backyard there could possibly have in common with Reid Park in Tucson.

The two spaces probably didn't have the same kinds of trees. So he tried to think about it practically, in what he calls a "lazy" way, as opposed to his usual pharmacological way. "I thought, well, trees are green. Grass is green. Maybe it's the color green. Maybe getting exposure to that color has some kind of effect."

This idea gave him an opportunity for a simpler, more specific scientific study. He bought LED lights, lots of them, in the entire spectrum: red, yellow, orange, purple, blue-green, amber, white. "If it's on the market, I got it," he says, and then he conducted an easy experiment. He started testing the different light colors on rats, turning his pharmacology lab into something that looked like a dance club. Each day, he tested a different color light. "People thought, what are you guys doing in there?"

Conducting a pain tolerance test, Ibrahim discovered that when rats had heat stimuli placed under their paws, they moved quickly off the heat source in all but one of the differently lighted environments. In the green light environment, they stayed put. "They didn't want to move," Dr. Ibrahim says. "We had to turn off the heat source, so we didn't damage their skin. And we thought, that is wild. This is unbelievable."

Several more studies confirmed those animal studies, and when the clinical trial for humans was launched, Dr. Ibrahim was thrilled to be able to open it to his own patients. "One of the most challenging conditions that I encounter in the clinic is seeing patients with mysterious conditions, such as fibromyalgia and migraine. Really tough, tough conditions that can ruin people's lives."

For the clinical trial, a typical course of treatment was two hours of green light exposure daily for ten weeks, with participants sitting in an otherwise dark room with only the therapeutic LED green light strip as a light source. They might listen to music, write, or read, but no TV or computer use was allowed, since it would add another light source. And just as with the animal studies, there was a measurable benefit in humans. The trials found that green light therapy not only reliably decreased chronic pain, as well as anxiety and depression; it also improved sleep in people with fibromyalgia and migraine.

Flip the Script: Conversation Starters for Healthier Self-Talk

Self-talk is the inner dialogue you have with yourself, often unconsciously, that can shape your mind-set and expectations about yourself, your circumstances, and your capacity to manage life's challenges, including pain. Remember: the person you talk to the most in your life is *you*. So be kind to yourself.

Health benefits of positive self-talk include lower rates of distress and pain, lower levels of depression, greater resistance to illness, and better coping skills during hardship and stressful times. In the inner dialogue about pain, positive self-talk can help rein in catastrophizing (focusing on the worst) and focus attention on your strengths and more optimistic possibilities.

To frame your inner conversation for the good, aim for these qualities:

- Show self-compassion.
- Emphasize your strengths.
- Tap memories of a time you faced adversity.
- Give yourself permission to step away, take a break, or take care of yourself.
- Encourage yourself.

Negative self-talk includes having our inner dialogue amplify fears, anger, resignation, and negative aspects of our experiences. Some common types of negative self-talk include these:

- Focusing on a situation's negative aspects while filtering out positive or potentially positive ones
- Magnifying, or interpreting minor problems as major ones
- Catastrophizing, or automatically assuming the worst, not only in the moment but also in thinking about the future

- Ruminating, or continually replaying upsetting thoughts
- Succumbing to all-or-nothing thinking, feeling that a situation has to go a certain way or else it's a failure—or you are

Negative self-talk trains the brain to predict and anticipate negative developments or outcomes, which in turn increases stress and can activate pain-related neurocircuitry that reinforces pain. As placebo science shows, negative expectations contribute to the "nocebo" effect—tipping the scale of intangible factors toward a disappointing outcome.

In "Working with Pain-Related Thoughts," a comprehensive online pain education resource put out by the Veterans Administration, a pain catastrophizing worksheet includes these examples of negative self-talk and the corresponding "Self-Encouragement and Coping Thoughts Worksheet" provides ways to flip the script.

STEP 1 Notice negative, catastrophizing self-talk statements you make—for example:

I will never be able to enjoy life again.

I can't be myself if I can't do these things the way I used to.

I have no control over my pain and never will.

I will never be able to manage my pain.

I am no good to anyone like this.

STEP 2 Challenge those statements to differentiate between facts and fears, feelings, or predictions.

STEP 3 Recognize that self-talk can amplify positive or negative aspects of your pain experience as it activates pain circuitry in the brain.

STEP 4 Choose to change the internal dialogue to messaging that is empowering, reframing the expectation to support self-encouragement and coping and potentially to shift the pain experience. For example:

This situation won't last forever. This pain flare too shall pass.

I can be anxious and still deal with the situation.

I may not like my pain, but I know that I can cope with it.
I'm strong enough to handle what's happening to me right now.
This is an opportunity for me to learn how to cope with my pain better.
I've survived other situations like this with my pain, and I'll survive this one too.
My pain/anxiety/fear/sadness won't kill me—it just doesn't feel good right now.
It's okay to feel sad/anxious/afraid sometimes.
My thoughts don't control my life. I do.
I am much more than my pain condition; my life has meaning.

"I was really surprised, because we thought we were just going to decrease pain, but green light did more than that," Dr. Ibrahim says. "Quality of life, which is the most important thing, also improved. People can be in severe pain, but if they have a good quality of life, they can cope very well. People can have no medical issues, they might be the richest people in the world, but if they don't have quality of life, they're miserable. So that was a very, very surprising thing, that the quality of life improved." If you're picking new wallpaper or paint, leaning toward the color green may be the "pain-friendly" choice.

New studies on the color green are now underway at the NIH and the Department of Defense. "The lab is growing, the projects are expanding, and we keep getting surprised with our findings," Dr. Ibrahim says. "I guess we are our biggest skeptics. But the data are wonderful. And that's the most exciting thing about science. You keep learning."

"With forest bathing, for instance, it might be a bit more complicated because you have more than one variable," he points out. "First, you're out walking. It's a quiet environment typically. People intentionally try to relax their minds and not think about work in the fresh air." Perhaps it is not surprising that such an activity would provide benefit. But the idea that the color green *alone* can provide such a strong treatment for pain is something the medical establishment is slowly starting to embrace.

LIVING IT

Rob Kyler

From Bicycle to Wheelchair in an Instant: Insights about Meditation and Pain

One summer day a few years back, I was invited to speak to the Chautauqua Institute, a creative, vibrant community full of lifelong adult learners in southwestern New York State. While seated at a table on a grassy lawn overlooking Chautauqua Lake, I was introduced to Rob Kyler. A radiation oncologist, Rob is handsome, in good physical shape, and projects a friendly smile. We started chatting about the gathering and the natural beauty of our surroundings. When we somehow pivoted to talking about pain, he shared that he suffers chronic pain in his legs.

Rob told me that years earlier, he had been involved in a terrible bicycling accident. A passionate cyclist, he'd been out for a typical two-hour wake-up ride through scenic farmland with his regular cycling partner, Jim. As they approached a long, steep downhill, a favorite place where Rob liked to surge ahead in a thrilling burst of speed, he did what he always did, racing ahead, his head down in an aerodynamic tuck. The road was paved, but one moment he was a blur of speed, and the next his bike veered off the road, hit some large stones in the culvert, and flipped over, leaving him on his back by the side of the road.

Jim was there in a flash, and he found Rob lying on his back on top of his bike, moaning but conscious. As many doctors do when they're injured, Rob was reflexively performing a self-neuro exam, and he didn't like the results. He couldn't feel or move his legs. At the hospital a few hours later, he received the kind of terrible news that he'd on occasion had to give to his own patients: Rob was paralyzed from the chest down, a paraplegic.

As Rob shared his story, I peered under the table and noticed for the first time that he was sitting in a wheelchair. The pain he'd been describing was in limbs that no longer had sensation. We ended up having a long conversation about neuropathic pain—the kind he experienced—and even whether an implanted spinal cord stimulator might alleviate it. But as Rob had already learned, that wasn't a good option for him, so he turned to another kind of treatment.

Years before his accident, Rob had trained in mindfulness-based stress reduction (MBSR) with Jon Kabat-Zinn, the father of the movement in the West. He had become an MBSR instructor himself, teaching the eight-week course and incorporating it into his medical practice. After the accident, he discovered how useful it could be in managing his own pain.

"Suffering = pain × resistance" goes the popular adage, and that mental math hit home as Dr. Kyler struggled to adjust to his new circumstances, including the unexpected and constant pain in his paralyzed lower body. "We all have pain, but the suffering is really magnified by our inability to accept it and our efforts to push it away—it's just the way we think about it," he told me. "In Buddhism, there's something called the second arrow of suffering. The first arrow is when something happens to us that we don't like that feels bad, and the second arrow is the self-inflicted wound when we go on and on about how could this happen to me? Why me? This is awful. When is it going to get better? How can I make it go away? All of that secondary is self-induced. And it's avoidable.

"I had intellectual understanding of the principle, but I've learned it again through hard-won experience, and I have learned that the more I resist, the more mental suffering there is," Dr. Kyler says. "So, I wouldn't say I ignore the pain; there are times when I just can't." But he now relies on two primary strategies to help alleviate it.

"One is just to distract myself with other things through work or recreation," he says. "But the other strategy, what I use when I'm lying in bed at night and there's really nothing that I can distract myself with and the pain is impossible to ignore, I actually try to pay attention to it. Instead of turning away from it, I'll turn toward it and with a little bit of curiosity, try to just lean into the sensations I've labeled as pain and examine them.

"So, what is it? All right, there's this burning and there's this vibration and now there's this pulsating, and you notice that it changes. Turning toward it and experiencing it and realizing that it's not this constant monolithic thing, that can be really helpful as well."

Digital Age Expands Horizons for Innovation

Much about these timeless practices of mindfulness, meditation, and attention-training has remained unchanged over centuries. Practiced the same way as they have been for the ages, they remain as powerful today as ever before, with the added credibility that Western science has brought to them.

The authors of a 2022 article, "The State of Science in the Use of Virtual Reality in the Treatment of Acute and Chronic Pain: A Systematic Scoping Review," reported on seventy studies representing 4,105 people. The review, which included forty-six acute pain studies, twenty-two chronic pain studies, and two that covered both, found something that Rob Kyler has learned as well: distraction was the most beneficial mechanism, followed by embodiment—leaning into and embodying the pain. Overall, participants experienced a greater than 70 percent reduction in the intensity of pain while they were using the VR technology.

With the caveat that research in this area is in the early stages, other favorable outcomes that have been reported are these:

- VR intervention reduced pain intensity and catastrophizing in people with chronic lower back pain. A study that involved two freely available VR programs reported that the intervention "also had high adherence and enjoyment," and the authors suggested it could be easily translated into clinical practice.

- A VR intervention for women during childbirth found that "despite expecting increasing pain intensity with labor progression, participants in the VR group reported less pain intensity and fear of labor pain compared to control subjects." The study showed a significant difference in pain score between the study groups and concluded that "virtual reality interventions can be regarded as a new non-pharmaceutical strategy to control labor pain and fear in pregnant women."
- Recent studies explored using VR with pediatric patients undergoing procedures ranging from laceration repair to dressing changes for burn wounds. Interacting with immersive VR might divert attention, the studies showed, leading to a slower response to incoming pain signals. A 2023 randomized clinical trial of 149 pediatric patients undergoing venipuncture, as in a blood draw or intravenous injection, showed that VR is effective in reducing the pain and anxiety young patients experience compared with standard care or other distraction methods.

Hypnosis

Hypnosis (also called hypnotherapy) has been studied for a number of conditions, including irritable bowel syndrome, anxiety (e.g., before medical procedures or surgeries), menopausal symptoms, hot flashes in breast cancer survivors, headaches, and post-traumatic stress disorder. It has also been studied for pain control and smoking cessation. (The term *clinical hypnosis* means the provider is a licensed health care professional with advanced degrees and training.) While increasing in popularity, the existing evidence is mixed, as you see below, according to the National Center for Complementary and Integrative Health.

- There is evidence that gut-directed hypnotherapy (a type of therapy in which practitioners use hypnosis to help the patient visualize their GI tract functioning normally) can help relieve symptoms and improve the quality of life in people with IBS. The idea is that the hypnosis addresses a fundamental miscommunication between the brain and the gut, and that suggestion, imagery, and relaxation techniques can help calm that brain-gut messaging.

- A growing body of evidence (albeit fairly low-quality evidence) suggests that hypnosis may help to manage other painful conditions as well.
- Some studies have shown promising results on hypnosis for anxiety related to medical or dental procedures, but the overall evidence is not conclusive.
- Studies of hypnosis to help with quitting smoking have had conflicting results.
- There is some evidence suggesting that hypnosis may help improve certain menopausal symptoms, such as hot flashes. A 2015 position paper from the North American Menopause Society recommended hypnosis for managing hot flashes but acknowledged that favorable evidence is limited.

PRACTICE

Tap the Positive Power of Suggestion: A Simple Anytime-Anywhere Self-Hypnosis Skill

We're all influenced by other people and the suggestions they offer us about ourselves, whether verbal (what they tell us) or nonverbal (what they communicate about their thoughts and feelings through, for example, facial expressions). We're even more strongly influenced by those we know and trust. We can use that in ways that support our best interests and are consistent with our values and goals, says Mark P. Jensen, professor at the University of Washington in Seattle.

As a clinician-scientist, Jensen develops and studies the efficacy of psychological pain treatments. With patients, he combines cognitive-behavioral, hypnotic, and motivational approaches.

Here are simple practices Jensen suggests you use anytime, anywhere, to tap into your own power of suggestion.

There are certain people who, when you're around them, you feel good about yourself. *Spend time with those people.*

You may be aware that there are other people who, when you're around them, you feel bad about yourself. *Spend as little time as possible around those people.* Remember that how you feel around others may affect your physical pain levels.

When you feel the need for an emotional buffer, Jensen recommends these self-hypnosis strategies:

You might visualize building a bubble around yourself, so that anything they say or do that's not useful to you just bounces right off. Words or nonverbal communications from others who deserve your attention can get through. Or you might imagine that their words are spoken in a language that you cannot understand, making it impossible for the words to have any negative effects. Just doing this simple visualization can help you avoid responding in a negative way.

Your Mind, Your Brain, Your Pain, Your Choice

As we've seen, meditation and mindfulness practices may provide a variety of health benefits and even help people improve the quality of their lives. Yet it's important to review the literature critically and spend the time interpreting the strength and validity of existing trials.

The bottom line is that we still have a long way to go. Much of the research on these topics has been preliminary or not sufficiently scientifically rigorous. That's not surprising, as these are difficult studies to conduct and control, and they're even harder to get funded. As I mentioned earlier, if there's no pill or procedure to be monetized, funding for these trials is harder to raise. And because the studies examine many different types of meditation and mindfulness techniques, the effects of those practices are hard to measure; results are difficult to analyze, and at times they may be interpreted too optimistically or pessimistically. Finally, the moving target in all of this is the subjective nature of pain for each person: the social and emotional colorations of their pain experience, their expectations and fears, and the variable imposition that pain presents them on any given day.

Suffice it to say that the evidence-based case is a work in progress. This includes the obvious fact that as with any other tool in the mix and depending on what style you use, mindfulness works better for some than for others, and it may even have potentially adverse effects for those who find it stressful to embody or focus on their pain. Although the psychological approaches studied for chronic pain have good safety records, that doesn't mean they're risk free for everyone. Your health and special circumstances (such as pregnancy) or underlying factors such as depression, anxiety, or chronic illnesses may affect the safety of these approaches.

I think back to Prasad Shirvalkar's point about how science and medicine are sometimes at odds in their objectives. Science aims at solutions that work at scale, broadly effective for large numbers of people. Medicine is aimed at relieving the suffering of one patient at a time.

For your own purposes, you are that "one." Now that you understand some basics about the way the brain creates pain, you can see why the mind may be one of the most powerful tools you can use to change your experience of it. Whatever techniques you pick to harness the power of your mind to influence your brain, remember this: you are the expert, and only you can choose how to use this extraordinary tool in the way that serves you best.

PRACTICE

Active Redirection: Using Cues to Disrupt, Refocus, Rewire for Relief

Whenever you notice a symptom you'd like to change, it's an opportunity to change the focus of your attention to something fun, meaningful, or connecting—and incompatible with pain processing—using the principles of neuroplasticity to help with chronic pain relief, says Eleanor Stein, a retired psychiatrist and clinical assistant professor at the University of Calgary. Stein, who teaches the principles of neuroplasticity for chronic pain relief, suggests one exercise you might use to cultivate your brain's capacity for change and strengthen the message over time with repetition. It starts with these steps.

- Be aware that change is possible. Hold this thought: All pain is created by the brain. Because the brain is neuroplastic, always changing, chronic pain can change. Each time you remember this, you're training your brain to anticipate this possibility.
- Use symptoms as a reminder. The brain unconsciously attaches negative emotions to unpleasant sensations. Since negative emotions strengthen learning even more than positive ones, this unconscious process has the potential to strengthen the very symptoms you don't want. To change this, use each awareness of pain as a reminder to redirect your attention to a new, rewarding activity or focus. Repetition can break the unconscious conditioning that sustains pain.
- Calm your nervous system. Neuroplasticity is more effective when the nervous system is regulated. So, as often as possible, use box breathing, self-hypnosis, and other evidence-based strategies to calm the nervous system so that your neuroplastic practice is most effective.
- Practice with your imagination. What experiences would you like to have more of? For the best chances of success, your goal should be something important to you, something worth working for, something that will maintain your motivation and sense of purpose. For example, imagine a body part moving with comfort and ease, an interpersonal interaction progressing successfully toward a desired outcome, or a task successfully completed.

- Take baby steps. Set small challenges for yourself using some of your goals. The best challenges are right on the edge of your capacity: hard enough that it takes focused attention but not so difficult to be demoralizing.
- Practice—and give it time. Practice includes any time you respond to a symptom cue by actively redirecting your thoughts and energy to something uplifting or that makes you feel better. A few examples include calming, elevating mood, imagining your future successes, doing creative activities, connecting with friends and loved ones, being grateful, maintaining hope.
- Rest or sleep after practice. Reward yourself with a restorative break. Put your feet up, close your eyes, and feel your body relax. Try listening to calming music or a self-hypnosis or relaxation audio. Both deep rest and sleep consolidate the mental messaging—so rest, sleep, and repeat!

CHAPTER 12

Befriend Your Body

When you say your back is "killing" you, you're setting up an adversarial relationship with your body, thinking of it as the enemy as opposed to an ally. This isn't a conducive dynamic for healing. Redefining that relationship between body and brain is a good place to start when it comes to dealing with pain. In this chapter, you'll learn all the ways to befriend your body, starting with getting on good terms with it. "Listen to your body" isn't a new idea, yet too often we forget to slow down and really pay attention to what our bodies are telling us. I'm going to give you a good approach to do just that.

I mentioned earlier that when patients are having trouble specifying where they feel pain, I'll sometimes ask them to close their eyes and think hard about the source of it. This can be tricky, however, because something like back pain can have a variety of triggers—anything from a spinal injury to a vitamin deficiency to a kidney problem. Even a simmering emotional burden can manifest as back pain.

My friend Renee Fleming, the opera singer, recently told me that she's been suffering with intermittent crippling back pain. Over the years, she has seen numerous doctors to try to diagnose the underlying problem, and yet when I asked her a few simple questions, she told me something fascinating. She believes her back pain is a result of her "emotional brain hijacking her thinking brain," acting as a sort of warning system. No surprise then that the onset of the pain is usually right before she starts a performance, and it nearly always resolves as soon as she's finished.

This means that the treatment for Renee's back pain would be very different than for most of my other neurosurgical patients, who often have physical causes such as slipped bones or herniated discs. And yet if she hadn't disclosed this waxing and waning nature of her back pain, she may have ended up with excessive testing and possibly even an unnecessary operation.

The truth is that even though back pain is one of the leading causes of ER visits, many times we have no idea what's causing it. Patients often complain of vague, unpleasant physical or emotional sensations, and enormous debates can swirl around how to treat them. Though we often start by asking the patient to try to identify the location of the pain, we also ask for any other contributing factors, such as the stage fright Renee described.

When I ask patients to close their eyes and think hard about the source of their pain, I'm actually asking them to focus specifically on where they are feeling the pain in that moment. This is a way to establish a fresh, more focused channel for communication between mind and body or between you and what pain experts describe as your "embodied" or somatic experience.

Think of it this way: Your brain creates the pain experience, but you don't feel the pain in your brain; you feel it in your body. This is true regardless of what type of pain we're talking about. So while all kinds of information about your pain are relevant for understanding and treating it, your ability to listen to your body's cues is absolutely fundamental to the process. Everything starts with that. And interestingly, it's a skill you can develop and sharpen through somatic practices such as the one I described above.

Even better, you can sharpen this skill for yourself through regular practice. One way is to do a body scan—not the medical imaging kind but the mental kind. Buddhist monk and peace activist Thich Nhat Hanh called this "experiencing the body in the body." No critical appraisals, thoughts of bettering yourself, or particular belief systems are required. It's just a way to introduce yourself to yourself. Mind, meet Body! This is the essence of somatic knowing, developing a relationship with your body that's friendly, accepting, respectful, collaborative, and intuitive.

The exercise is simple. Get in a comfortable position, close your eyes, and focus your attention inward on your muscles and bones, head to toe. My medical orientation to anatomy means I'm visualizing dozens of different muscles in the back alone, along with twenty-four individual vertebrae connected through flexible joints called facets. It takes time and energy to take stock of all that, and my method is perhaps more detailed than necessary to be therapeutic for others. Any level of detail that works for you is good.

The idea of body scanning has been used widely in different approaches to mind-body health—some oriented toward self-regulation, others with a spiritual intention. In medical settings, the exercise is used to achieve the relaxation response, a physical state of deep relaxation that occurs when your body releases chemicals that slow your breathing and heart rate. It's also often used in cardiac or pain rehabilitation, to help reduce acute and chronic pain.

Dr. Harvey Rich, the doctor whose life's work is exploring traditional healing cultures in postwar countries, tells a story from closer to home. Early in his career, he saw a hospitalized patient who was in terrible pain, unable to urinate following a medical procedure. The typical plan in a situation like this is to place a catheter into the patient's bladder, but despite his pain, the patient didn't want it. As a psychiatrist, Dr. Rich routinely considers how mind and body might work together, so he offered to guide the patient through progressive muscle relaxation. "It took several minutes, and along the way we performed the equivalent of a body scan," he told me. "The patient slowly relaxed and ultimately [urinated]. No meds. No catheter."

Calling on a psychiatrist for a patient in pain was a novel intervention at the time, so the story spread through the wards. Even now, it's still rare in hospital settings, though there is increased awareness that a simple conversation with our body is a powerful tool in our box. It allows not only a clearer diagnosis—as was the case with Renee Fleming—but also a chance to heal in noninvasive ways.

The mental body scan becomes its own resource, something like a compass you can use to identify pain or discomfort. That may help you then target specific treatments for relief. One of my favorites, which often gets overlooked, is myofascial release.

Nine Things You Should Know about Chronic Pain and Complementary Health Approaches

Some complementary health approaches have been shown to have modest benefits for chronic pain, but the amount and quality of evidence varies for different approaches and pain conditions.

1. In general, research on complementary approaches for fibromyalgia is preliminary. However, there's encouraging evidence that practices such as tai chi, qi gong, massage therapy, acupuncture, and balneotherapy (spa therapy) may help relieve some fibromyalgia symptoms.
2. Some mind and body practices, such as relaxation training, biofeedback, acupuncture, and spinal manipulation have been found to be helpful for headaches and migraines. Preliminary studies suggest that certain dietary supplements, including the herb feverfew, the vitamin riboflavin, the mineral magnesium, and coenzyme Q10, may also be helpful for migraines. The herb butterbur seems to reduce migraine frequency, but serious concerns have been raised about its possible liver toxicity.
3. There haven't been many large, well-designed studies on complementary approaches for irritable bowel syndrome, but some evidence now suggests that peppermint oil may have modest, short-term benefits and that gut-directed hypnotherapy is a helpful form of psychological therapy. Some studies have examined probiotics for irritable bowel syndrome, but the current

evidence does not clearly show which types of probiotics might be most helpful.

4. There's low- or moderate-quality evidence that a variety of psychological or physical complementary health approaches, including acupuncture, electromyography biofeedback, low-level laser therapy, mindfulness-based stress reduction, progressive muscle relaxation, spinal manipulation, tai chi, and yoga, may be helpful for chronic low-back pain. Topical preparations of the herb cayenne may also help to relieve low-back pain.
5. Evidence suggests that acupuncture has been helpful for neck pain. Spinal manipulation might also be helpful, but much of the research on this practice has been of low quality. Massage therapy has also been shown to be helpful for neck pain, but the effects may only last for a short time.
6. Tai chi may be helpful for pain from osteoarthritis of the knee or hip. Other complementary approaches that have shown promise for osteoarthritis include acupuncture and yoga.
7. Psychological and physical approaches—such as relaxation, mindfulness meditation, tai chi, and yoga—may be beneficial additions to rheumatoid arthritis treatment plans, but they can do more to improve other aspects of patients' health (such as quality of life) than to relieve pain. For example, tai chi may improve mood and overall physical function, and mindfulness meditation is likely to improve patients' ability to cope with pain. Dietary supplements containing omega-3 fatty acids, gamma-linolenic acid, or the herb *Tripterygium wilfordii*, also known as thunder god vine, have been shown to relieve some rheumatoid arthritis symptoms.
8. Acupuncture, reflexology, or acupressure may be helpful for cancer pain, and acupuncture has also been shown to relieve joint pain caused by treatment with aromatase inhibitors. Massage therapy can be helpful for patients who have pain during palliative or hospice care.

9. As with any treatment, it's important to consider safety before using complementary health approaches. If you're considering a complementary approach to help manage your chronic pain, talk with your health care providers first. You can find more information on the NCCIH's website about the safe use of complementary health products and practices.

Source: Courtesy of the National Institutes of Health, Complementary and Integrative Health, https://www.nccih.nih.gov/health/tips/things-you-should-know-about-chronic-pain-and-complementary-health-approaches.

New Focus on the Fascia

As an amateur athlete for most of my life, I've been pretty diligent about strengthening and stretching my muscles and tendons, avoiding injuries, and caring for my body as best I can. It was only a few years ago, however, that I came to appreciate the value of taking care of my myofascia.

The fascia is the thin casing of tough, flexible connective tissue that surrounds, separates, and/or holds together muscles, organs, joints, tendons, and ligaments. It's like a full body suit around those structures, holding everything in place. Over time, with age and use, the fascia can start to thicken, become less flexible, and even apply pressure on those internal structures. And just like the rest of your body, when your fascia is stressed, it tightens up. This can cause pain just about anywhere in your body—and it may have been a contributing factor to Renee Fleming's preperformance back pain.

Myofascial release is a manual therapy focused on the "myo," or muscle component, of fascial release, a specialized kind of massage in which hands-on pressure is applied to improve circulation, release muscles, and improve joint mobility. Fair warning: it can be painful. But for many people, the pain is worth it.

Helene Langevin, MD, director of the National Institute for Complementary and Integrative Medicine, says she doesn't play favorites with the array of approaches under the integrative medicine umbrella. Yet for most of her career, her work as a scientist has been devoted to the study of connective tissue, and she has been particularly outspoken for a long time on the need to pay more attention to the fascia.

"It's been neglected—the whole of what we call the soft tissue—not the stuff you see on X-rays and MRIs, not the cartilage, the bone, the discs, but the other stuff that is harder to see," she says. "That includes the muscles, but also the connective tissues around the muscles, the ligaments, the capsules around the joints, all of those things." That overlooked tissue has sensory nerves that can generate the sensation of pain, but the signals are often ignored by doctors trained to look elsewhere. This is beginning to change. The NIH HEAL initiative has funded seven fascia-related studies to determine how to measure different aspects of the fascia, as well as how to measure the effect of an intervention.

We've long known that a poorly functioning fascial system has a negative impact on performance in exercise and sports, which is why serious athletes take time to focus on the fascia. More recently, we've learned about the impact of fascia on the development of musculoskeletal disorders, including that ever-vague lower back pain. Many now believe that "releasing" or loosening the fascia can reduce the chance that mild to moderate muscle inflammation—say, from a challenging workout—will become painful.

One of many theories now being explored in the NIH HEAL studies is that easing the tension and opening up that fascia may create more room for the soft tissue. The problem is that it's hard to measure how much muscles get "stuck" by the fascia and how much you can actually "unstick" them with a release. For now, we mostly rely on the patients themselves to do a body scan pre- and post-myofascial release or massage and self-report whether they feel better. Many do, including me.

When it comes to myofascial release, the tools of the trade vary. People use solid balls in different sizes, or even golf balls. Foam rollers, wooden rods, sticks, and blocks are commonly used as well.

If you've ever had plantar fasciitis—an inflammation of the connective tissue, or plantar fascia, that runs along the sole of your foot from heel to toe—you know how painful it can be. Because it's often worse in the morning, one treatment is using night splints to flex the foot while you sleep. Myofascial release is another effective treatment. When I developed plantar fasciitis a few years ago, my physical therapist showed me how to carefully roll the sole of my foot over a golf ball. She told me that while it shouldn't be *too* painful, like a lot of myofascial release therapy, it would probably cause a little discomfort.

In a study of sixty-six patients with plantar fasciitis, those who underwent myofascial release similar to the kind I did had a 72 percent reduction in symptoms, compared with just 7 percent in the control group. As with many new pain modalities, it will take time to collect data and make the case for whether regular myofascial massage will help prevent or treat chronic pain. But even so, many doctors, orthopedic surgeons, physical therapists, and yoga instructors already recommend it regularly. And you can safely perform it at home with hardly any risk—as long as you don't overdo it. Using a simple foam roller is a good start for helping release your fascia and increasing range of motion. And, of course, make sure you do a self-assessing body scan before and after. The tighter the fascia, the more painful the therapy is likely to be, as the deep pressure can stimulate and even initially aggravate sensitive areas in the fascia and underlying muscle. When I underwent the therapy, the pain alternated between discomfort and sharp pain. It took a few days for that to subside but ultimately was worth it.

To prevent myofascial pain syndrome in the first place, Dr. Langevin suggests focusing on areas of concern by starting with slow, gentle movements within the range of comfort, then gradually increasing the range of movement as tolerated. If there's an area of tightness or a place where the fascia feels stuck, focus more attention there. Learning how to pay close attention to your body and move safely can be challenging, so take it slow—mindfully.

Acupuncture: Needles Notwithstanding, a "Gentle Tool"

Let's be honest: The idea that inserting fine needles into your skin can deliver pain relief is, to some people, pretty far-fetched. And yet we now have good evidence that it's true.

A few years ago, I visited a traditional acupuncturist in Japan who also happens to be blind. I had read a story about the seventeenth-century father of Japanese acupuncture, Waichi Sugiyama, who lost his sight at a young age, learned acupuncture, and then created a school to teach others his skills. Nearly four hundred years later, blind acupuncturists still use Sugiyama's techniques to sense disruptions in vital energy or qi (or chi) before opening up those areas with specially designed needles, placed through a guide tube. By feeling my limbs and torso while asking me questions, my blind acupuncturist ascertained within seconds where to place the needles: in my upper back and just below my left knee, at the location of an old injury, even though I had not disclosed that injury ahead of time.

While the exact science behind acupuncture is still a bit mysterious to me—and also to the practitioner when I asked him about it—there's little question that it has withstood the test of time. Originally a Chinese medicinal practice, it has been in use in some form for at least twenty-five hundred years and has gained popularity worldwide since the 1970s. According to the World Health Organization, acupuncture is used in 103 of the 129 countries that reported data, and a US National Health Interview Survey showed a 50 percent increase in the number of acupuncture users between 2002 and 2012. In 2012, the most recent year for which statistics are available, 6.4 percent of US adults reported they had used acupuncture at least once in their lives, and 1.7 percent reported they had used it in the past twelve months. National survey data indicate that in the United States, acupuncture is most commonly used for pain, such as back, joint, or neck pain.

None of this surprises Dr. Richard Harris, the Susan and Henry Samueli Endowed Chair in the Department of Anesthesiology and Perioperative Care in the School of Medicine at the University of California at Irvine. A copresident for the Society for Acupuncture Research, Harris hails from a background in genetics and molecular and cell biology, graduated with a PhD from UC Berkeley, completed a postdoctoral fellowship at NIH, and along the way graduated from the Maryland Institute of Traditional Chinese Medicine and earned a master's degree in clinical research design and statistical analysis at the University of Michigan. For the past twenty years, he has been studying the central neurobiological components of pain, specifically fibromyalgia and other neuroplastic pain conditions, in addition to using acupuncture and acupressure as ways to reduce pain.

Steeped in both Western science and traditional Chinese medicine, Harris is conversant in both, helpfully bilingual when it comes to talking about how acupuncture works. From a Western biomedical perspective, he says, acupuncture has multiple effects on the body. The most obvious one is that it affects the nervous system. "It's very clear that when you get stuck with the acupuncture needle and you get that chi sensation, you feel it. That's because it causes a change in the nervous system. We've shown that those changes are related to changes in neurotransmitter concentration"—specifically, increasing the amount of gamma-aminobutyric acid (GABA) in the insular cortex region of the brain, which then inhibits pain.

Think of it as a system of pipes in your house, he explains. "Water's flowing in those pipes, and you can direct that flow based on turning the faucet, anywhere in the house. There's a spot where you can do that, and in Chinese medicine, the acupuncturist goes into a spot"—called the acupoint—"and then either turns up or turns down that chi, regulates that flow so that it's more balanced." The needles are inserted and manipulated at specific locations across the body surface to improve the flow of chi.

In Chinese medicine, chi and blood are the body's basic components; blood is matter, derived from food and water, that delivers nourishment throughout the body in addition to carrying chi, which is energy, considered the vital life force. From the traditional East Asian medicine perspective, acupuncture works by mobilizing chi and increasing blood flow by stimulating the release of certain compounds that dilate blood vessels, Harris explains. Blood and chi are yin and yang—they balance each other out—and "when the body is out of balance, then you get illness."

Picture a flowchart. Like blood, which moves through vessels, chi is thought to pass along channels, called meridians. "Western medicine hasn't really defined them or found them [and] we're not really quite sure how to define that from a Western biomedical perspective," Harris says. "My guess is that it's probably neurobiological, but we don't know for sure."

Regardless, when the chi flow and blood flow aren't balanced—when you have too much or you have too little—"then you get disharmony," he says. "You need to have a good balance."

I was so fascinated by acupuncture and the ways in which it might work that after returning from Japan, I decided to invite a practitioner to perform acupuncture on me on live TV. My goal was to demystify the practice for our television audience—and afterward, we received thousands of emails from people wanting to learn more.

Tapping into the Chi: How it's Done

During an acupuncture session, a practitioner inserts hair-thin needles into acupoints on the body, where they intersect with the energy flow in muscles, nerves, and connective tissue. Depending on the type of treatment, the needles may stay in place for anywhere from ten to thirty minutes, after which they're removed.

Needles can be stimulated by either manual twirling or applying a small electrical current, and lasers are sometimes used instead of needles to stimulate acupuncture points. Because acupuncture needles are extremely fine, they don't hurt going in like an injection does. You may not even notice that a needle has been inserted. That said, some acupuncturists aim to produce a sensation called *de qi*—a sense of heaviness, soreness, or numbness at the point of needling. This is thought to be a sign that an acupuncture point has been correctly stimulated.

As Western medicine has advanced its understanding, Harris is hopeful for increased adoption of these kinds of pain treatments for certain chronic pain conditions. "It's funny. I often like to joke about this," he says. "When I started my career, I was doing acupuncture in fibromyalgia patients. This was the late nineties, and at the time, physicians didn't believe that fibromyalgia was a real condition. . . . They thought I was studying a fake condition with acupuncture, which they considered just a placebo. So, I was using a fake treatment to treat a fictitious disease." A few decades later, we now know that fibromyalgia is real and that there's evidence that acupuncture can help alleviate its symptoms.

"It's important to realize that what we call 'integrative' here in the US is more traditional in China and Japan and Korea," he notes. "These things have been around. They've been tested for a long time, pragmatically at least, if not objectively, with randomized control trials. There's now a lot of data out there that acupuncture works. It's not just made up. And it's been really refreshing to see that."

Harris also echoed a theme that came up many times while I was conducting interviews for this book. "We need to expand the toolbox of options, and for many patients, it requires many tools to get relief, a mix," he told me. "Usually with a chronic pain condition, it's complex, and you can't do just one thing and you're done. You may have to use multiple tools to get your symptoms under control, and acupuncture is just one of those additional tools."

With the usual caveats—acupuncture isn't effective for everyone and even its low risks should be taken seriously—Harris underscores its relative appeal as a pain management option: "It's nice that it's not addictive. It's nice that it doesn't have side effects. It's nice that it can be added to almost anything. It's nice that the effects last a long time—meaning you can get four or five treatments of acupuncture over the course of a month or two months and then you might not need to come back for a long time. Or maybe you need to come back monthly for a tune-up. It's really nice that it helps the body's own system correct itself." And, he added, it's gentle. "Sometimes those gentle tools are what's needed. You don't need to take a sledgehammer on something that you don't need to take a sledgehammer on."

PRACTICE

Progressive Muscle Relaxation

Progressive muscle relaxation (PMR) is a relaxation technique targeting tension associated with anxiety. It involves tensing and then releasing muscles progressively throughout the body, with the focus on achieving relaxation in the muscle release phase. PMR can be practiced individually or with the support of a narrator. I often act as a narrator for my three teenage daughters to help them relax before a big exam or after a long day.

STEP 1: Sit or lie down comfortably, ideally in a space with minimal distractions. Pay attention to the order and progression of the muscle relaxation. During the release after every step, make sure to focus all your attention on the alleviation of tension and the experience of relaxation.

STEP 2: Curl your toes under, and tense the muscles in your foot. Hold for 5 seconds, then slowly release for 10 seconds. Focus on the sensation of release, then relaxation.

STEP 3: Tense the muscles in your lower legs. Hold for 5 seconds, then slowly release for 10 seconds. Release . . . relaxation.

STEP 4: Tense the muscles in your hips and buttocks. Hold for 5 seconds, then slowly release for 10 seconds. Release . . . relaxation.

STEP 5: Tense the muscles in your stomach and chest. Hold for

5 seconds, then slowly release for 10 seconds. Release . . . relaxation.

STEP 6: Tense the muscles in your shoulders. Hold for 5 seconds, then slowly release for 10 seconds. Release . . . relaxation.

STEP 7: Tense the muscles in your face (e.g., squeezing your eyes shut). Hold for 5 seconds, then slowly release for 10 seconds. Release . . . relaxation.

STEP 8: Tense the muscles in your hand, creating a fist. Hold for 5 seconds, then slowly release for 10 seconds. Release . . . relaxation.

Be careful not to tense to the point of physical pain, and be mindful to take slow, deep breaths throughout the exercise.

—Samantha Norelli, Ashley Long, Jeffrey Krepps, Stat Pearls.

PRACTICE

Caring Touch and Gentle Massage

Simple caring touch such as hand-holding, gentle massage, or light stroking on the skin has been shown to reduce pain or change the pain experience in positive ways. In studies of the effects of so-called affective touch, scientists have found that these benefits point to promising candidates for new interventions for both acute and chronic pain in a variety of patient groups. You can try them yourself, adjusting pressure and movement for the best effect.

- Gentle stroking activates the C-tactile (CT) nerve receptors found under the skin that signal positive touch.

- CT-optimal touch is a slightly more specific gentle stroking that activates small, unmyelinated CT nerves. It can be activated by stroking at an optimal speed of about one inch per second, with a soft brush or hand.
- Hand-holding involves medium to light pressure and primarily stimulates the smooth, hairless skin of the palm, where there are no CT fibers. Hand-holding can increase physiological and neural synchrony, and it can reduce pain expression in the brain and in self-reports.
- Massage activates receptors sensitive to deep pressure and may enact pain relief by stimulating nerve fibers competing with nociceptors.
- Pain and affective touch depend on partially overlapping neural mechanisms, and this shared circuitry in the neural process may explain how affective touch influences pain processing and the pain experience.

The latest research shows that acupuncture may be most effective for specific pain conditions, including back or neck pain, knee pain associated with osteoarthritis, and postoperative pain. It may also help relieve joint pain associated with the use of aromatase inhibitors, which are drugs used to treat breast cancer. While the NIH notes that relatively few complications from using acupuncture have been reported, complications have resulted from use of nonsterile needles and improper placement of needles, which can cause serious problems including infections, punctured organs, and injury to the central nervous system. That's why the FDA regulates acupuncture needles as medical devices, requiring them to be sterile and labeled for single use only. (One way to find a credentialed acupuncturist in your area is to check the National Certification Commission for Acupuncture Medicine [nccaom.org], and click on "find the practitioner" or check the American Academy of Medical Acupuncture patient referral directory.)

Health insurance coverage varies, but some plans do cover a limited number of treatments.

To help bridge the gap between medical cultures, Harris and a team of colleagues are compiling a "topological atlas" for an open-access, Web-based portal and database incorporating both traditional East Asian medicine and conventional Western biological nomenclature systems. Imagine anatomical atlases, curated by an expert committee, of male and female human bodies (and one for rats, for research purposes)—each with a standardized three-dimensional coordinate system and a searchable database of relevant acupoints. The hope, Harris says, is that greater clarity on the biological basis of acupoints will increase integration into clinical care.

Heed Cues, or Court the Consequences

All seven of the pain-smart strategies we're now exploring represent concrete ways to befriend your body. In the pages ahead, when you think about exercise and movement, nutrition, sleep, social connection, and savoring, remember that you can choose what you use to make those strategies work for you. Think of progressive muscle relaxation, the golf balls or rollers used for myofascial release, or acupuncture needles. You can choose ways to implement them and decide how to turn ideas into actions. Your world is full of choices, from identifying favorite healthy foods for snacking to creating an inviting sleep environment, preferably one without screen distractions. You can keep notes in a journal, use an app to ping you with motivating or affirming messages, or follow through on plans to call a friend or send a note of appreciation or encouragement to someone.

As a closing thought, I encourage you to carry the body scan idea forward. Think of it as a continuing dialogue with your body, heavy on the listening part, that will help you pick up on cues your body is giving you. Also remember that your body may sometimes send out a signal of pain as a warning light, as Renee Fleming's did for her. This doesn't necessarily mean there's anything structurally wrong with your body or that you need medications or a procedure. In the same way my young children would occasionally act out when they wanted attention, your body may do the same. It's worth paying attention. And as you practice working with your body each day, instead of just pushing it to the limit and hating that you can't do more, you'll begin to feel the rewards. Your body will thank you.

CHAPTER 13

Move More

Consider this: There's no such thing as a universally recommended medication. Diets are not universally agreed on, procedures have potential risks, and the benefits of treatments must always be weighed against their side effects. Yet there is one thing that every health care practitioner recommends: movement. Everything can be improved by keeping your body in motion. From chronic back pain to arthritis, where rheumatologists preach that "motion is lotion," we're constantly told to get up and get moving—and for good reason.

When it comes to your joints, simply moving more can increase not only blood flow but also the critically important and nourishing synovial fluid that provides lubrication to your joints. And when it comes to your back, pelvic tilts and double knee hugs can go a long way toward loosening large muscles and reducing compression on spinal nerves. Remember that beyond your muscles, movement and exercise work at a systems level, changing your chemistry, adjusting the levers and dials that can reduce pain and prevent it. In the pursuit of keeping pain free, you should be moving as much as possible.

A Buff Brain Brings Its Best Game to Tame Pain

About twenty years ago, schools around the country began cutting back on the length of recess and physical education classes in favor of basic curriculum courses. The shift was partly triggered by a dip in standardized test scores in the United States, which were lagging far behind those of other countries. "More math and less recreation" became the rallying cry.

When I began investigating what impact these policy changes had on learning, what I found was unmistakable. In places where students spent more time and energy engaging in sports, there was a positive impact on learning. But in places where sports had been cut back, the opposite was true. For many people, this came as a surprise. For me, it was a revelation. It marked the first time I started to think of exercise as a way of improving not only the physical body but the mind as well.

Truth is, even though anecdotal evidence going back millennia revealed the many benefits of exercise, it wasn't until the mid-twentieth century that large-scale studies revealed that physical fitness prevented illness and protected health. Exercise used to be seen as mainly a form of leisure, but then exercise physiology became a bona fide field of study. Fast-forward to today, and a new study emerges seemingly every week showing the neuro-protective benefits of exercise. Conversely, it also shows that sedentarism (aka couch potato syndrome) appears to cause the brain to atrophy while simultaneously increasing the risk for Alzheimer's disease and other types of dementia.

After following 334,000 European men and women for more than twelve years, researchers found inactivity was twice as deadly as being obese. Read that again. Even if you are thin, inactivity is a significant risk factor for all sorts of health problems, including pain. If you've been keeping up with the latest health news, you've likely come across headlines calling couch potatoes "smokers"—as in, "sitting is the new smoking." To be fair, that's a somewhat misleading overstatement, because smoking is a much worse habit. But the headlines highlight an important fact: prolonged sitting—more than eight hours a day with zero physical activity—is a huge risk factor and can lead to an early death. But here is the good news: regardless of what you currently weigh, movement alone can counteract many of the detrimental health impacts of being overweight.

Most of the damage is metabolic. Here's what happens: When you're immobile, your circulation slows and your body uses less of your blood sugar. This means more sugar is circulating, which can be toxic to blood vessels and organs. Being motionless also has a negative impact on high-density lipoprotein (the good cholesterol), resting blood pressure, and the satiety hormone leptin (which tells you when to stop eating). Think about that: prolonged sitting can actually stimulate you to eat more, even though you aren't burning that many calories.

Sitting too much also puts muscles into a sort of dormant state where their electrical activity is diminished, leading to atrophy and breakdown. Additionally, the production of lipoprotein lipase, the enzyme that breaks down fat molecules in the blood, is shut down, leading to more fat circulating. And your metabolic rate plummets, which means you stop burning as many calories as possible at rest. When you sit too much, it's as if you're sending a message to your body and brain that you have given up, and the process of cell death and destruction can begin.

The healthiest and happiest societies in the world share many common elements, and a big one is regular movement. It's not that people go to the gym every day; many of these places don't even have gyms. It's that movement is incorporated into people's daily lives—such as walking to the grocery store instead of driving and walking regularly after meals. This is probably why, in many places around the world, it's often elderly people you see sitting. Interestingly, one of the benefits of regular walking is that it simply decreases the time you spend sitting.

The good news is that if you're active, even a few minutes in motion will counter the effects of being on your butt too much. A 2015 study out of the University of Utah School of Medicine showed that getting up for light activity—something as simple as walking—for two minutes every hour was associated with a 33 percent lower chance of dying over a three-year period. Two minutes! That's a big boost in prevention for a very short investment of time. A mere 120 seconds each hour can help offset the damaging effects that prolonged sitting has on the body, including the likelihood of chronic pain later in life. As I also often tell my students, the human body wasn't designed to move for an hour and then sit or lie down for twenty-three hours every day. Whatever you do, space out your movement so that your body is in more perpetual motion rather than stationary.

Research on people who maintain an active lifestyle indicates that exercise can inhibit certain pain pathways without drugs and also reduce the impact of chronic pain on the brain. In her 2023 talk "Beyond Opioids: Engaging Endogenous Pain Modulation in the Brain," Catherine Bushnell noted that thirty years of research shows:

- We have systems in the brain that modulate pain; opioids and other drugs activate these systems.
- We've long known that we can also independently activate these systems through our focus, emotions, and psychological outlook.
- Most recently, we have learned that these systems are automatically triggered through an active lifestyle, meaning more movement now results in less chronic pain later.

When you're in pain, moving may be the last thing you want to do. But now that you know the immediate and direct impact that movement has on all the pain pathways you've learned about, it may inspire you to start getting your body in motion—even a little bit. This isn't about losing weight; it's about changing your brain to withstand pain much more easily.

Bushnell noted that a meta-analysis has shown yoga to be particularly beneficial for people with hard-to-treat low-back pain and chronic low-back pain.

Looking at people who had practiced for at least six years and at least a couple of times a week, she said, "They weren't like crazy yogis, but people who practiced it regularly . . . had a much higher pain tolerance than the control subjects." When anatomical brain imaging was done on the yoga practitioners versus the healthy controls, the researchers found that "the yoga practitioners actually had more gray matter in multiple parts of the brain, including regions involved in pain modulation."

She continued, "So, whereas chronic pain patients show all these regions with reduced gray matter . . . the people who have been practicing yoga actually had widespread areas of increased gray matter." This helped explain findings she had spoken about more than a decade earlier, describing "a nice correlation" between the size, amount, and thickness of the gray matter in the insula and how long they've practiced yoga, "suggesting that it's possible that the yoga practice itself is having a protective effect"—not just on the body but also on the brain. Simply put, she has since concluded: "There seems to be less chronic pain when they're practicing yoga than not."

PRACTICE

Purposeful, Pleasurable Pain-Fighting Moves to Add to Your Toolbox

Different types of physical activity deliver different benefits for pain management and prevention. Aim for a mix that suits your particular needs, preferences, and capabilities. The "best" exercise is the one you'll do, so be sure to include activities that you enjoy!

- Aerobic exercise: Can help with weight loss, reducing pressure on joints and musculoskeletal system
- Resistance exercise: Can help improve musculature, relieving stiffness and providing some pain relief
- Balance and flexibility training: Can reduce the risk of falls and further pain or injury
- Motor control exercise: Can help restore coordination of core muscles
- Yoga: In addition to stress reduction, certain yoga poses, including cat-cow, lotus, and triangle pose, may help strengthen and relax muscles, which can help back pain. Yoga also leads to gray matter changes that are protective against chronic pain.

- Stretching: Light stretches before exercise and deeper stretches after work differently to prevent or reduce pain
- Tai chi: May be helpful in reducing pain in people with low-back pain, fibromyalgia, and knee osteoarthritis. May also improve walking function and posture control in older adults with knee osteoarthritis
- Dance and creative movement: Enhances mind-body integration of cognitive, emotional, physical, and social aspects of pain management, promoting physical and psychological health and social well-being. Has been shown to improve pain coping and acceptance, particularly when performed for 60 to 150`minutes weekly.

To add somatic mind-body benefits to any exercise, pay close attention to how you use your body in the activity, how that feels, and how it changes if you alter or slow the movements. This is crucially important because it gives you time to do muscle releases (tensing, then relaxing the muscles) and change your posture. Notice where in your body you're holding tension and focus on releasing it. This is also the perfect opportunity to do a body scan, noticing how your body feels and making adjustments.

You can continue to tinker to adapt movements based on how your body feels or natural fluctuations in your energy. The goal is not to go for the burn or exhaust your inner resources. The goal is to work with your body.

Whatever exercise plan you choose, the key is sticking with it, says Dr. Sluka, the University of Iowa pain scientist, whose earlier career as a physical therapist motivated her to go into research to find better ways to treat pain. Whether you want to do yoga, tai chi, walk around the block, run, or go to the gym and do some strength training, she says, "the most effective exercise program that someone can do is the one that they will do. Because if you don't do the exercise . . . it cannot work."

Sluka also strongly recommends sensible pacing of whatever you choose, adjusting for variable days to stay active without overdoing it. She speaks from experience, having lived with rheumatoid arthritis herself for years.

An Action Plan to Prevent Back Pain

Aim for 150 minutes a week of moderate-intensity aerobic activity.

- If you weren't physically active before or you haven't been active in a while, start slowly. Even five minutes of physical activity has health benefits, and you can build up to more over time. Try to move throughout the day, as opposed to concentrating all your movement in a short period.
- Choose activities that get your heart beating faster, like walking fast, dancing, swimming, or raking leaves.
- Tell your doctor if you have shortness of breath, chest pain, or unplanned weight loss.
- Do muscle-strengthening activities at least two days a week, no matter your age. Simply adjust for your fitness level.
- Try using exercise bands or lifting hand weights. You can also use books or cans of food as weights or try bodyweight activities like squats or lunges.
- Don't forget to breathe! Holding your breath can cause unsafe changes in your blood pressure.
- Do balance exercises:
    - Practice standing on one foot; you can hold on to a chair if you're feeling unsteady.
    - Walk backward or sideways.
    - Try tai chi, a mind-body exercise that improves balance.
- Sign up for a yoga class or try out a yoga video at home.

Talk with your doctor if you have questions. You might have questions about getting active, especially if you have a health problem such as chronic pain, heart disease, diabetes, or obesity. You can ask:

What activities would you recommend for me?

Can you refer me to a trained physical activity specialist, such as a physical therapist or personal trainer? (A trained physical activity specialist can help you plan a routine that fits your needs and helps you feel your best, both physically and mentally.)

If you're taking any medicine, be sure to ask if it can affect how your body responds to physical activity.

Source: US Department of Health and Human Services, Office of Disease Prevention and Health Promotion.

Steady, Sane Pace Wins the Day

Many people view movement in one of two ways: as recreation or as a way to lose body weight. Sometimes the goal is both. Yet we now know that simple movement also has enormous and measurable impacts on the brain. It helps the brain generate new neuronal growth and preferentially thickens the brain in many areas, including those associated with reducing chronic pain. Simply moving sends your brain a signal that you are still very much alive, functioning and wanting to be pain free. Steady and sane wins the day.

Aim for a Mix

Consider different types of movement and exercise to round out the benefits—strength and flexibility exercises to reduce pain and improve function. Make sure to include mood boosters, such as time in nature or with friends to tap the power of pleasure for psychological benefits. Combine activities to boost the benefits. Consider salsa dancing, raking leaves, a water aerobics class, or a walk that includes breakout segments for stretches or resistance exercise. Individualize your plan to make it enjoyable, related to your personal goals, and flexible. Recently I've started using a weighted vest on all my walks to add a little more challenge.

Recognize and Value/Celebrate Incremental Progress

Each person's activity and exercise "prescription" will be different. But whatever you choose to do, start slowly and gradually increase the intensity and duration of any workouts. The same goes for routine physical activity, especially if you're looking to build up. On errands, park a little farther from the store door each time. Walk an extra aisle or two before checking out. Add a block to your walk. Incorporate short movement and exercise "snacks" throughout the day with extra repetitions of a favorite exercise or a few cleansing or calming breaths. It all adds up quickly.

Take It Slow and Low

Choose low-impact activities that won't put too much stress on your joints and muscles. Warm up before exercising, and cool down after. Savor the feeling of this mindful kind of "body building"; remember, this isn't just muscles but also mental strength and resilience.

Listen to Your Body

Stop or pause if you experience pain. Some physical therapy movements and exercises may be designed to work in a way that creates some predictable discomfort—but beyond that, unexpected pain is a signal to get your attention. Close your eyes and use your body scan practice to home in on the location and nature of the pain. Let that inform your next step. Perhaps all that's needed is a break and gentler action as you resume.

Pair Commitment with Action

This is how you take a good idea and turn it into a reality for yourself. Aim for consistent effort. That doesn't mean doing the same exercises for the same length of time and intensity every day. It means doing something that continues your practice in some way every day. *Do what you can when you can.* Pace yourself for sustainable progress. Again, steady and sane: that's a winning streak you can extend forever.

Connect the Dots for Synergy

Each of the seven strategies boosts the benefits of the others. Look for ways to use them together. Exercise with a friend or group, whether that's on the ground, on Zoom, or in an online community. In your mix of activities, choose some you find especially relaxing to reduce stress and support a good night's sleep. Time your exercise and meals, along with mindful food choices to optimize your body's use of food as fuel. (See chapter 15, "Eat Well.") Stay hydrated throughout!

CHAPTER 14

Sleep Well

Pain often gets the blame for a poor night's sleep. But a closer look shows the reverse might be true: by improving your sleep, you may in fact be able to alleviate pain.

A body of evidence suggests that pain often disrupts sleep, which shouldn't come as a surprise to you. But what *is* surprising is that there is now "stronger evidence to suggest that poor sleep quality predicts pain to a greater extent than pain is a predictor of poor sleep," according to Dr. Carla York, a board-certified behavioral sleep medicine specialist in the Washington, DC, area. This is a fundamental shift in how we look at the relationship between sleep and pain.

I realize that this may be hard to believe, particularly if pain has made it difficult for you to fall asleep or awakened you in the night. But what Dr. York and other experts in pain and sleep are saying is that once good sleep habits are in place, the resulting better sleep is likely to lead to improvement in pain.

"A robust body of research supports an interaction between sleep and pain," says York. Because the relationship is bidirectional, however, "pain can influence or worsen sleep problems, and sleep problems can influence or worsen pain." But the more significant takeaways are that poor sleep has a negative impact on a range of health factors, and these upstream factors make us more sensitive to pain.

Much of our understanding about the link between pain and sleep changed when a 2018 systematic review showed that a decline in sleep quality and quantity was associated with a two- to threefold increase in the risk of developing a pain condition, elevations in levels of inflammatory markers, and a decline in self-reported physical health status. For the first time, sleep problems were specifically linked to the development of chronic pain rather than occurring solely as a secondary symptom to chronic pain. The authors of a 2022 study put it more bluntly, declaring that "we are currently in the midst of a sleep crisis." We've normalized poor sleep habits, they said, and it's showing in a cascade of health problems. "Sleep deprivation is an even greater issue for people with musculoskeletal conditions and with chronic pain," they went on, concluding that improving sleep in people living with those conditions had the potential to "deliver great benefit to many."

So, if you need a reason to take your sleep habits seriously, this is it. We live in a sleep-starved culture, and it's not just making us tired; it makes us hurt. So with all this in mind, the next question is, what can you do about it?

For starters, Dr. York says, shift your mind-set. She hears statements like these a lot:

> "I started having sleep problems around the time the pain started."
> "It takes a long time to fall asleep because I can't get comfortable."
> "The pain wakes me up at night."

She doesn't question the veracity of the statements, but a significant strategy she uses is to shift the mind-set that assumes that everything hinges on a cure for the pain and anything short of that is bound to fail. Thanks to this newly described bidirectional relationship between sleep and pain, we know that's not the case, and that's something York reinforces to her patients. Focus on getting better sleep first, and better pain relief will follow.

An Active Day Promotes Better Sleep at Night

Another important sleep factor that has been long overlooked has nothing to do with what happens at night but how active you are during the day.

The 2022 Sleep in America poll highlighted the association between exercise and better sleep, noting that physical activity promotes deeper sleep at night.

Here's how it works: A person who's physically active during the day has a higher amount of the naturally occurring molecule adenosine by bedtime. Adenosine promotes the start of sleep and subsequent deep sleep stages. So exercisers, compared with nonexercisers, are more likely to report falling asleep more easily, as well as higher levels of restorative sleep. At the same time, poor sleep makes us less likely to exercise, which in turn leads to relative difficulty falling asleep, or falling back asleep in the middle of the night and waking up too early.

The result? An exhausting cycle of reduced physical activity and reduced sleep. The solution is not to let regular exercise and movement get sidelined, even if you have a poor night's sleep. Adding that activity to your day will increase the chances of a good night's sleep, helping to break that cycle.

Food for Thought—and Sound Sleep

Meals can act as important cues to help regulate your sleep/wake cycle. The problem is that four in ten Americans take meals at irregular times, another tiring loop: poor diet contributes to poor sleep, and poor sleep contributes to poor diet. We've long known that the quality of our food choices and how much we consume specific nutrients can affect regulatory hormonal pathways that influence the quality and quantity of our sleep. But simply becoming more diligent about when you eat can also make a huge difference in your sleep, and therefore on your likelihood of pain.

I admit that I sometimes reach for my cache of comfort foods—crunchy, salty snacks or a bowl of ice cream before bedtime. Before researching and writing this book, I hadn't fully appreciated how that habit might be setting me up for not only poor sleep but also an increased likelihood of aches and pains.

"You Are What You Eat" Extends to Sleep Quality Too

Dietary composition, with a focus on specific dietary components, is known to influence sleep duration, quality, and behaviors. In studies analyzing the role of macronutrients (carbohydrates, fats, proteins), micronutrients (vitamins, minerals), and whole foods on sleep, researchers found evidence that suggests changes in daily dietary composition and eating behaviors can subsequently affect elements of sleep. Findings from across studies include the following:

- Eating low fiber, high-saturated fat, and sugar are associated with lighter, less restorative sleep.
- A high-carbohydrate, low-fat diet is associated with poorer sleep quality versus a low-carbohydrate/high-fat diet.
- Protein and carbohydrate deficiencies are also associated with shorter sleep duration.
- Consuming high-glycemic index carbohydrate meals (white bread, white rice or pasta, mashed potatoes, sugary drinks, processed snack foods) approximately four hours before bedtime decreases sleep latency, which means it takes you less time to fall asleep. (I've heard people refer to this as the "carb coma" effect.) It doesn't necessarily mean your quality of sleep will improve.
- Coffee and other beverages containing stimulants affect adenosine, the hormone that regulates sleep/wake cycles, altering sleep patterns.
- Evening dietary increases in tryptophan, an amino acid building block in the sleep-regulating hormone serotonin, improved sleep in adults with sleep disturbances and enhanced alertness in the morning, most likely as a result of improved sleep quality. Most people think of turkey as tryptophan-containing food,

but all animal proteins, along with most plant proteins, have some.

- Certain whole foods, such as milk, fatty fish, cherries, and kiwis, are associated with beneficial effects on sleep outcomes, perhaps due in some cases to relatively high tryptophan content. Bread, pulses (dried seeds of plants in the legume family, such as beans, peas, chickpeas, and lentils), and fish and shellfish are positively correlated with sleep duration.

Source: Sarah Frank, Kelli Gonzalez, Lorraine Lee-Ang, Marielle C. Young, Martha Tamez, and Josiemer Matteit. "Diet and Sleep Physiology: Public Health and Clinical Implications." Frontiers in Neurology *11, no. 8 (2017).*

Many other factors adversely affect good sleep. For example, while appropriate light exposure—including bright light during the day and dim light at night—helps regulate the circadian rhythm (the natural sleep/wake process behind healthy sleep), nearly half of Americans say they're not exposed to bright light indoors in the morning and afternoon, and most indulge in screen time too close to bedtime. But these habits are easily modifiable. The first thing I do every morning is let the outside light hit my face, preferably outside, but even if it's just through a window. I stand there for a minute and let the natural light flood my brain and set my internal clock. The key is to make sure you do this before looking at the blue light from your phone.

Sleep Specialists Can Help Smooth Your Way to Better Sleep

If you're in pain and not sleeping well, I encourage you to seek out a sleep specialist. These are medical professionals with special training in treating sleep disorders, including insomnia, sleep apnea, and pain-related sleep problems. Many are psychologists or psychiatrists who draw from cognitive behavioral therapy and other therapies, as well as from the broader array of behavioral medicine approaches. Sleep specialists also include neurologists and pulmonologists, among others. You should check for sleep specialists who are board certified by the American Board of Sleep Medicine (ABSM) or the American Board of Medical Specialists.

If You Wake Up in the Night

If waking up in the middle of the night is a problem for you, try activating your parasympathetic nervous system with a simple breathing practice. Slow, deep breathing is the key.

- Inhale slowly, to a count of four.
- Then exhale even more slowly, to a count of eight.
- Repeat this pattern for as long as you need to.

This kind of breathing specifically targets the vagus nerve, which carries signals from your brain to your heart and your gut, controlling everything from your heart rate to your digestion. It is the major nerve of your parasympathetic nervous system—which means it can help calm you down quickly.

Another way to activate this nerve is humming (which you can do quietly if someone else is in your bed). Humming activates the muscles in your throat and vocal cord, which will stimulate your vagus nerve and increase your heart rate variability, lowering stress levels.

The Best Bedtime Starts Well before Bedtime

Most of us have had worries that kept us up at night, and we know that worrying only makes it harder to relax, fall asleep, and stay asleep. So let's turn to the strategies that the experts say can help make bedtime sleep time.

- Keep a regular sleep schedule. Going to bed and waking up at about the same time each day establishes a natural sleep cycle. Experts recommend between seven and nine hours of sleep a night, but quality counts, so don't lose sleep fretting about the clock. Take steps to make the hours you get as relaxed and restorative as possible.

- Use your bed for sleep and not for casual hanging out, reading, eating, or working. If your home office is in your bedroom, try to keep your workspace and materials separate from your sleeping space—especially your bed. You want to train your brain to associate bed with sleep, and those boundaries will help.
- Improve the environmental factors in your sleep space that disturb your sleep. These include noise (inside and outside), light, temperature, and an uncomfortable mattress. The best room temperature for sleep is about 65 degrees Fahrenheit (18.3 Celsius). That can vary a bit according to personal preference, and of course your comfort is what counts. But aim for between 65 and 68 degrees Fahrenheit (18.3 to 20 degrees Celsius). And if outdoor lighting shines into your room at night, consider window coverings to block it.
- Develop evening rituals that include time to relax and wind down your day. Aim for soothing activities such as a bath or shower, listening to quiet music, journaling, or meditation.
- Try mindfulness meditation or a visualization exercise. This can calm stress pathways and counteract the stress response that typically prevails through a demanding day. The stress response involves rapid heart rate, faster breathing, and other physiological changes—none of them conducive to sleep. It's well established that mindfulness meditation can engage the relaxation response that calms breathing, settles the nervous system, reduces heart rate and blood pressure, and slows brain waves, acting as antidotes to the stress response so your body can prepare for sleep.
- Dim the lights, and pull the plug on screen time. Limit exposure to bright light in the evenings. And turn off electronic devices at least thirty minutes before bedtime. I know how tempting it is to check

> email or news updates one last time, but it's rare that anything you find there will be soothing for your brain or spirit. More likely, what you choose to view or see by chance will just stir up your mental state and leave you less relaxed as you try to fall asleep.

For the last two decades, I have been a world-class sleeper. My wife often jokes that I'll say good night, put my head down, and immediately fall asleep. If she says anything even a few seconds later, she doesn't get a reply because I'm already out. I once did a sleep study for a documentary I was making, and even with all the bright lights on my face for filming and the gadgets all over my head for measuring, I still fell asleep almost immediately—to the surprise of the sleep researchers, who were monitoring my brain waves from a different control room.

It wasn't always this way, but one basic act really helped me: keeping a notepad next to my bed. The problem for me—and maybe for you as well—was that there were too many things swirling around in my head as I got ready to fall asleep. The simple act of writing them down—not typing them on my phone but physically writing—allowed me to outsource them from my brain to the paper.

Every night I still spend a few minutes reflecting on my day and planning the next one, paper and pen in hand. And every person I've recommended this to has thanked me, even my teenage daughters! Hope it helps you as well.

PRACTICE

A Sample Meditation for Sleep

It takes practice to master the art of relaxing and letting the mind be at peace. A good place to start is with a simple meditation exercise that involves breathing exercises for sleep.

1. Turn off the lights and phone notifications, set the thermostat to a comfortable temperature, and sit upright in a chair with your feet on the floor or lie comfortably in bed facing up. Place one hand on your chest, the other on your midsection.
2. Breathe in slowly through the nose. The hand on your midsection should rise, while the hand on your chest should stay still. This is called diaphragmatic breathing.
3. Breathe out slowly. Repeat ten calm, controlled breaths, always making sure to use your diaphragm instead of the chest muscles.
4. Clear your mind and focus on breathing. Try not to become anxious if negative thoughts appear. Acknowledge them, then let them go and return to a place of peace.

Source: Sleep Foundation. "Meditation for Sleep," December 16, 2022. https://www.sleepfoundation.org/meditation-for-sleep.

CHAPTER 15

Eat Well

A few years ago, my wife Rebecca was diagnosed with an autoimmune disease. Some days, the pain was so bad she had to wait for me to carry her up the stairs from the family room couch to the bedroom. I remember lying in bed with her one early morning, asking her to point to the site of her pain. As she did her own body scan, I realized she could barely point to a single place on her body that *didn't* hurt.

These days, she's doing a lot better, even able to do daily yoga and brisk walks with our dogs. But in those scary early days, I was surprised to find that even as a doctor, not to mention an investigative journalist, I found it challenging to navigate the system and figure out the best therapies for her.

One thing that every doctor recommended was an anti-inflammatory diet. Reduce the level of inflammation, we were told, and that will help mitigate the crippling pain. She started with an elimination diet, with the goal of trying to find specific triggers for her symptoms. Then we transitioned to an anti-inflammatory, low-histamine diet—mostly plain whole grains, fruits and vegetables, and occasionally some baked chicken, but no cheese, tomatoes, or citrus. Rebecca and I both ate these meals, as I had joined my wife in the restrictive diet as a show of solidarity. But over time, something extraordinary happened to me as well.

Even though I hadn't had any specific ongoing pains before starting the diet, I had noticed an increasing number of minor aches—not unusual for a man in his mid-fifties. My heel might hurt longer than it used to after I missed a step on the stairs. Getting out of bed in the morning, I'd notice muscle stiffness that I hadn't felt a couple of decades earlier. Things I'd bounce back from easily in the past would become an annoyance for several days. But a few weeks into diligently abiding by that anti-inflammatory diet, I noticed one day that I was more limber, performing better in yoga, and not suffering as much from the usual aches and pains of midlife. And the diet was the only thing I'd changed.

Many people consider starting an anti-inflammatory diet only to address an underlying problem, like my wife did with her illness. Yet even for me—someone with no underlying problem—it helped enormously. Over time, we figured out how to make tastier and more diverse options. Within a few months, even my three teenage daughters were asking to join in on our meals.

Nutrition is considered the top modifiable lifestyle factor for pain. What you eat and drink can enhance the function of your nervous, immune, and endocrine systems, all of which directly affect pain experiences. Your food choices can provide protective benefits against pain and greater resilience if pain comes your way. What's more, evidence from systematic reviews of pain science literature shows that optimizing the quality of your diet to include foods containing anti-inflammatory nutrients such as fruits, vegetables, long chain and monounsaturated fats (olive, soybean, and other plant-based oils, avocados, and oily fish), antioxidants, and fiber leads to reduction in pain severity.

I often tell people that what we decide to eat is the one signal that we consciously send from our outside world to our inside world—from our environment to the cells located deep in our bodies. We should be incredibly thoughtful about that decision.

A systematic review of more than seventy studies, investigating the impact of a variety of nutrition interventions on self-reported pain severity in adults with chronic pain, concluded with three major findings.

1. A healthy diet helps pain medications work as they should, as well as helping to reduce side effects.
2. A body dealing with pain imposes a serious demand on energy. Your food is your fuel to get you through those times.

3. There's a strong link, as Rebecca learned, between diet and systemic inflammation. Incorporating foods containing anti-inflammatory nutrients leads to reduction in pain severity.

Looking through the kaleidoscope of pain-related mechanisms, studies have specifically traced the intricate linkages between diet and oxidative stress, which is the state in which cells basically become overwhelmed by the toxic cleanup task. According to the authors of a 2020 study, oxidative stress may play a relevant role in pain processing and can cause long-term damage to the central nervous system.

While oxidative stress is known to be influenced by various stimuli, including exercise, it is perhaps most fundamentally influenced by the food we eat. And because oxidative stress, chronic inflammation, and pain are all closely linked, diet can play a critical role in reducing all of them.

A recent animal study underscored the point that high-fat or high-carbohydrate diets are most associated with oxidative stress. Healthy diets, however, play a crucial role in maintaining cell and tissue balance, reducing oxidative stress, and inhibiting inflammation.

The point is that our food choices don't just boil down to pounds gained or lost on a scale. They affect every aspect of our health, including our resistance or resilience to pain. The individual nature of our food choices are an especially potent access point for meaningful, mindful, personalized action. Here are ways to customize yours for the best food fit.

The Personalized Pain-Smart Pantry

Customize to Keep Your Best Healthy Choices Handy

The simplest way to start tailoring your diet to optimize inflammation-fighting foods is to keep those foods handy and plentiful for meal making and snacks. But what should those foods be? General recommendations are a great start, and you'll find some here. But for a plan to really work for you, you'll want to personalize the list to reflect your specific health needs and preferences. This includes any health conditions you may have, medications you take, or food sensitivities that should guide your choices.

For instance, if a recommended food is a trigger for your migraines or other pain, hard for you to digest, or conflicts with medications you're taking, then it's obviously not a healthy choice for you. As you go through this exercise, it will help to keep a food journal and pay close attention to how you feel after eating certain foods. If you have special considerations, I encourage you to seek out a nutritionist or dietician because they are typically much easier to access than pain doctors, and ask for recommendations on how to customize your anti-inflammatory pantry.

The list that follows generally supports the two most popular anti-inflammatory diets, the Mediterranean diet and DASH (dietary approaches to stop hypertension). These two diets share a focus on fresh, whole (unprocessed) foods, predominantly plant-based though not exclusively so, that have a low glycemic load, rich antioxidant content, and limited sugar. Both are rich in fresh fruits and vegetables, cereals (preferably wholegrain, low-sugar), pulses, and nuts. The Mediterranean diet has a higher fat content compared to the DASH diet, which has a low fat content, ideally around 27 percent. A third eating plan, the MIND (Mediterranean-DASH intervention for neurodegenerative delay) diet, combines elements from the traditional Mediterranean diet and the DASH diet, also emphasizing anti-inflammatory foods.

The following foods are generally recommended for their anti-inflammatory properties:

- Deep orange, yellow and red, and dark green foods, such as pumpkin, sweet bell peppers, tomatoes, carrots, kale, spinach, Swiss chard, arugula, and endive
- Deep blue or purple foods, such as blueberries, blackberries, plums, and Concord grapes
- Cruciferous vegetables including broccoli, cauliflower, and cabbage
- Onions
- Citrus fruits, such as oranges, grapefruits, and pomelos

- Whole grains, such as wheat, oats, rye, buckwheat, millet, quinoa, and brown rice
- Plant-based proteins, including dried beans, lentils, lentil pasta, tofu, and other soy products
- Nuts, including walnuts and almonds, and seeds like chia, flax, and hemp
- Spices and herbs, including ginger, garlic, turmeric, cardamom, black pepper, cinnamon, and rosemary
- Beverages such as water, herbal and green teas, and coffee

What's in Your Mix?

I grew up in a home filled with the wonderful aromas of spices and herbs. My mom was a practitioner of the traditional Indian Ayurvedic diet, so every weekend we traveled to the farmers' market to get whole fresh foods and vegetables. We ate hardly any processed foods, and if we ate meat at all, it was mostly chicken and fish. Given that both my parents worked full-time jobs, it was most remarkable that we almost always ate at fixed times, sitting down to dinner promptly at 6:30 p.m.

As I was writing this book I realized that, no surprise, my mom was ahead of her time. In later years, I came to learn that the diet she prepared for us was tailored for our specific body type—our *dosha*. In Ayurvedic medicine, there are three categories of dosha: Vata, Pitta, and Kapha. Each has its own characteristics and its own recommended dietary guidelines.

Everyone in my family is pretty lean and a little restless, so we fit into the category of Vata Dosha. For my mom, that meant choosing certain spices thought to be more calming, such as ashwagandha, turmeric, ginger, and cumin. She also emphasized that we should never eat in a hurry or when we were stressed. As a result, there was always a lot of joy surrounding our meals. Also, the diet provided all the raw minerals and vitamins we needed and even to this day, I make a point of getting all the necessary ingredients from my food, taking no additional pills.

Cooking Up Health

Plant. Prep. Plate.

3 Ps to Anti-Inflammatory Eats

Melinda R. Ring, MD, executive director of the Osher Center for Integrative Health at Northwestern University and Tina Trott Professor of Integrative Health at Northwestern University's Feinberg School of Medicine, teaches "culinary medicine" to medical students because, she says, "Combining the art of cooking with the science of medicine beats pills and prescriptions." She encourages all of us to use these three distilled principles of culinary medicine on a daily basis, embracing an anti-inflammatory diet "to be your own first best doctor."

How to do it? She offers this "3 Ps" advice: plant, prep, and plate.

Plant

There's no getting around it: if you don't eat plants, you are shortchanging your health. No matter what diet you subscribe to—Mediterranean, keto, intermittent fasting—it needs to be built on abundant vegetables and fruit, because plants are rich in phytonutrients that fight all the root causes of disease. Besides fighting inflammation, they are potent antioxidants. They support a healthy gut microbiome. They detoxify the body from cancer-causing compounds. The next time you're at the grocery store, get at least three colors of fruits and vegetables—rainbow colors of red, orange, yellow, green, blue, even purple—because each color has its own unique phytonutrients.

Prep

Sharpen your knife skills so you're comfortable slicing and dicing all of those colorful vegetables and fruits. If you're thinking, "Who has time to prep with everything else I have to do?" the good news is there are shortcuts to cuts. You can buy packaged precut vegetables and fruit, then put them at eye level in your refrigerator so they're the first thing you and your family members see when reaching for a snack. Prepping foods, whether you do it yourself or buy it that way, makes the healthy choice the easy choice.

Plate

Your goal with every plate is to make it half plant. It's time to ditch "Where's the beef?" and start asking, "Where's the plant?" So when you're at the store, ask yourself, *Where's the plant?* When you're eating out at a restaurant or pulling through a drive-thru, ask yourself, *Where's the plant?* At home, making your plate for breakfast, lunch, or dinner, ask yourself, *Where's the plant?*

Doing these three pieces—plant, prep, and plate—on a daily basis will make a tangible difference to your health. You will never regret doing the three Ps. You will only regret not doing them sooner!

Water Works Wonders—Stay Hydrated!

When you're well hydrated, you think better, sleep better, move better, and are providing your brain and body with the fluid necessary to work better in every way. Poor hydration can worsen headaches and other pain; cause constipation, fatigue, dizziness, and confusion; and affect your body's ability to keep your temperature and other vitals stable. Cognitive and physical performance is impaired by just a 2 percent decrease in hydration. A diet rich in fruits and vegetables with high water content can help, and milk and other beverages (preferably unsweetened) can too.

Proper hydration is important in pain management to keep joints lubricated and cushioned, support healthy muscle function, carry nutrients and oxygen to cells, and remove toxins, promote overall cell health and cell-to-cell signaling, and support a range of anti-inflammatory actions throughout the body.

Some medications and chronic diseases, such as diabetes or chronic kidney disease, can affect how often you urinate and can lead to fluid loss. Fever, vomiting, and diarrhea obviously require extra fluids to rehydrate. Other factors include sweaty exercise, hot or humid weather (or high altitudes), whether you're pregnant or breastfeeding, your overall health, and your diet.

PRACTICE

Steady Sipping for Optimal Hydration

Keep your water glass full. Drink up, then fill up again so it's easy to sip throughout the day. Although individual factors affect precisely how much is right for you, experts generally recommend about nine 8-ounce cups of fluids a day for women and thirteen cups for men on average. Aim for a steady pace that's easy to remember, such as wake-up time, pegging meals or snack times for a water break, and keeping a water bottle nearby at all times. It is better to drink consistently throughout the day, rather than chugging water only occasionally.

The Anti-Inflammatory Diet: Top 10 Suggestions

Pay attention to proteins. If you get most of your proteins from plants such as beans, whole grains, and nuts, your levels of inflammation will be lower. If you eat red meat, it is best to eat grass-fed meat or wild game rather than grain-fed beef. Wild-caught (as opposed to farmed) fish can be a better source of protein. As journalist Michael Pollan says in his book *Food Rules*, "The fewer the feet, the better the meat."

Eat more fiber. Fiber, a form of carbohydrate, lowers inflammation. Read food labels. Different groups suggest different daily amounts, but try for the following:

- Women 19–50 years old: 25 grams daily
- Men 19–50: 38 grams daily
- Women over 50: 21 grams daily
- Men over 50: 30 grams daily

Good sources of fiber include whole grains, oatmeal, nuts, berries, beans, vegetables, brown rice, and popcorn. Potato skins have a lot of fiber. If you don't already eat much fiber, increase your intake of these foods slowly to avoid bowel discomfort.

Eat your vegetables and fruits. When it comes to ideas for healthier eating, eating more fruit and vegetables is at the top of the list. In addition to their many other benefits, vegetables and fruits reduce inflammation. Berries and cherries are especially good options. Fruit juice is not usually a good choice because it is high in sugars and low in fiber. Making your own smoothies is a good idea. Choose dark-colored produce that's many different colors. Plants get their colors from phytonutrients, helpful compounds that are anti-inflammatory. Strive for a minimum of five cups of vegetables and fruits per day. And if you have diabetes or pre-diabetes, emphasize nonstarchy vegetables over fruits.

Use more anti-inflammatory herbs and spices. A 2012 study found that the best anti-inflammatory spices to eat, in order, are paprika, rosemary, ginger, turmeric, sage, and cumin. An earlier study looked at other chemical properties of spices and found that cloves, ground Jamaican allspice, cinnamon, sage, marjoram, and tarragon are also great choices.

Note that the guidelines below are related to fats. In the body, different types of fats are processed in different ways, which can either increase or decrease inflammation.

Avoid trans fats. Trans fats, which are added to foods to increase their shelf life, can add to the body's inflammation. Avoid foods that have labels saying they have "partially hydrogenated" oils. Foods that often have trans fats include baked goods (e.g., cakes, pie crusts, frozen pizza, and cookies) and fried foods (e.g., doughnuts, fries).

Limit saturated fats. Most (not all) saturated fats also promote inflammation. These fats mostly come from animal sources such as meats (lamb, pork, chicken with skin, fatty beef) and dairy products like milk, cheese, cream, and butter. If you eat meat, a good general rule is to try to eat white meats, fish, and other seafood.

Balance omega-6s and omega-3s. You may have heard about essential fatty acids. These are types of polyunsaturated fats that your body can't make on its own; you have to get them from your diet. You need both omega-6 and omega-3 fats for your body to work properly, but they need to be in the right balance. The problem is that eating high amounts of omega 6s compared to omega-3s can increase inflammation. And unfortunately, that's exactly what most Americans do. Our ancestors ate twice as much omega-6 fat as omega-3. But now, most Americans eat fourteen to twenty-five times as much omega-6.

Omega-6s come from plant oils like corn oil, soybean oil, and sunflower oil, as well as nuts and seeds. Omega-3s are found in fatty fish like salmon, tuna, and mackerel. Try to eat at least two servings of fish (3 to 4 ounces each) weekly. Fish oil supplements are also useful, and they're widely available. A usual dose is 1,000 to 2,000 mg per day. If you're taking blood thinners, however, talk to your doctor before you start taking fish oil. Omega-3s are also found in whole grains, walnuts, and green leafy vegetables. Finally, eating a Mediterranean diet will give you a much healthier balance of omega-6s and omega-3s than the average American diet.

Eat monounsaturated fats. One of the monounsaturated fats, olive oil, is known to reduce inflammation, blood pressure, bad cholesterol, and blood sugar levels. Other sources of this type of fat are canola, peanut, safflower, and sesame oils. Avocados are another good source.

Some experts suggest you get one-fourth of your fat from saturated fats, one-fourth from polyunsaturated, and one-half from monounsaturated. Many diets recommend that total fats add up to about one-third of all the calories you eat. You have to explore what works best for you.

Eat some dark chocolate. Most people like this suggestion! To help with inflammation, dark chocolate should be at least 70 percent cocoa mass—check the label for the cocoa percentage. One and a half ounces daily decreases inflammation and also lowers blood pressure.

If you choose to drink alcohol, choose red wine. Of course, don't take up drinking to get this benefit. Having said that, there is some evidence that red wine can decrease inflammation. One study found that drinking wine and cooking with olive oil worked together to lower inflammation as well. Even one drink of alcohol a day may slightly increase the risk of breast cancer. Other beverages, like grape juice, have been found to have some benefits, too, though more studies are needed to see how different beverages compare.

—From the Veterans Administration Whole Health Library.

INCREASE

Fruits & Vegetables

- Red: berries, cherries, peppers
- Orange-Yellow: Sweet potato, pineapple, yellow pepper, squash, peaches
- Green: Dark leafy greens, broccoli, cabbage, green beans, Brussels sprouts
- Blue/Purple/Black: blueberries, blackberries, grapes, eggplant, olives, plums, purple cabbage

Fiber

- Whole grains, oatmeal, bran cereal, nuts, berries, beans, brown rice, popcorn, potato skins
- Vegetables
- Fruits

Proteins

- Plant-based (beans, grains, nuts, seeds)
- Grass-fed or wild meat and fish

Herbs & Spices

- Paprika, rosemary, ginger, turmeric, sage, cumin, cloves, Jamaican allspice, cinnamon, marjoram, tarragon, green and black tea

Omega-3's

- Fatty fish (salmon, tuna, mackerel)
- Fish oil
- Whole grains, walnuts, green vegetables
- *Eat more Omega-3's than Omega-6's*

Monounsaturated Fats

- Oils (olive, canola, peanut, safflower, sesame)
- Avacados

Desserts /Snacks

- Dark chocolate (70% of cocoa or more)

DECREASE

Proteins

- Grain-fed beef
- Processed means (lunch/deli meats, hot dogs, bacon, sausage)

Trans fats

- Partially hydrogenated oils
- Baked goods (cakes, pie crusts, frozen pizza, cookies)
- Fried foods (donuts, fries)

Saturated fats

- Meats (lamb, pork, fatty beef, chicken with skin)
- Dairy products (milk, cheese, cream, butter)
- Fruit juice

What's the Scoop on Intermittent Fasting?

Not only what but when you eat can matter. Intermittent fasting involves alternating periods of eating with periods of fasting (not eating). It has been shown to have beneficial cellular, physiological, and system-wide effects in animal and human studies, and it may have a promising role in chronic pain treatment, report the authors of "Intermittent Fasting: Potential Utility in the Treatment of Chronic Pain across the Clinical Spectrum," published in 2022 in the journal *Nutrients*. The fasting need not be for an extreme period of time; a common intermittent fasting schedule takes place in a twenty-four-hour day, with an eight-to-twelve-hour span for eating, and the remaining hours, including your sleep time, abstaining from food.

In the overview of research on intermittent fasting and various health conditions, the authors found that intermittent fasting provided benefits in the management of inflammatory and autoimmune diseases including rheumatoid arthritis, psoriasis, psoriatic arthritis, ankylosing spondylitis, multiple sclerosis, asthma, and type 1 diabetes, in addition to chronic pain. To be clear, fasting is not for everyone. Children, pregnant women, and the elderly in particular should be cautious about the possible effects.

You Pick the Best Strategies to Make Pain-Smart Choices a Habit

When it comes to strategies for turning new choices into a habit, what works best for you? Lists with detailed options? Short tips? A slow shift to new behavior works best for some; others prefer to go cold turkey (so to speak) and never look back (or, if not "never," then at least only when they're at a safe distance from the Twinkies).

Whatever you prefer, you can find lots of free, excellent coaching tips online from respected sources like Mayo Clinic, Harvard Medical School, and Cleveland Clinic health information sites, as well as patient advocacy organizations with specialized grounding in particular pain conditions.

Here are a few styles you may find helpful.

The first is to go "whole" and reach for fresh, whole foods instead of processed foods and, especially, ultraprocessed foods. As Harvard Health explains:

> *Stay away from "ultra-processed" foods, which include just about anything that comes in a package—like microwaveable dinners, hot dogs, chicken nuggets, dehydrated soups, baked goods, sugary cereals, processed meats, biscuits, and sauces. These foods have little nutritional value. Worse, they're high in salt, added sugars (which can spike your blood sugar), and saturated fat (which can increase your "bad" LDL cholesterol).*
>
> *All these ingredients are associated with promoting inflammation in the body. The biggest offender is anything with added sweeteners, whether that means cane sugar, or any compounds used to add sweetness, including some artificial sweeteners.*
>
> *A report published in December 2019 in* Nature Medicine *notes that sugars, grains, and extra salt in ultraprocessed foods can change the bacteria in your gut, damage the gut's lining, and switch on inflammatory genes in cells.*

Swap or substitute food items that you eat now but that you could easily trade for healthier, anti-inflammatory options. Johns Hopkins Medicine advises starting gradually, using a substitution strategy to find alternatives to foods that cause inflammation. Its "One Meal at a Time" strategy suggests these substitutions:

Instead of...	**Try...**
Charcuterie boards	Vegetable slices with hummus
French fries	Baked sweet potatoes
Sauces with butter or cheese	Olive oil, vinegar, and herbs
Grilled burgers	Grilled eggplant or portobello mushrooms
Bakery cakes and pies	Dark chocolate with raspberries or grilled peaches

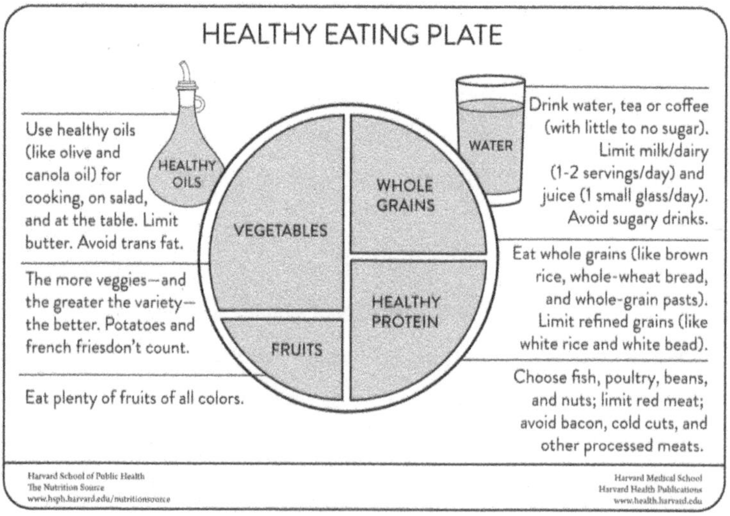
HEALTHY EATING PLATE
Use healthy oils (like olive and canola oil) for cooking, on salad, and at the table. Limit butter. Avoid trans fat.
HEALTHY OILS
The more veggies—and the greater the variety—the better. Potatoes and french friesdon't count.
Eat plenty of fruits of all colors.
VEGETABLES
FRUITS
WHOLE GRAINS
HEALTHY PROTEIN
WATER
Drink water, tea or coffee (with little to no sugar). Limit milk/dairy (1-2 servings/day) and juice (1 small glass/day). Avoid sugary drinks.
Eat whole grains (like brown rice, whole-wheat bread, and whole-grain pasts). Limit refined grains (like white rice and white bead).
Choose fish, poultry, beans, and nuts; limit red meat; avoid bacon, cold cuts, and other processed meats.
Harvard School of Public Health
The Nutrition Source
www.hsph.harvard.edu/nutritionsource
Harvard Medical School
Harvard Health Publications
www.health.harvard.edu

CHAPTER 16

Cultivate Connection

Many years ago, I participated in a group tai chi class at a beautiful park in Hong Kong. It was a blistering hot day, and I was pretty nervous—mostly worried that I would sweat too much and embarrass myself.

But the thing about finding your rhythm, or even entering a flow state, is that it can transform a very personal, almost isolated experience into feeling that you're part of something much larger. While I wasn't in physical contact with any of the other participants, I could sense their energy; I felt the buzz, and I knew they could feel mine. My instructor referred to tai chi as "meditation in motion." As I spread my "wings" like a white crane and simulated movements from martial arts, I knew what she meant; it was magical.

We don't necessarily move through daily life aware of those kinds of shared energies, but our relationships, everyday social interactions, and sense of connection through community act in much the same way. We need the chi of social connection to thrive, and there's plenty of evidence to bear that out. A look at the data shows that enjoying close ties to friends and family, as well as participating in meaningful social activities, provides a buffer against the harmful effects of stress on the brain and its contribution to pain. People with chronic pain are more vulnerable to social isolation, and the experience of rejection and disconnection reliably amplifies pain.

Nearly every day in my work as a neurosurgeon, I've seen the anecdotal evidence for both sides of this cause and effect. The people I meet who are the most joyful and pain free, regardless of age or health complications, are the ones who have high-quality friendships, loving families, and expansive, dynamic social networks. My heart sinks when I meet a patient who has no immediate family and no close friends. There's nothing more heartbreaking than watching someone suffer through chronic pain alone.

Even people who have caring friends, loving family, and a thriving social network might find that pain isolates them physically and emotionally. It can strain relationships to the breaking point. I have seen how pain shreds social connections, prompting people to scuttle plans, avoid activities, or shrink away from engaging with others in ways they once enjoyed.

In the isolation that chronic pain imposes, it can be hard to imagine how things might ever change for the better. But in cases like this, we need to remember everything we have learned so far. Nature provides the perfect coach to shepherd us through: the brain itself, master networker, creator of relationships, and reducer of pain.

Take the Connection Challenge

STEP 1 Commit to connect. Think of five different ways to connect with people in your life. It might be a lunch date, pickle ball game, an email to express gratitude, an offer of support, or a request for help.

STEP 2 Connect each day for five days in a row.

To learn more or access resources, visit https://www.hhs.gov/surgeongeneral/priorities/connection/challenge/index.html.

You've already learned how the brain's pain-processing system engages multiple distinct but interrelated neural networks, which draw from experiences, emotions, beliefs, and interactions with others. When focused on pain relief, these shared roots include healing rituals, memories, and pleasurable experiences—especially those we share with others. We can choose to access or create them in even the smallest ways.

And as we've seen, the brain's reward center recognizes a pleasurable experience with (among other things) a burst of dopamine that reinforces the importance of that pleasurable experience and makes you want to repeat it. This means that with each small step toward healing, you boost your inclination and desire for the next, especially when it comes to social relationships, which are the connective tissue of life.

LIVING IT

Marsha Garcia

Racing for the Joy of It—and Community

When Marsha Garcia tightens the strap on her TN Warrior–branded racing helmet, greets fans and track friends, then roars out across the Arizona desert on her all-terrain vehicle (ATV), she's part of a pack of weekend racers, most of them men. Though the guys aren't big on small talk, they are nonetheless a kind of brotherly band, and their howdies and hugs make for a sense of a family that includes friendly sibling rivalry for making the finish line first.

There was a time, maybe ten years ago, when Garcia raced to win, and she was no stranger to the winner's circle. "I wanted the trophy and the bragging rights," she says. "I raced with *fierceness*." Then a mysterious and excruciating head pain set in, for no apparent reason. "It didn't start with a shock—that came later," she recalls, "but just real bad head pain on the left side." Her head became extremely sensitive and painful to the touch, and when the pain flared, it felt volcanic. Fierce. It made her ability to work as a bank manager unpredictable and stressful. She never knew when the pain would strike, which it did with increasing frequency. And, she says, "This was no 'let me go sit in the back room for a minute' kind of head pain." It was debilitating.

Doctors didn't initially know what to make of it. Some told her the concussions she'd suffered while racing might be to blame. Others told her it was the dust and grit from the desert tracks and warned that she should stop racing altogether. She did cut back, but the head pain only grew worse. She began spending less time with her small, closely knit family, including her rambunctious young grandsons. The pain persisted, and one day about three years into her ordeal, it struck hard as she got ready to leave for work. She crumpled to the floor, then couldn't get up.

More doctors, more tests, more bills, more pain followed. Eventually the pain won; Garcia, then in her late forties, was forced to leave her job of fifteen years.

"It closed my world off," she recalls. "You know, you're part of the community, whether it's at work or your friends and family. Once you start dealing with the pain and you close yourself off for days at a time, you kind of lose yourself. You're free to make plans, the intentions are there, but nine times out of ten, you're going to cancel them. People keep asking you out, kind of like a formality—they don't want you to feel left out. But they eventually stop. The pain wins." As bad as the pain itself was, as she pulled back from family, friends, and her wider community, she found that the disconnect added a devastating new dimension of hurt.

After five years of mixed results from medications and procedures, Garcia was finally diagnosed with trigeminal neuralgia (TN). Lacking the funds to pay for other costly medical interventions not covered by her insurance, she turned her pragmatic, problem-solving energy to ways she could manage on her own. She was determined not to let the pain keep her at arm's length from her grandsons, from racing, and from the sense of belonging she found in the track community.

As her desire to reconnect became a powerful motivator—almost as great as her desire to tame the pain—she expanded her search for pain self-management options, adding some nonmedical approaches that she'd never considered before. She explored mindfulness-based practices, sound therapy with particular frequencies that she'd been told might promote healing, and dry needling, an acupuncture-like treatment (with a practitioner) that targets pain points. Meditation was especially helpful with both the physical pain and the anguish she felt at her isolation.

When she finally was able to return to racing, she rediscovered the joy she'd always felt roaring across the desert, as well as the embrace of that community. She also had an epiphany about where she wanted to channel her energy going forward: in raising awareness of TN, advocating for others struggling with their own pain conditions, continuing to confront her fears, and encouraging others to do so too. She launched an organization called TN Warrior Racing to help make this happen. As an African American woman on the ATV racing circuit, she says she also wanted to encourage others, and more women in general, to try racing. But even more important, she urged people to challenge themselves to move beyond fear and to seek out strength in community, as she has.

"I've raised a family and I've done all these things, I've won championships, but this is like a life goal for me," she says. "I feel like God just said, 'Well, here you go. This is your job. This is what you're going to do. Because you have trigeminal neuralgia, and you can't work a nine to five. So, hey, let's advocate. For other people.' So that's where I am."

The Need to Feel Acknowledged, Accepted, Affirmed

Social connection isn't just a practical or superficial trapping of human behavior; it's a core biological imperative reflecting the hardwired human need to feel safe. "We intuitively believe social and physical pain are radically different kinds of experiences, yet the way our brains treat them suggests that they are more similar than we imagine," writes Matthew D. Lieberman in

Social: Why Our Brains Are Wired to Connect. Simply put, humans are social because it hurts to be nonsocial.

At the heart of all of this is something even more fundamental, a basic need to be acknowledged. A Purdue University study found that people who simply made eye contact with strangers reported feeling less pain than those who felt as if people looked right through them. Reaching out, even in the smallest ways, can prevent much of the damage that social isolation causes. People with larger social networks are less likely to get sick, have sharper memories, and yes, even less physical pain.

A remarkable study led by Naomi Eisenberger, PhD, an associate professor of social psychology at UCLA, gave us an idea of how it works. She performed an fMRI study of people in a virtual ball-tossing game who were progressively excluded from receiving the ball. She found that the same areas of the brain responsible for physical pain—the anterior cingulate cortex, for example—lit up in those who'd been excluded. No surprise, then, that people feel real pain from the emotional loss of a loved one or rejection by their social group. Even animals experience pain and distress when they're separated. Though it might not leave a mark, being cast out of the tribe hurts physically.

From an evolutionary perspective, this makes sense; our prehistoric ancestors relied on social groups not just for companionship but also for survival. Staying close to the tribe brought access to shelter, food, and protection. Separation from the group meant danger.

And keep in mind that loneliness doesn't discriminate—it can affect the single and the attached, the city dweller and the suburbanite. And what's missing can be different for everyone.

I've seen this phenomenon firsthand in the stories I've covered during my own investigative work on loneliness. Some have stopped me cold, in part because they came from people with no outward hint of a problem, but mostly because the descriptions of their sense of isolation were so heartbreaking: "It's unceasing, toxic, brutal." "I feel invisible." "It's like living with a hole smack in the center of your chest—a hollow feeling." "My loneliness magnifies every pain in my body."

At any given time, at least one in five people, or roughly sixty million Americans, suffers from loneliness. By loneliness, I mean both the acute bouts of melancholy we all occasionally feel, as well as a chronic lack of intimacy—a yearning for someone to truly know you, get you, see you—that can leave people feeling deeply unmoored.

The *pain* of loneliness is what really captured my attention. It's worth pointing out that the 20 percent of Americans who suffer from loneliness have significant overlap with the approximately 20 percent of people who suffer chronic pain. For Eisenberger, that overlap presented an opportunity to try and address both issues.

In a study she coauthored, when women in long-term romantic relationships were asked to rate the pain they felt from heat applied to their arms, they reported lower levels of discomfort when looking at pictures of their partners. Simply cultivating connection through images and imagination reduced physical pain. (Lamaze, or prepared childbirth, with its focus on the supporting role of the partner, recognizes the value of this calming connection.)

I encourage you to try a version of the experiment above—without adding the painful stimulus, of course. The next time you're preparing for something uncomfortable or troubling, try sharing the experience with someone you trust to be caring and supportive. You're likely to feel some extra courage, not to mention increased pain tolerance.

Loneliness Predicts Long-Term Physical Health Consequences

A wave of new research suggests that the effects of isolation aren't only painful; they're bad for our bodies. Our physiology actually suffers. People with fewer social connections have disrupted sleep patterns, altered immune systems, more inflammation, and higher levels of stress hormones—already dominant issues for those with chronic pain. Research has found that severe loneliness is an independent predictor of pain, fatigue, depression, and the cluster of all three symptoms years later.

Calling the crisis of loneliness and isolation "one of our generation's greatest challenges," former US surgeon general Vivek Murthy declared it a national health crisis in 2023. Upon launching a national public health initiative that year, Murthy wrote in an editorial in the *New York Times* that he had suffered a dark period of deep loneliness in his own life between his first term as US surgeon general and the second. "During one of my lowest lows, the people in my life patched me up with their acts of love and connection," he wrote.

In his book *Together: The Healing Power of Human Connection in a Sometimes Lonely World*, Murthy points to the lack of training on the subject in medical schools, and the gap this creates in treating loneliness and social isolation as the serious health concern it is. The dawning recognition of social connection as a "vital sign" is crucial if we're to address it not only in community efforts but also as an important personal health issue.

Your Brain Is Ready to Network: Follow That Lead

In the conversation about pain, we talk a lot about the calming effect of connection. But just to be clear, calm isn't the only benefit of a strong connection. You are likely to have more curiosity, fun, emotional expression, and physical adventure. Spiritual connection contributes to resilience—whether that might be a feeling of connection to a higher presence or to a faith that accepts and affirms you.

The beauty of this is that opportunities for healing connection are all around us. You'll find them as soon as you begin to look—and there's no end to them. Make yourself available for the experience, whether it's initiating something as simple as eye contact or a friendly hello, responding to someone else's overture, or watching for opportunities to be supportive when others face challenges.

As the work of Eisenberger and others shows, there are shared neural pathways connecting physical and social pain, suggesting a substantial overlap between the two. And as we've seen so often in the brain's pain-processing system, the fact that this shared circuity can work both ways means that if we can ease our social pain, it may also help relieve physical pain.

Rx: Write Your Own Social Prescription

Where to start? Consider the shared roots of human connection I mentioned earlier: rituals, celebrations, past moving experiences. Each offers opportunities to share something you can tailor to your physical capabilities. If attending a birthday party is too much, you can extend an invitation for a low-key event at home, a walk, or even a video chat to connect. The point isn't the hoopla or the venue; it's to share some one-on-one time together.

Revisit the four frames identity model we explored in chapter 5, but now use the frames to identify social spheres that offer opportunities to strengthen or expand your social interactions. For example, the relational frame would include existing relationships that would benefit from some extra attention, or potential new ones from among people who may share your interests or hobbies. The communal frame would focus outward to community groups, perhaps organizations, that interest you, and offer a way to engage with others in your local community or beyond.

In practical terms, the frames serve as a tool for self-review, a prompt for reflection on strengths, vulnerabilities, obstacles, and opportunities; a window on what's working well and what you'd like to change or build on. With a clearer understanding of how pain is shaping your engagement with other people and your own interests, you can take steps to shape that part of your life.

As I've mentioned in each of the seven strategies thus far, look for opportunities for synergy. Try a cooking class that involves types of food you can enjoy, adding the element of some culinary camaraderie. Look for ways to add a low-stress buddy component to something you already enjoy doing, mixing your solo sessions with those who put you in good company. I've found that I really enjoy being in the presence of another person, even if we're doing our own things. Nowadays this often means sitting in the family room with one of my daughters, each of us immersed in our own reading. Just having someone there provides a sense of comfort, physically and emotionally.

Tips for Cultivating Social and Emotional Connections

Spending more time with friends and family can help you better manage chronic pain. Socializing calms your nervous system and decreases stress levels. It can also help alleviate feelings of depression and loneliness. As that emotional distress lessens, the severity of your pain may also decline. But what should you do if your chronic pain seems to get in the way of socializing? Here are a few tips.

Take advantage of days when pain is low. If your symptoms seem to be easing, prioritize being social on those days.

Extend an invitation. Rather than wait for an invite, take the initiative and reach out to family, friends, and acquaintances. In-person interactions have the best effect on your mood, so invite people over to your home for a visit. If you go out to socialize, suggest outings that won't aggravate your pain. For example, if you suffer from migraines, you might want to avoid loud bars or concerts.

Open up about your chronic pain. If you feel comfortable doing so, let friends and family members know about your condition and how pain affects you. If you need to cancel or reschedule plans due to a pain flare-up, they won't take it personally.

Join a support group. Online or in-person support groups can help you connect with people who are dealing with similar pain issues. These groups can provide social support, and you might learn new coping strategies from other members.

Use technology when necessary. On days when you're incapacitated by pain, consider calling, texting, or video-chatting with friends. Virtual connections aren't a perfect substitute for face-to-face interactions, but they can still help you feel connected to those you love.

Source: "Chronic Pain and Mental Health: HelpGuide.Org," May 16, 2022, https://www.helpguide.org/wellness/health-conditions/chronic-pain-and-mental-health.

CHAPTER 17

Savor Moments and Memories

Much of what you've read so far has explored how pain is manufactured in the body, where it is processed in the brain, and what you can do about it. By now, you're certainly aware that it's possible to dramatically reduce your chances of developing chronic pain and to shorten or alter the pain experience when it does arise. And yet, as so often happens when pain is the focus, there's a forgotten part of the conversation: the possibility for life not just free of pain but still full of joy.

That is where I wanted to end this book: with a reminder to *savor* as the seventh and final pain-smart strategy. The reminder to savor isn't simply the idea of diverting your attention from pain but also actively focusing on something pleasant. This isn't about distraction; it's about immersion—"Like water seeping into the soil," as Eric Garland instructs clinical trial participants in the savoring segment of MORE (mindfulness-oriented recovery enhancement).

The brain is always thirsty for a good soaking, the kind you might get by looking up into a magnificently starry sky and feeling the sense of overwhelming awe that most of us get only a few times in our life. But here's the thing: your brain is capable of producing that feeling on command. You don't have to wait for a clear night with a satin sky and the stars in alignment to have a transcendent experience.

Savoring isn't a passive emotion; it's an action. It's something you do, and you can do it with greater intention for even greater effect. You can savor every day. You can gaze at great art, listen intently to music or a bird's song, taste every morsel of your favorite meal. Take time to see something familiar with fresh eyes or even reassess the unlovely or unwelcome with fresh appreciation.

Carpe diem—"seize the day"—is one of the oldest philosophical nuggets in Western history. This two-word phrase is actually drawn from a longer passage written by the Roman poet Horace in 23 BC: *carpe diem quam minimum credula postero,* translated as "seize the day, trusting as little as possible in the next one."

This phrase has special relevance in light of modern pain science and what it tells us about the brain and our capacity to rewire our neurocircuitry to manage pain. We know that mindfulness meditation changes the brain in ways that can reduce pain or change our experience of it. Think of savoring as a special kind of mindful attention, an evidence-based therapeutic technique that intensifies the beneficial effects of positive emotional experience in the brain.

As a tool in your pain management toolbox, it is cost-free, accessible, nonpharmacological, noninvasive, and you control every aspect of it yourself. The capacity to consciously direct your attention, to choose what you target and how you titrate your focus—you own that. We can, as psychologist Albert Bandura encouraged, assert ourselves as "producers as well as products" of our lives.

"When we make a conscious choice to seize the day, even when our options are limited by circumstance, we are making a commitment to being active rather than passive beings, to pursuing our own path rather than one determined for us, to living in this moment rather than waiting for the next," writes the social philosopher Roman Krznaric in his book *Carpe Diem Regained: The Vanishing Art of Seizing the Day.* "And through that act of decision, we gain a sense of purpose by becoming the author of our own life. I choose, therefore I am."

Over twenty-five years of working as a journalist while traveling to more than a hundred countries, I have seen people at their very worst and their very best. As a trauma neurosurgeon, I have seen people rise up in impossible situations and live longer, healthier lives than I thought possible. In the personal stories shared by others in this book, this has been a recurring theme: even among those dealing day in and day out with intractable chronic pain conditions, when asked what, if anything, is a source of joy for them, they never hesitate long before smiling and naming a person or a place, or perhaps recalling a pet, or another memory—maybe a quality they discovered about themselves or witnessed in others.

They're able to be the best and bravest versions of themselves in part because of their ability to deeply engage and give meaning to these positive aspects of life. That sense of awe and connection is there for most of us, just under the surface; sometimes we just need to dig a little bit deeper to find it. When you savor, things don't feel as bleak—perhaps because you're tapping into something deeper and richer than you previously recognized.

I'm reminded of a particular stretch of high desert in South Dakota—a sprawling, roughly four-hundred-square-mile area of eroded buttes, bluffs, and pinnacles that Native American tribes are said to have named *mako sika*, which translates as "badlands." This geological aberration cuts a sudden, stark, forbidding swath across the otherwise calm expanse of the Great Plains, grassy fields abruptly giving way to a haunting moonscape. Coming upon the badlands for the first time from any direction, you might think you were at the ends of the Earth. But once you slow down and pay attention, you can see the natural boundaries of that harsh terrain and something more hospitable and even beautiful inside it. With that perspective, even the badlands can be savored.

Closer to home, look to the laboratory of childhood to find the hardwiring for elementary savoring skills. Watch kids play. For them, the world is always new and worthy of intense exploration and attention. As adults, we have the capacity for metacognition (thinking about how we think) and meta-awareness (thinking about our own consciousness), but we're often too jaded or too hurried to use it.

We lose some of our ability to sit with the full sensory experience of what's right in front of us: the subtle hues of a flower, a child's delight, a stranger's kind word, or a neighbor's helping hand. We dwell on past disappointments and dampen our expectations of the future rather than allow ourselves to simply savor the pleasure of anticipation. We become less willing to try new things outside our comfort zone. After all, when was the last time you did something for the *first* time?

Beauty and the Brain: Training the Eye of the Beholder

Fred Bryant, PhD, professor in the department of psychology at Loyola University in Chicago, and his late collaborator Joseph Veroff, wrote the seminal book *Savoring: A New Model of Positive Experience.* Now, nearly twenty years later, savoring is a core concept in positive psychology. But if you're tempted to think of positive psychology as "psychology lite," or savoring as nothing more than a "stop to smell the flowers" bumper sticker, the research literature and extensive evidence in gold-standard clinical trials and treatments like the MORE program show otherwise. Bryant himself shared an overview just a few years ago of the concept's evolution, directions he sees for future research, and, most helpful for our purposes, the mechanisms that make savoring work and how we can get the most out of it.

The essence of savoring is surprisingly simple, Bryant notes, quoting the seventeenth-century French writer François de La Rochefoucauld: "Happiness does not consist in things themselves but in the relish we have of them."

Savoring: Three Steps, Plus Our Own Strategies, Rewire the Neurocircuitry of Rewards

Three essential components mark the pathways into the extended positive experience of savoring.

Savoring the past, or reminiscence—for example, remembering a special moment with a friend or loved one, a favorite trip, or a memorable meal.

Savoring the present, or being in the moment as it unfolds. You might focus on a meal as you eat, taking in the smells, taste, and textures of the food. Or on a walk outdoors, focus your attention on the sensory experience of the sights, sounds, and smells around you.

Savoring the future, or *anticipation*. You might visualize an upcoming event, vacation, or a personal milestone and how you plan to celebrate.

Different savoring strategies might include sharing memories with others, creating occasions for memory making, congratulating yourself on an accomplishment, celebrating qualities you feel good about, or simply counting your blessings.

Don't underestimate the positive experience of repetition. Remember, repetition is the way we learn anything new, whether that's a dance step, a physical therapy exercise, a craft skill, a practice like diaphragmatic breathing or mindful meditation. Practice makes possible the incremental gains toward mastery, and there can be incredible joy in that.

"We are prone to neglect pleasurable situational nuances that we can discover only through continued exposure," Bryant says, adding that in some contexts, repetition can be equally or more enjoyable than a novel experience. In fact, the ability to savor repetition may be the mark of mastery, he suggests: "Those who are more skilled at savoring are better able to seek out, find, and appreciate the unforeseen pleasures that await discovery in repeating familiar positive experiences."

Explore ways to heighten your sensory perception of different types of positive stimuli. For example, concentrating your gaze can boost the impact of visual stimuli, whether you're looking at a rose or merely a photograph of one. Closing your eyes can intensify the pleasure of physical sensations or of listening to music. Stretch your savoring repertoire to include not only reactive savoring, which occurs spontaneously when something presents itself, but also proactive savoring, or deliberately seeking out or creating the positive experience.

The more strategies in the mix, the better. Studies have found that "the happiest individuals generally have a wider range of savoring strategies that they use across a greater variety of situations," Bryant notes. "Having a broader savoring repertoire and knowing when and how to use optimal combinations of various savoring strategies seems most beneficial."

Although you don't have to be an expert to practice savoring in this way, you may find it helpful to consult one for specific coaching regarding pain management. Psychologists and others who work with the therapeutic principles of positive psychology have developed savoring strategies and interventions they can tailor to your more specific circumstances, as Garland has done in the MORE protocol to reduce pain and opioid misuse risk.

Some of these address pain directly, as you'll see below in the rheumatoid arthritis study. Others may improve pain through strengthening resiliency, boosting a sense of agency, buffering the negative effects of chronic illness on a sense of well-being, or food-related behaviors that increase people's consumption of healthy foods, decrease overeating, and promote a healthy relationship with food. As you know by now, all of these are relevant in managing or preventing pain.

The Rheumatoid Arthritis Trial

When I first saw savoring as a specific piece of Garland's mindfulness-based MORE therapy protocol (see chapter 10), I was intrigued by the data. The fact that the intervention has been effective in the opioid reduction effort was encouraging enough. But on top of that, I found the possibility that mindfulness-based savoring meditation could directly reduce pain—in a measurable way—really exciting.

Garland joined colleagues on a multidisciplinary team from the University of Virginia, Johns Hopkins, the University of Maryland, the University of California, San Diego, and Western University in Ontario to find out how it might all work. The 2023 randomized, controlled trial to study the mechanism of savoring meditation in people with rheumatoid arthritis found that the practice:

- Produced a meaningful analgesic effect in response to experimental pain stimuli.
- Increased activation and functional connectivity of the ventromedial prefrontal cortex, which plays a key role in a range of functions that include not only emotion regulation but also social cognition, memory, and decision making.
- Increased the experience of positive emotions.
- Reduced anhedonic symptoms, or the inability to experience pleasure in normally pleasurable things.

Participants in the trial were forty-four patients diagnosed with rheumatoid arthritis who were randomized to either a savoring meditation or a slow-breathing control group. The savoring participants were trained to generate positive emotional memories, enjoy a multisensory experience of positive emotions arising from those memories, and maintain attention toward that positive emotional state during periods of elevated pain. The approach was derived in part from the mindfulness-based savoring skills taught in MORE, as well as prior experimental work on positive autobiographical memories.

Both meditation interventions were brief (four twenty-minute sessions), and afterward the participants practiced the meditation technique on which they had been trained while exposed to nonpainful and painful heat stimuli in an fMRI scanner.

The researchers found that savoring significantly reduced the experimental pain intensity ratings. Participants in the savoring group also reported significantly increased positive emotions, as well as reduced symptoms of the flat response to normally pleasurable things. And finally, savoring was found to recruit reward-enhancing brain circuits when the body is confronted with pain.

Slow Down, Press Pause, Linger

The good news is that despite its neurocomplexity, savoring is simple. The challenge, if you can call it that, is that it requires you to slow down, even if only for an impromptu minute, to listen to the birds, study the ripples of color in tulip petals, or just focus on the feel of a breeze on your skin. Don't multitask. And remember that the active ingredient of savoring involves not just the awareness of pleasure, but also a conscious attention to the experience of pleasure.

If you're naturally inclined to this kind of reflection but have never tried a focused exercise like this, I recommend it. Purposefully holding your gaze or your thought in that positive energy just a little longer than you might ordinarily do can yield some surprising sensations.

Here's a simple way to start:

- Focus your attention on what is pleasant, beautiful, and good in your life: pleasurable sights, sounds, smells, textures, or memories that evoke those sensations.
- Let positive emotions and pleasurable body sensations emerge from that experience, thought, or memory.
- If there's a "badlands" equivalent in your experience, turn your sustained attention to a positive reappraisal.
- Recognize positive emotions in your mind or sensations of pleasure in the body.
- Turn your attention inward to savor the positive inner feeling.
- Imagine breathing it into the center of your being. Or as Garland puts it, picture it like water seeping into the soil.

More suggestions, distilling the wisdom from dozens of sources including mental health professionals, friends, family, colleagues, and of course my mother and father, include these:

- Focus on something specific and set the rest aside.
- Share experiences and memories with others.
- Take a mental picture. Use your mind's eye and your own sensory "apps" to take in colors, light and dark, and other aspects of the subject.

- Don't overthink it. Save analytical or critical reflection for later.
- Appreciate the bittersweet and other emotional textures of life. Beauty is there too.

Stick to savoring. Let the rest wait.

- Don't turn to your to-do list or succumb to distraction. Stick to savoring for the time you've planned.
- Don't give traction to negative, critical, or worrisome thoughts if they arise. Just observe them, and set them aside, or practice using them as a cue to refocus your attention on the savoring experience.
- Don't be a killjoy, dismissing this pleasurable exercise as naive or a waste of time. It isn't. You're actively rewiring your brain to counter pain in ways that strengthen with practice. This is nature's evolutionary gift to you. Seize the moment!

The poet and author Ross Gay says that he sets out in his work "to investigate what practices, habits, rituals, and understandings—you know, the stuff we do and think and believe—make joy more available to us. What in our lives prepares the ground for joy . . . what *incites* joy," he writes in his book of essays of the same name. "But what happens," he posits, "if joy is not separate from pain? What if joy and pain are fundamentally tangled up with one another?" Such was the case with my mom and me.

I'm sitting on the second floor of my parents' condominium in Fort Myers, Florida. Three months have passed since my mom had her fall and experienced the worst pain in her life—a pain that made her want to stop living. Looking out the window, I see her walking hand in hand with my dad. In his right hand he has a cane, and with his left, he's gripping my mother's hand tightly, seeming almost scared to let her go.

As is often the case with Indian immigrants of their age, my parents hardly ever displayed affection, and I'm not sure I ever heard them say "I love you" to one another. Even holding hands was considered too much

PDA. But now here they are, fingers intertwined, ambling along as my mom's face lights up in a smile. I can almost hear her schoolgirlish giggling all the way up here.

I would never wish the pain my mother experienced on anyone. And yet that pain is what ultimately brought her to a new place. She underwent surgery, which helped tremendously. But she also learned to scan her body in ways she had never done before. Never particularly self-reflective, my mother became a master of analytical meditation. And now, as I silently watched my parents walk together, I saw her savor life in a way I'd never seen before. With her face turned up to the sun, her hand clutching that of the man she loves, she was absorbing every moment, not only helping to free her from pain but also filling her with joy.

Acknowledgments

For the countless people who came forward to share their deeply personal stories during the most vulnerable times in their lives. Through highs and lows, and some incredibly painful days, you were willing to talk, with the hope your experience could help others.

And for the pain specialists who dedicate their lives to alleviate suffering. You inspired me to write this book. For years, pain was thought to be a necessary consequence of living, but these scientists convinced me otherwise. They often spend their days caring for patients who too often feel forgotten or neglected, and in the process they have developed simple, effective, and sometimes revolutionary ways to deal with pain. I greatly appreciate your candor and your willingness to share your stories and translate the remarkable new developments in the world of pain science.

Priscilla Painton is one of the great giants of the publishing world. Her editorial skills are unparalleled, simply the best. Clean, seamless, and purposeful. I may be a brain surgeon, but she is a master surgeon of the literary world. I am so honored and lucky to work alongside you.

One of the wonderful things about working with Simon & Schuster is that it feels like family. Johanna Li feels like a sibling now, always making sure I took care of myself while making our deadlines.

We should all be so lucky to have a Jonathan Karp in our lives. He is a constant reminder that these books matter more than ever, and he will always be a protector of their legacy. Bob Barnett is my lawyer, and the day he agreed to take me on as a client was one of the best days of my life. I am still not sure how I made his list, considering he represents presidents, pundits, and even the pope.

Lisa Dickey, you are the closer we all need in our lives, helping smooth out the rough edges, offering up lovely suggestions and providing doses of enthusiasm at the exact right moments.

From design to delivery into readers' hands, my gratitude to senior production editor Yvette Grant, copyeditor Bev Miller, book interior designer Joy O'Meara, cover designer Jackie Seow, publicist Elizabeth Herman, and marketing specialist Elizabeth Venere for their masterful work.

AARP's partnership has been invaluable, thanks to Leah Miller, AARP director of publishing, and fact-checkers Stephanie Abramson and Claudia Bloom.

Also indispensable, Steve Weiner, Becca Barker, Aaron Weiner, and Leslie Rowan, through Readmore Communications, Inc.

And, Teresa Barker. You have been a world-class collaborator and I greatly appreciate your time and energy. You dealt with my sudden bursts of new ideas with unfaltering patience, and always kept the Pain Train moving forward. This book would not have been possible without you. Collectively, we offered up a reminder for millions of people around the world that as difficult as life may be, there is still hope, and it doesn't have to hurt.

Notes

Introduction

xiii **"It puts you":** Bess Talbot interviews with Teresa Barker, November 20, 2023; January 8, May 18, November 8, 20, 2024; January 27, 2025.

xv **"Genetics put the":** Joel Saper interviews with Teresa Barker, August 15, 2023; February 16, July 25, 2024.

xvii **Nearly one-quarter:** Lucas, Jacqueline W., and Sohi, Inderbier. *Chronic Pain and High-Impact Chronic Pain in US Adults, 2023.* National Center for Health Statistics, US Centers for Disease Control and Prevention. November 21, 2024. https://doi.org/10.15620/cdc/.

xvii **Among those who:** Rikard, S. Michaela, Andrea E. Strahan, Kristine M. Schmit, and Gery P. Guy Jr. "Chronic Pain among Adults—United States, 2019–2021." *Morbidity and Mortality Weekly Report* 72 (2023), https://doi.org/10.15585/mmwr.mm7215a1.

xviii **In its 2022 survey report:** US Pain Foundation. *A Chronic Pain Crisis: 2022 Survey Report.* 2022. https://uspainfoundation.org/wp-content/uploads/2022/07/A-Chronic-Pain-Crisis-US-Pain-2022-FINAL.pdf.

xix **In some cases:** Devitt, James. "Memories Are Not Only in the Brain." NYU, November 7, 2024. http://www.nyu.edu/content/nyu/en/about/news-publications/news/2024/november/memories-are-not-only-in-the-brain--new-research-finds.

xix **Yet this hasn't:** Parser, Parveen, Pinar Ozcan, and Kathryn L. Terry. "Endometriosis: Epidemiology, Diagnosis and Clinical Management." *Current Obstetrics and Gynecology Reports* 6, no. 1 (March 2017): 34–41. https://doi.org/10.1007/s13669-017-0187-1.

xx **This amid a flurry:** Blades, Nicole. "How We Recover from Minor Injuries Is Changing." *Wall Street Journal*, January 25, 2025. https://www.wsj.com/lifestyle/fitness/injury-recovery-ice-rest-exercise-science-ca1c1774; Collins, Lauren. "PEACE and LOVE; the NEW Acronym for the Management of Acute Soft Tissue

Injuries." Berwick Family Osteopathy and Spinal Clinic, January 12, 2022. https://www.berwickfamilyosteopathy.com.au/peace-and-love-the-new-acronym-for-the-management-of-acute-soft-tissue-injuries/; Rawson, Ben. "Recovery from Athletic Injuries: Is MEAT Better Than RICE?," Center for Healing and Regenerative Medicine, May 10, 2021. https://charmaustin.com/recovery-from-athletic-injuries-meat-over-rice/; Physiopedia. "Soft Tissue Injuries." Revised March 22, 2025. https://www.physio-pedia.com/Soft_Tissue_Injuries.

xxi **A consortium pain:** Tick, Heather, Arya Nielsen, Kenneth R. Pelletier, Robert Bonakdar, Samantha Simmons, Ronald Glick, et al. "Evidence-Based Nonpharmacologic Strategies for Comprehensive Pain Care: The Consortium Pain Task Force White Paper." *Explore* 14, no. 3 (2018): 177–211. https://doi.org/10.1016/j.explore.2018.02.001.

Chapter 2 Tell Me about Your Pain

13 **As she talked:** Wendy Miller interviews with Teresa Barker, May 29, 2023; March 3, 2024; email interviews with Teresa Barker, August–September 2023; March 2, March 19, March 28, June 7, July 31, 2024.

13 **I was reminded of:** Frida Kahlo (website). Accessed December 9, 2024. https://www.fridakahlo.org.

13 **Just forty-seven when she died:** Lawson-Tancred, Jo. "Does Frida Kahlo's Art Hold the Key to a Hidden Medical Condition?" Artnet, October 25, 2024. https://news.artnet.com/art-world/frida-kahlo-new-diagnosis-2558956; Institut Guttmann. "Frida Kahlo: Diagnosis 70 Years after Her Death." October 9, 2024. https://www.guttmann.com/en/news/frida-kahlo-diagnosis-70-years-after-her-death; Arslantas, Oyku, Sergiu Albu, Josep Valls-Sole, and Hatice Kumru. "Frida Kahlo Could Have Had Cauda Equina Syndrome: A Case Report." *Journal of Neurology* 271, no. 12 (December 2024): 7619–7621. https://doi.org/10.1007/s00415-024-12695-5.

13 **Kahlo was often:** Gracia, Peyton. Laura. "Inside the Fantastical World of Frida Kahlo." *MSU Denver RED,* April 8, 2022. https://red.msudenver.edu/2022/inside-the-fantastical-world-of-frida-kahlo/.

14 **"I don't paint":** Frida Kahlo (website). Accessed December 9, 2024. https://www.fridakahlo.org.

15 **quick-list questionnaire called WILDA:** Fink, Regina. "Pain Assessment: The Cornerstone to Optimal Pain Management." *Proceedings (Baylor University. Medical Center)* 13, no. 3 (July 2000): 236–239. https://doi.org/10.1080/08998280.2000.11927681.

16 **A pocket card:** Murray, Patti, and Donna Barker. "C4 An Institutional Comprehensive Pain Assessment: WILDA Revised." *Pain Management Nursing* 19, no. 2 (April 1, 2018): 106. https://doi.org/10.1016/j.pmn.2018.02.043.

20 **Some of these distinctions:** National Institute of Neurological Disorders and Stroke. "Pain." National Institutes of Health (NIH). Reviewed February 12, 2025. https://www.ninds.nih.gov/health-information/disorders/pain.

20 **So is gout:** Fenando, Ardy, Manjeera Rednam, Rahul Gujarathi, and Jason Widrich. "Gout." In *StatPearls [Internet]*. StatPearls Publishing, 2024. https://www.ncbi.nlm.nih.gov/books/NBK546606/.

23 **"This is one":** Roger Fillingim interview with Teresa Barker, February 23, 2024.

24 **"Most people are":** Carmen Green interview with Sanjay Gupta, November 30, 2021.

25 **In 2016, a University of Virginia:** Hoffman, Kelly M., Sophie Trawalter, Jordan R. Axt, and M. Norman Oliver. "Racial Bias in Pain Assessment and Treatment Recommendations, and False Beliefs about Biological Differences Between Blacks and Whites." *Proceedings of the National Academy of Sciences of the United States of America* 113, no. 16 (April 4, 2016): 4296. https://doi.org/10.1073/pnas.1516047113.

25 **minority women were 52 percent:** Anderson, Karen O., Carmen R. Green, and Richard Payne. "Racial and Ethnic Disparities in Pain: Causes and Consequences of Unequal Care." *Journal of Pain* 10, no. 12 (December 1, 2009): 1187–1204. https://doi.org/10.1016/j.jpain.2009.10.002.

28 **But other forms of acute:** Casale, Roberto, Fabiola Atzeni, Laura Bazzichi, Giovanna Beretta, Elisabetta Costantini, et al. "Pain in Women: A Perspective Review on a Relevant Clinical Issue That Deserves Prioritization." *Pain and Therapy* 10, no. 1 (June 2021): 287–314. https://doi.org/10.1007/s40122-021-00244-1.

28 **anxiety, depression, and sleep issues:** Brown, Donnamay, Sabrina Schenk, Dunja Genent, Boris Zernikow, and Julia Wager. "A Scoping Review of Chronic Pain in Emerging Adults." *PAIN Reports* 6, no. 1 (April 1, 2021): e920. https://doi.org/10.1097/PR9.0000000000000920; Lunde, Claire E., Emma Fisher, Elizabeth Donovan, Danijela Serbic, and Christine B. Sieberg. "Cutting the Cord? Parenting Emerging Adults with Chronic Pain." *Paediatric and Neonatal Pain* 4, no. 3 (2022): 136–147. https://doi.org/10.1002/pne2.12072; McLean, Carmen P., Anu Asnaani, Brett T. Litz, and Stefan G. Hofmann. "Gender Differences in Anxiety Disorders: Prevalence, Course of Illness, Comorbidity and Burden of Illness." *Journal of Psychiatric Research* 45, no. 8 (August 2011): 1027–1035. https://doi.org/10.1016/j.jpsychires.2011.03.006.

28 **Only in 2024:** Wright, Vonda J., Jonathan D. Schwartzman, Rafael Itinoche, and Jocelyn Wittstein. "The Musculoskeletal Syndrome of Menopause." *Climacteric: Journal of the International Menopause Society* 27, no. 5 (October 2024): 466–472. https://doi.org/10.1080/13697137.2024.2380363.

29 **This social media campaign:** Wu, Jenny, Esmé Trahair, Megan Happ, and Jonas Swartz. "TikTok, #IUD, and User Experience with Intrauterine Devices Reported on Social Media." *Obstetrics and Gynecology* 141, no. 1 (January 2023): 215. https://doi.org/10.1097/AOG.0000000000005027; Bever, Lindsey. "IUD Placement

Can Be Painful. These Women Used Their Phones to Record It." *Washington Post*, March 25, 2024. https://www.washingtonpost.com/wellness/2024/03/25/tiktok-iud-birth-control-pain/.

29 **While the CDC action:** Curtis, Kathryn M., Antoinette T. Nguyen, Naomi K. Tepper, Lauren B. Zapata, Emily M. Snyder, Kendra Hatfield-Timajchy, Katherine Kortsmit, Megan A. Cohen, and Maura K. Whiteman. "U.S. Selected Practice Recommendations for Contraceptive Use, 2024." *Morbidity and Mortality Weekly Report* 73, no. 3 (August 8, 2024): 1–77. http://dx.doi.org/10.15585/mmwr.rr7303a1.

29 **women were overmedicated:** Zucker, Irving, and Brian J. Prendergast. "Sex Differences in Pharmacokinetics Predict Adverse Drug Reactions in Women." *Biology of Sex Differences* 11 (June 5, 2020): 32. https://doi.org/10.1186/s13293-020-00308-5.

30 **"need to immediately reevaluate":** Lemer, Louise. "Women Are Overmedicated Because Drug Dosage Trials Are Done on Men, Study Finds." UChicago News, June 22, 2020. https://news.uchicago.edu/story/women-are-overmedicated-because-drug-dosage-trials-are-done-men-study-finds.

30 **physicians respond to pain differently:** Weisse, Carol S., Paul C. Sorum, Kafi N. Sanders, and Beth L. Syat. "Do Gender and Race Affect Decisions about Pain Management?" *Journal of General Internal Medicine* 16, no. 4 (April 2001): 211–217. https://doi.org/10.1046/j.1525-1497.2001.016004211.x.

30 **their own sex or race:** Schulman, Kevin A., Jesse A. Berlin, William Harless, Jon F. Kerner, Shyrl Sistrunk, et al. "The Effect of Race and Sex on Physicians' Recommendations for Cardiac Catheterization." *New England Journal of Medicine* 340, no. 8 (February 25, 1999): 618–626. https://doi.org/10.1056/NEJM199902253400806.

31 **Not wanting the clinician:** Levy, Andrea Gurmankin, Aaron M. Scherer, Brian J. Zikmund-Fisher, Knoll Larkin, Geoffrey D. Barnes, and Angela Fagerlin. "Prevalence of and Factors Associated with Patient Nondisclosure of Medically Relevant Information to Clinicians." *JAMA Network Open* 1, no. 7 (November 30, 2018): e185293. https://doi.org/10.100SIDEBAR1/jamanetworkopen.2018.5293.

31 **Many already feel stigmatized:** Devitt, Michael. "Many Patients Hide Life-Threatening Issues from Clinicians." American Academy of Family Physicians, September 10, 2019. https://www.aafp.org/news/health-of-the-public/20190910withhholdinfo.html; Politi, Mary C., Melissa A. Clark, Gene Armstrong, Kelly A. McGarry, and Christopher N. Sciamanna. "Patient–Provider Communication about Sexual Health among Unmarried Middle-Aged and Older Women." *Journal of General Internal Medicine* 24, no. 4 (February 14, 2009): 511. https://doi org/10.1007/s11606-009-0930-z; Yang, Xin, Jason Parton, Dwight Lewis, Ning Yang, and Matthew Hudnall. "Effect of Patient-Physician Relationship on Withholding Information Behavior: Analysis of Health Information National Trends Survey

(2011–2018) Data." *Journal of Medical Internet Research* 22, no. 1 (January 29, 2020): e16713. https://doi.org/10.2196/16713.

31 **"the whole long Covid thing":** Yale Medicine. "Long COVID (Post-COVID Conditions, PCC)." Accessed February 27, 2025. https://www.yalemedicine.org/conditions/long-covid-post-covid-conditions-pcc; CDC. "Long COVID Basics." February 3, 2025. https://www.cdc.gov/covid/long-term-effects/index.html.

31 **One major survey:** Gavin, Kara. "Aching Joints Make Older Adults Reach for Many Forms of Pain Relief—but Health Risks Could Follow." Michigan Medicine, University of Michigan. September 12, 2022. https://www.michiganmedicine.org/health-lab/aching-joints-make-older-adults-reach-many-forms-pain-relief-health-risks-could-follow.

32 **Why Patients Lie:** Levy, Andrea Gurmankin, Aaron M. Scherer, Brian J. Zikmund-Fisher, Knoll Larkin, Geoffrey D. Barnes, and Angela Fagerlin. "Prevalence of and Factors Associated with Patient Nondisclosure of Medically Relevant Information to Clinicians." *JAMA Network Open* 1, no. 7 (November 30, 2018): e185293. https://doi.org/10.1001/jamanetworkopen.2018.5293.

33 **"I would hear the stories":** Eve Valera interview with Teresa Barker, March 4, 2024, and emails.

34 **head injuries or strangulation:** St. Ivany, Amanda, and Donna Schminkey. "Intimate Partner Violence and Traumatic Brain Injury: State of the Science and Next Steps." *Family and Community Health* 39, no. 2 (2016): 129–137. https://doi.org/10.1097/FCH.0000000000000094.

34 **The early years:** Boserup, Brad, Mark McKenney, and Adel Elkbuli. "Alarming Trends in US Domestic Violence during the COVID-19 Pandemic." *American Journal of Emergency Medicine* 38, no. 12 (December 2020): 2753–2755. https://doi.org/10.1016/j.ajem.2020.04.077; Valera, Eve. "Intimate Partner Violence and Brain Injury: A Selective Overview." Brain Injury Professional, June 13, 2023. https://braininjuryprofessional.com/intimate-partner-violence-and-brain-injury-a-selective-overview/.

35 **"'why don't you try'":** Linda Porter interview with Teresa Barker, January 23, 2024.

Chapter 3 Mastermind: The Brain as Pain Maker

38 **mood, emotions, mind-set:** Buckingham, Ashley, and Elizabeth J. Richardson. "The Relationship Between Psychological Resilience and Pain Threshold and Tolerance: Optimism and Grit as Moderators." *Journal of Clinical Psychology in Medical Settings* 28, no. 3 (September 1, 2021): 518–528. https://doi.org/10.1007/s10880-020-09731-7; Coen, Steven J., Lidia Yágüez, Qasim Aziz, Martina T. Mitterschiffthaler, Mick Brammer, Steven C. R. Williams, and Lloyd J. Gregory. "Negative Mood Affects Brain Processing of Visceral Sensation." *Gastroenterology* 137, no. 1 (July 1,

2009): 253–261.e2. https://doi.org/10.1053/j.gastro.2009.02.052; Nielsen, Christopher S., Roland Staud, and Donald D. Price. "Individual Differences in Pain Sensitivity: Measurement, Causation, and Consequences." *The Journal of Pain* 10, no. 3 (March 1, 2009): 231–237. https://doi.org/10.1016/j.jpain.2008.09.010.

40 **"It's not at all":** Clifford Woolf interview with Teresa Barker, February 8, 2024.

41 **"labor simulator" experience:** Grassullo, Stephanie. "Men Take Part in Simulated Labor Experience and Their Reactions Are Priceless." *The Bump*. Updated November 26, 2018. https://www.thebump.com/news/labor-pain-experience-ultrasound-babyface.

42 **Fibromyalgia, chronic and often intense:** Bhargava, Juhi, and John A. Hurley. "Fibromyalgia." In *StatPearls [Internet]*. StatPearls Publishing, 2024. http://www.ncbi.nlm.nih.gov/books/NBK540974/.

43 **One simple model:** Chen, Qiliang, and Mary M. Heinricher. "Shifting the Balance: How Top-Down and Bottom-Up Input Modulate Pain via the Rostral Ventromedial Medulla." *Frontiers in Pain Research* 3 (June 28, 2022): 932476. https://doi.org/10.3389/fpain.2022.932476.

45 **Sensory neurons:** Science Direct. "Nociception." Accessed August 30, 2024. https://www.sciencedirect.com/topics/neuroscience/nociception.

45 **The revised definition:** Raja, Srinivasa N., Daniel B. Carr, Milton Cohen, Nanna B. Finnerup, Herta Flor, Stephen Gibson, Francis J. Keefe, et al. "The Revised International Association for the Study of Pain Definition of Pain: Concepts, Challenges, and Compromises." *Pain* 161, no. 9 (September 1, 2020): 1976–1982. https://doi.org/10.1097/j.pain.0000000000001939.

45 **a moot point to the brain:** Garland, Eric L. "Pain Processing in the Human Nervous System." *Primary Care: Clinics in Office Practice* 39, no. 3 (September 2012): 561–571. https://doi.org/10.1016/j.pop.2012.06.013.

47 **All of that shapes:** Mackey, Sean. "Pain and the Brain." Stanford Pain Medicine, 2016. https://www.facebook.com/watch/?v=1313293282022746.

50 **"We can chat":** Randolph Nesse interview with Teresa Barker, March 11, 2024.

51 **So if you simply believe:** Barnes, Kirsten, Nicolas A. McNair, Justin A. Harris, Louise Sharpe, and Ben Colagiuri. "In Anticipation of Pain: Expectancy Modulates Corticospinal Excitability, Autonomic Response, and Pain Perception." *Pain* 162, no. 8 (August 1, 2021): 2287–2296. https://doi.org/10.1097/j.pain.0000000000002222.

51 **The famous "rubber hand":** Garner, Brit, host. "How Well Do You Know Your Own Hand?" *SciShow Psych*, April 13, 2017. https://www.youtube.com/watch?v=E7qpQiwxv1A.

52 **Canadian psychologist Donald O. Hebb:** Langille, Jesse J., and Richard E. Brown. "The Synaptic Theory of Memory: A Historical Survey and Reconciliation of Recent Opposition." *Frontiers in Systems Neuroscience* 12 (October 26, 2018): 52. https://doi.org/10.3389/fnsys.2018.00052.

53 **Merzenich, considered:** Merzenich, Michael. *Soft-Wired: How the New Science of Brain Plasticity Can Change Your Life*. Parnassus Publishing, 2013, 236–237.

53 **It's not only the most:** Fitzcharles, Mary-Ann, Steven P. Cohen, Daniel J. Clauw, Geoffrey Littlejohn, Chie Usui, and Winfried Häuser. "Nociplastic Pain: Towards an Understanding of Prevalent Pain Conditions." *The Lancet* 397, no. 10289 (May 29, 2021): 2098–2110. https://doi.org/10.1016/S0140-6736(21)00392-5.

56 **"How do you take them":** Linda Porter interview with Teresa Barker, January 23, 2024.

56 **Many healing traditions:** Bautista-Valarezo, Estefanía, Víctor Duque, Adriana Elizabeth Verdugo Sánchez, Viviana Dávalos-Batallas, Nele R. M. Michels, Kristin Hendrickx, and Veronique Verhoeven, et al. "Towards an Indigenous Definition of Health: An Explorative Study to Understand the Indigenous Ecuadorian People's Health and Illness Concepts." *International Journal for Equity in Health* 19, no. 1 (June 22, 2020): 101. https://doi.org/10.1186/s12939-020-1142-8; Lewis, Gwyn N., Nusratnaaz Shaikh, Grace Wang, Shikha Chaudhary, Debbie J. Bean, and Gareth Terry. "Chinese and Indian Interpretations of Pain: A Qualitative Evidence Synthesis to Facilitate Chronic Pain Management." *Pain Practice* 23, no. 6 (July 2023): 647–663. https://doi.org/10.1111/papr.13226; Ding, Zuoqi, and Furong Li. "Publications in Integrative and Complementary Medicine: A Ten-Year Bibliometric Survey in the Field of ICM." *Evidence-Based Complementary and Alternative Medicine: eCAM* 2020 (October 6, 2020): 4821950. https://doi.org/10.1155/2020/4821950; Ogbu, Chukwuemeka E., Chisa Oparanma, Stella C. Ogbu, Otobo I. Ujah, Menkeoma L. Okoli, and Russell S. Kirby. "Trends in the Use of Complementary and Alternative Therapies among US Adults with Current Asthma." *Epidemiologia* 4, no. 1 (March 21, 2023): 94–105. https://doi.org/10.3390/epidemiologia4010010.

59 **But when these mediators:** Juhn, Steven K., Min-Kyo Jung, Mark D. Hoffman, Brian R. Drew, Diego A. Preciado, Nicholas J. Sausen, Timothy T. K. Jung, et al. "The Role of Inflammatory Mediators in the Pathogenesis of Otitis Media and Sequelae." *Clinical and Experimental Otorhinolaryngology* 1, no. 3 (September 2008): 117. https://doi.org/10.3342/ceo.2008.1.3.117; Chen, Linlin, Huidan Deng, Hengmin Cui, Jing Fang, Zhicai Zuo, Junliang Deng, Yinglun Li, Xun Wang, and Ling Zhao. "Inflammatory Responses and Inflammation-Associated Diseases in Organs." *Oncotarget* 9, no. 6 (December 14, 2017): 7204–7218. https://doi.org/10.18632/oncotarget.23208.

59 **Some have even suggested:** Omoigui, Sota. "The Biochemical Origin of Pain—Proposing a New Law of Pain: The Origin of All Pain Is Inflammation and the Inflammatory Response. Part 1 of 3—A Unifying Law of Pain." *Medical Hypotheses* 69, no. 1 (2007): 70–82. https://doi.org/10.1016/j.mehy.2006.11.028.

60 **When researchers silenced:** Jin, Hao, Mengtong Li, Eric Jeong, Felipe Castro-Martinez, and Charles S. Zuker. "A Body–Brain Circuit That Regulates Body In-

flammatory Responses." *Nature* 630, no. 8017 (June 2024): 695–703. https://doi.org/10.1038/s41586-024-07469-y.

60 **"The results suggest":** Guglielmi, Giorgia. "Found: The Dial in the Brain That Controls the Immune System." *Nature,* May 1, 2024. https://doi.org/10.1038/d41586-024-01259-2.

Chapter 4 Hot-Wired: What Trips the Switch for Chronic Pain?

63 **Looked at from:** De La Rosa, Jennifer S., Benjamin R. Brady, Mohab M. Ibrahim, Katherine E. Herder, Jessica S. Wallace, Alyssa R. Padilla, and Todd W. Vanderah. "Co-Occurrence of Chronic Pain and Anxiety/Depression Symptoms in U.S. Adults: Prevalence, Functional Impacts, and Opportunities." *Pain* 165, no. 3 (March 2024): 666–673. https://doi.org/10.1097/j.pain.0000000000003056.

63 **A recent study:** De La Rosa, et al. "Co-Occurrence of Chronic Pain," 666.

64 **When these conditions coexist:** Surah, A., G. Baranidharan, and S. Morley. "Chronic Pain and Depression." *Continuing Education in Anaesthesia, Critical Care and Pain* 14, no. 2 (April 1, 2014): 85–89. https://doi.org/10.1093/bjaceaccp/mkt046.

65 **"Sometimes, it's fear":** Howard Schubiner email interview with Teresa Barker, May 28, 2024.

65 **Living It: Courtney Putnam:** Courtney Putnam interview with Teresa Barker, December 20, 2023.

66 **"In a very simple":** Vania Apkarian interview with Teresa Barker, March 27, 2024.

67 **"With the networked":** Mansour, A. R., M. A. Farmer, M. N. Baliki, and A. Vania Apkarian. "Chronic Pain: The Role of Learning and Brain Plasticity." *Restorative Neurology and Neuroscience* 32, no. 1 (2014): 129–139. https://doi.org/10.3233/RNN-139003.

68 **McGill University geneticist:** Parisien, Marc, Lucas V. Lima, Concetta Dagostino, Nehme El-Hachem, Gillian L. Drury, Audrey V. Grant, Jonathan Huising, et al. "Acute Inflammatory Response via Neutrophil Activation Protects Against the Development of Chronic Pain." *Science Translational Medicine* 14, no. 644 (May 11, 2022): eabj9954. https://doi.org/10.1126/scitranslmed.abj9954.

68 **It was as if:** Luda Diatchenko interview with Teresa Barker, January 19, 2024.

68 **This finding:** Mast, Jason. "In Radical Claim, Study Suggests Inflammation Wards Off Chronic Pain Instead of Causing It." *STAT,* May 11, 2022. https://www.statnews.com/2022/05/11/study-suggests-inflammation-wards-off-chronic-pain/.

69 **Over a hundred years ago:** Osler, Sir William. *The Quotable Osler.* ACP Press, 2008.

69 **This reverse translational research:** Barroso, Joana, Paulo Branco, and Apkar Vania Apkarian. "Brain Mechanisms of Chronic Pain: Critical Role of Translational Approach." *Translational Research: The Journal of Laboratory and Clinical Medicine* 238 (December 2021): 76–89. https://doi.org/10.1016/j.trsl.2021.06.004.

70 **In 2023, his team was able:** Shirvalkar, P., J. Prosky, G. Chin, P. Ahmadipour, O. Sani, M. Desai, et al. "First-in-Human Prediction of Chronic Pain State Using In-

tracranial Neural Biomarkers." *Nature Neuroscience* 26 (2023): 1090–1099. https://doi.org/10.1038/s41593-023-01338-z.

71 **"The findings represent":** Fontaine, Denys, Valentin Vielzeuf, Philippe Genestier, Pascal Limeux, Serena Santucci-Sivilotto, Emmanuel Mory, Nelly Darmon, et al. "Artificial Intelligence to Evaluate Postoperative Pain Based on Facial Expression Recognition." *European Journal of Pain* 26, no. 6 (2022): 1282–1291. https://doi.org/10.1002/ejp.1948.

71 **anesthesiologists at the Leiden University:** Wal, Imeen van der, Fleur Meijer, Rivka Fuica, Zmira Silman, Martijn Boon, Chris Martini, Monique van Velzen, Albert Dahan, Marieke Niesters, and Yaacov Gozal. "Intraoperative Use of the Machine Learning-Derived Nociception Level Monitor Results in Less Pain in the First 90 Min after Surgery." *Frontiers in Pain Research* 3 (January 9, 2023): 1086862. https://doi.org/10.3389/fpain.2022.1086862.

72 **data taken from Mowery's brain:** The Helping to End Addiction Long-Term® Initiative. *5th Annual NIH HEAL Initiative Scientific Meeting Part 3*. NIH, February 8, 2024. https://videocast.nih.gov/watch=54148.

73 **CRPS can occur:** National Institute of Neurological Disorders and Stroke. "Complex Regional Pain Syndrome." NIH. Reviewed August 16, 2024. https://www.ninds.nih.gov/health-information/disorders/complex-regional-pain-syndrome.

75 **"I felt I had no":** Ed Mowery interview with Teresa Barker, November 13, 2024; email interviews with Teresa Barker, June 29, August 5, September 17, 2024; February 16, 2025.

82 **We're so much better:** Wang, Ying, Bo Hu, Yuxue Zhao, Guofang Kuang, Yaling Zhao, Qingwei Liu, and Xiuli Zhu. "Applications of System Dynamics Models in Chronic Disease Prevention: A Systematic Review." *Preventing Chronic Disease* 18 (December 23, 2021): E103. https://doi.org/10.5888/pcd18.210175.

Chapter 5 My Pain, My Self: A Hostile Takeover

86 **"I felt really good":** "Elsa S." interviews with Teresa Barker, September 20, October 20, December 8, 2023; January 8, 31, April 30, 2024, May 23, 2024, September 11, November 4, 2024.

87 **Following shingles came:** National Health Service, United Kingdom. "Post-Herpetic Neuralgia." Reviewed February 24, 2025. https://www.nhs.uk/conditions/post-herpetic-neuralgia/.

87 **long-term nerve damage:** CDC. "Shingles Symptoms and Complications." April 19, 2024. https://www.cdc.gov/shingles/signs-symptoms/index.html.

88 **I never really thought:** Kelly, David. "The Ego Death of Bran Stark (Why He's Weird)." HeadStuff, May 17, 2019. https://headstuff.org/topical/science/ego-death-bran-stark/.

88 **Through this "pathological interweaving":** Reddan, Marianne C., and Tor D. Wager. "Brain Systems at the Intersection of Chronic Pain and Self-Regulation." *Neuroscience Letters* 702 (May 29, 2019): 24–33. https://doi.org/10.1016/j.neulet.2018.11.047.

88 **"There's a very neurologic":** Timothy Furnish interview with Teresa Barker, March 19, 2024.

90 **This sense of identity paralysis:** Toubiana, Madeline, Trish Ruebottom, and Luciana Turchick Hakak. "When a Major Life Change Upends Your Sense of Self." *Harvard Business Review*, January 28, 2022. https://hbr.org/2022/01/when-a-major-life-change-upends-your-sense-of-self.

91 **"At some point":** Heather Voorhees interview with Teresa Barker, January 15, 2024; subsequent email exchanges.

91 **Voorhees describes interviewing:** Voorhees, Heather L. "'I Was Literally Just Not Myself': How Chronic Pain Changes Multiple Frames of Identity." *Health Communication* 38, no. 8 (July 3, 2023): 1641–1653. https://doi.org/10.1080/10410236.2022.2025702.

93 **"I was constantly":** Joe Arcidiacono email interview with Teresa Barker, March 20, 2024.

93 **In a 2022 study:** Hecht, Michael L. "2002—a Research Odyssey: Toward the Development of a Communication Theory of Identity." *Communication Monographs* 60, no. 1 (1993): 76–82. https://doi.org/10.1080/03637759309376297.

94 **Voorhees describes each:** Heather Voorhees interview with Teresa Barker, January 15, 2024.

96 **But when the conversation:** Herbert, Matthew S., Burel R. Goodin, Samuel T. Pero IV, Jessica K. Schmidt, Adriana Sotolongo, Hailey W. Bulls, Toni L. Glover, et al. "Pain Hypervigilance Is Associated with Greater Clinical Pain Severity and Enhanced Experimental Pain Sensitivity among Adults with Symptomatic Knee Osteoarthritis." *Annals of Behavioral Medicine* 48, no. 1 (August 1, 2014): 50–60. https://doi.org/10.1007/s12160-013-9563-x.

97 **Hypervigilance and its anxious twin:** Herbert, Matthew S., Burel R. Goodin, Samuel T. Pero IV, Jessica K. Schmidt, Adriana Sotolongo, Hailey W. Bulls, Toni L. Glover, et al. "Pain Hypervigilance Is Associated with Greater Clinical Pain Severity and Enhanced Experimental Pain Sensitivity among Adults with Symptomatic Knee Osteoarthritis." *Annals of Behavioral Medicine* 48, no. 1 (August 1, 2014): 50–60. https://doi.org/10.1007/s12160-013-9563-x.

97 **and the risk of postoperative pain:** Horn-Hofmann, C., J. Scheel, V. Dimova, A. Parthum, R. Carbon, N. Griessinger, R. Sittl, and S. Lautenbacher. "Prediction of Persistent Post-Operative Pain: Pain-Specific Psychological Variables Compared with Acute Post-Operative Pain and General Psychological Variables." *European Journal of Pain* 22, no. 1 (2018): 191–202. https://doi.org/10.1002/ejp.1115.

97 **They can affect sleep quality:** Poluha, Rodrigo Lorenzi, Giancarlo De la Torre Canales, Dyna Mara Ferreira, Juliana Stuginski-Barbosa, and Paulo César Rodrigues

Conti. "Catastrophizing and Hypervigilance Influence Subjective Sleep Quality in Painful TMD Patients." *Journal of Oral and Facial Pain and Headache* 37, no. 1 (2023): 47–53. https://doi.org/10.11607/ofph.3269.

97 **increase negative thinking:** WebMD Editorial Contributors and Smitha Bhandari. "What Is Hypervigilance?" WebMD. February 25, 2024. https://www.webmd.com/mental-health/what-is-hypervigilance.

97 **increase avoidance behaviors:** Science Direct. "Fear-Avoidance Model." Accessed March 3, 2025. https://www.sciencedirect.com/topics/medicine-and-dentistry/fear-avoidance-model.

97 **narrow cognitive focus:** Sturgeon, John A., and Alex J. Zautra. "Psychological Resilience, Pain Catastrophizing, and Positive Emotions: Perspectives on Comprehensive Modeling of Individual Pain Adaptation." *Current Pain and Headache Reports* 17, no. 3 (March 2013): 317. https://doi.org/10.1007/s11916-012-0317-4.

99 **"And that is what keeps me going":** Amy Tomasulo interview with Teresa Barker, October 5, 2023, and email or text correspondence May 9, 22, 2024; February 26, 2025.

Chapter 6 From Hope to Healing: An Argument for Optimism

105 **"It was yelling":** Scott G. Weiner interview with Steve Weiner, June 3, 2024.

106 **In fact, follow-up:** Gazelka, Halena M., Casey M. Clements, Julie L. Cunningham, Holly L. Geyer, Jenna K. Lovely, Cheri L. Olson, et al. "An Institutional Approach to Managing the Opioid Crisis." *Mayo Clinic Proceedings* 95, no. 5 (May 1, 2020): 968–981. https://doi.org/10.1016/j.mayocp.2019.11.019.

106 **In one notable:** Cohen, Victor, Sergey Motov, Bradley Rockoff, Andrew Smith, Christian Fromm, Dimitri Bosoy, et al. "Development of an Opioid Reduction Protocol in an Emergency Department." *American Journal of Health-System Pharmacy* 72, no. 23 (December 1, 2015): 2080–2086. https://doi.org/10.2146/ajhp140903; Cisewski, David H., and Sergey M. Motov. "Essential Pharmacologic Options for Acute Pain Management in the Emergency Setting." *Turkish Journal of Emergency Medicine* 19, no. 1 (December 10, 2018): 1–11. https://doi.org/10.1016/j.tjem.2018.11.003.

109 **"But we have had widespread culture change":** Interview with Sandeep Kapoor, James Dwyer, and Eugene Vortsman, with Steven Weiner, April 8, 2024.

110 **"It was just a matter":** Alexis LaPietra interview with Steven Weiner, May 24, 2024.

111 **"But we have the power":** Kim Burchiel interview with Teresa Barker, September 14, 2023; January 4, 2024.

Chapter 7 Reset

115 **Don't forget that lifestyle changes:** Niederberger, Ellen, and Michael J. Parnham. "The Impact of Diet and Exercise on Drug Responses." *International Journal*

of Molecular Sciences 22, no. 14 (July 19, 2021): 7692. https://doi.org/10.3390/ijms22147692.

116 **This isn't a new idea:** Antonovsky, Aaron. "The Salutogenic Perspective: Toward a New View of Health and Illness." *Advances* 4, no. 1 (1987): 47–55; Antonovsky, Aaron. "The Salutogenic Model as a Theory to Guide Health Promotion." *Health Promotion International* 11, no. 1 (March 1, 1996): 11–18. https://doi.org/10.1093/heapro/11.1.11.

116 **Albert Bandura, an eminent:** Bandura, A. "Self-Efficacy: Toward a Unifying Theory of Behavioral Change." *Psychological Review* 84, no. 2 (March 1977): 191–215. https://doi.org/10.1037//0033-295x.84.2.191.

116 **"Given that individuals":** Bandura, Albert. "Toward a Psychology of Human Agency." *Perspectives on Psychological Science* 1, no. 2 (June 2006): 164–180. https://doi.org/10.1111/j.1745-6916.2006.00011.x.

117 **Patients who reported higher:** Sturgeon, John A., and Alex J. Zautra. "Resilience: A New Paradigm for Adaptation to Chronic Pain." *Current Pain and Headache Reports* 14, no. 2 (April 2010): 105–112. https://doi.org/10.1007/s11916-010-0095-9; Jackson, Todd, Yalei Wang, Yang Wang, and Huiyong Fan. "Self-Efficacy and Chronic Pain Outcomes: A Meta-Analytic Review." *The Journal of Pain* 15, no. 8 (August 1, 2014): 800–814. https://doi.org/10.1016/j.jpain.2014.05.002.

117 **These beliefs can be internal:** Palmiter, David, Mary Alvord, Rosalind Dorlen, Lillian Comas-Diaz, Suniya S. Luthar, Salvatore R. Maddi, H. Katherine (Kit) O'Neill, Karen W. Saakvitne, and Richard Glenn Tedeschi. "Building Your Resilience." American Psychological Association. Updated February 1, 2020. https://www.apa.org/topics/resilience/building-your-resilience.

118 **Maintaining a healthy lifestyle:** Nijs, Jo, and Felipe Reis. "The Key Role of Lifestyle Factors in Perpetuating Chronic Pain: Towards Precision Pain Medicine." *Journal of Clinical Medicine* 11, no. 10 (May 12, 2022): 2732. https://doi.org/10.3390/jcm11102732; Vasic, Verica, and Mirko H. H. Schmidt. "Resilience and Vulnerability to Pain and Inflammation in the Hippocampus." *International Journal of Molecular Sciences* 18, no. 4 (April 2017): 739. https://doi.org/10.3390/ijms18040739; Sturgeon, John A., and Alex J. Zautra. "Resilience: A New Paradigm for Adaptation to Chronic Pain." *Current Pain and Headache Reports* 14, no. 2 (April 2010): 105–112. https://doi.org/10.1007/s11916-010-0095-9.

118 **This is about more:** Sluka, Kathleen. "The Science of Exercise for Pain Control." San Diego Pain Summit, November 1, 2023. https://www.youtube.com/watch?v=PDB5b2Pf2LY.

119 **Besides quickly improving mental health:** Geneen, Louise J., R. Andrew Moore, Clare Clarke, Denis Martin, Lesley A. Colvin, and Blair H. Smith. "Physical Activity and Exercise for Chronic Pain in Adults: An Overview of Cochrane Reviews." *Cochrane Database of Systematic Reviews* 2017, no. 4 (April 24, 2017): CD011279. https://doi.org/10.1002/14651858.CD011279.pub3; Sluka, Kathleen A., James M. O'Donnell, Jessica Danielson, and Lynn A. Rasmussen. "Regular Physical Activity

Prevents Development of Chronic Pain and Activation of Central Neurons." *Journal of Applied Physiology* 114, no. 6 (March 15, 2013): 725–733. https://doi.org/10.1152/japplphysiol.01317.2012; Palmiter, et al. "Building Your Resilience"; Berardi, Giovanni, Laura Frey-Law, Kathleen A. Sluka, Emine O. Bayman, Christopher S. Coffey, Dixie Ecklund, Carol G. T. Vance, et al. "Multi-Site Observational Study to Assess Biomarkers for Susceptibility or Resilience to Chronic Pain: The Acute to Chronic Pain Signatures (A2CPS) Study Protocol." *Frontiers in Medicine* (Lausanne) 25, no. 9 (April 25, 2022), 849214. http://doi.org/10.3389/fmed.2022.849214; Vasic, Verica, and Mirko H. H. Schmidt. "Resilience and Vulnerability to Pain and Inflammation in the Hippocampus." *International Journal of Molecular Sciences* 18, no. 4 (April 2017): 739. https://doi.org/10.3390/ijms18040739; Sturgeon, John A., and Alex J. Zautra. "Resilience: A New Paradigm for Adaptation to Chronic Pain." *Current Pain and Headache Reports* 14, no. 2 (April 2010): 105–112. https://doi.org/10.1007/s11916-010-0095-9; Sturgeon, John A., and Alex J. Zautra. "Social Pain and Physical Pain: Shared Paths to Resilience." *Pain Management* 6, no. 1 (January 2016): 63–74. https://doi.org/10.2217/pmt.15.56; Náfrádi, Lilla, Zlatina Kostova, Kent Nakamoto, and Peter J. Schulz. "The Doctor-Patient Relationship and Patient Resilience in Chronic Pain: A Qualitative Approach to Patients' Perspectives." *Chronic Illness* 14, no. 4 (December 2018): 256–270. https://doi.org/10.1177/1742395317739961; Buckingham, Ashley, and Elizabeth J. Richardson. "The Relationship Between Psychological Resilience and Pain Threshold and Tolerance: Optimism and Grit as Moderators." *Journal of Clinical Psychology in Medical Settings* 28, no. 3 (September 1, 2021): 518–528. https://doi.org/10.1007/s10880-020-09731-7.

120 **Think of resilience as strength training:** Berardi, et al. "Multi-Site Observational Study"; Palmiter, et al. "Building Your Resilience"; Hemington, Kasey S., Joshua C. Cheng, Rachael L. Bosma, Anton Rogachov, Junseok A. Kim, and Karen D. Davis. "Beyond Negative Pain-Related Psychological Factors: Resilience Is Related to Lower Pain Affect in Healthy Adults." *Journal of Pain* 18, no. 9 (September 1, 2017): 1117–1128. https://doi.org/10.1016/j.jpain.2017.04.009.

121 **Resilience is defined:** Sturgeon, John A., and Alex J. Zautra. "Psychological Resilience, Pain Catastrophizing, and Positive Emotions: Perspectives on Comprehensive Modeling of Individual Pain Adaptation." *Current Pain and Headache Reports* 17, no. 3 (March 2013): 317. https://doi.org/10.1007/s11916-012-0317-4.

121 **Reasons you might seek:** Payne, et al. "Patient-Initiated Second Opinions."

122 **The more informed you are:** Van Such, Monica, Robert Lohr, Thomas Beckman, and James M. Naessens. "Extent of Diagnostic Agreement among Medical Referrals." *Journal of Evaluation in Clinical Practice* 23, no. 4 (2017): 870–874. https://doi.org/10.1111/jep.12747000.

122 **Studies show that feeling comfortable:** Agarwal, Vinita. "Patient Communication of Chronic Pain in the Complementary and Alternative Medicine Therapeutic Relationship." *Journal of Patient Experience* 7, no. 2 (April 2020): 238–244. https://doi

.org/10.1177/2374373519826137; Wampold, Bruce E. "Healing in a Social Context: The Importance of Clinician and Patient Relationship." *Frontiers in Pain Research* 2 (2021). https://www.frontiersin.org/articles/10.3389/fpain.2021.684768.

122 **intangibles like their communication:** Payne, Velma L., Hardeep Singh, Ashley N. D. Meyer, Lewis Levy, David Harrison, and Mark L. Graber. "Patient-Initiated Second Opinions: Systematic Review of Characteristics and Impact on Diagnosis, Treatment, and Satisfaction." *Mayo Clinic Proceedings* 89, no. 5 (May 2014): 687–696. https://doi.org/10.1016/j.mayocp.2014.02.015.

122 **"With complex pain":** Jane Ballantyne interview with Teresa Barker, February 6, 2024.

122 **"The study, led by University of Illinois Urbana-Champaign":** Thompson, Charee M., Manuel D. Pulido, Suma Gangidi, and Paul Arnold. "How Chronic Pain Patients' and Physicians' Communication Influences Patients' Uncertainty: A Pre- and Post-Consultation Study." *Journal of Health Communication* 29, no. 5 (May 2024): 357–370. https://doi.org/10.1080/10810730.2024.2352556.

123 **Thompson suggests four ways:** Charee Thompson email interview with Teresa Barker, March 2, 2025.

124 **You may have to keep searching:** "Bess Talbot" interviews with Teresa Barker, November 20, 2023; January 8, May 18, November 8, 20, 2024; January 27, 2025.

125 **"Engaging in the ritual":** LeWine, Howard E. "The Power of the Placebo Effect." Harvard Health Publishing, July 22, 2024. https://www.health.harvard.edu/newsletter_article/the-power-of-the-placebo-effect.

126 **"Moment by moment, we choose":** Merzenich, Michael. *Soft-Wired: How the New Science of Brain Plasticity Can Change Your Life*. Parnassus Publishing, 2013.

Chapter 8 Pain Relief: What's in Your Toolbox?

129 **Keep in mind:** Holden, Janean E., Younhee Jeong, and Jeannine M. Forrest. "The Endogenous Opioid System and Clinical Pain Management." *AACN Clinical Issues* 16, no. 3 (2005): 291–301. https://doi.org/10.1097/00044067-200507000-00003.

129 **Opioids, whether endogenous:** Science Direct. "Opioid Receptor." Accessed September 6, 2024. https://www.sciencedirect.com/topics/biochemistry-genetics-and-molecular-biology/opioid-receptor.

129 **Like molecular keys in locks:** MedLine Plus Genetics. "OPRM1 Gene." National Library of Medicine. Updated November 1, 2017. https://medlineplus.gov/genetics/gene/oprm1/.

129 **This prevents some:** Corder, Gregory, Daniel C. Castro, Michael R. Bruchas, and Grégory Scherrer. "Endogenous and Exogenous Opioids in Pain." *Annual Review of Neuroscience* 41 (July 7, 2018): 453. https://doi.org/10.1146/annurev-neuro-080317-061522.

129 **Nature even added:** Dafny, Nachum. "Pain Modulation and Mechanisms." In *Neuroscience Online: An Electronic Textbook for the Neurosciences*. Department of Neu-

robiology and Anatomy, University of Texas Health Science Center at Houston, McGovern Medical School. Revised October 7, 2020. https://nba.uth.tmc.edu/neuroscience/m/s2/chapter08.html.

130 **Having devoted her career:** Daniela Salvemini interview with Teresa Barker, November 2023.

130 **A variety of stressors:** Butler, Ryan K., and David P. Finn. "Stress-Induced Analgesia." *Progress in Neurobiology* 88, no. 3 (July 1, 2009): 184–202. https://doi.org/10.1016/j.pneurobio.2009.04.003; Vaughan, Christopher W. "Stressed-Out Endogenous Cannabinoids Relieve Pain." *Trends in Pharmacological Sciences* 27, no. 2 (February 2006): 69–71. https://doi.org/10.1016/j.tips.2005.11.011.

131 **Recognizing a placebo's intrinsic value:** Medoff, Zev M., and Luana Colloca. "Placebo Analgesia: Understanding the Mechanisms." *Pain Management* 5, no. 2 (March 2015): 89–96. https://doi.org/10.2217/pmt.15.3.

132 **The concept of RICE:** Scialoia, Domenic, and Adam J. Swartzendruber. "The R.I.C.E Protocol Is a MYTH: A Review and Recommendations." *Sport Journal*. US Sports Academy, October 30, 2020. https://thesportjournal.org/article/the-r-i-c-e-protocol-is-a-myth-a-review-and-recommendations/.

132 **What I see as most compelling:** Rawson, Ben. "Recovery from Athletic Injuries: Is MEAT Better Than RICE?." Center for Healing and Regenerative Medicine. May 10, 2021. https://charmaustin.com/recovery-from-athletic-injuries-meat-over-rice/.

134 **The practice continues:** Espeland, Didrik, Louis de Weerd, and James B. Mercer. "Health Effects of Voluntary Exposure to Cold Water—a Continuing Subject of Debate." *International Journal of Circumpolar Health* 81, no. 1 (2022): 2111789. https://doi.org/10.1080/22423982.2022.2111789; Williamson, Laura. "You're Not a Polar Bear: The Plunge into Cold Water Comes with Risks." American Heart Association, December 9, 2022. https://www.heart.org/en/news/2022/12/09/youre-not-a-polar-bear-the-plunge-into-cold-water-comes-with-risks.

135 **These nonprescription medications:** Cleveland Clinic. "NSAIDs (Non-Steroidal Anti-Inflammatory Drugs)." Updated July 24, 2023. https://my.clevelandclinic.org/health/treatments/11086-non-steroidal-anti-inflammatory-medicines-nsaids; Wirth, Theo, Pierre Lafforgue, and Thao Pham. "NSAID: Current Limits to Prescription." *Joint Bone Spine* 91, no. 4 (July 1, 2024): 105685. https://doi.org/10.1016/j.jbspin.2023.105685.

135 **For decades, aspirin:** Huang, Athena L., Ann Marie Navar, Colby Ayers, Anand Rohatgi, Erin D. Michos, Salim S. Virani, Parag Joshi, Eric D. Peterson, and Amit Khera. "US Population Qualifying for Aspirin Use for Primary Prevention of Cardiovascular Disease." *American Journal of Preventive Cardiology* 18 (June 2024): 100669. https://doi.org/10.1016/j.ajpc.2024.100669.

136 **But in general, many:** US Preventive Services Task Force. "Aspirin Use to Prevent Cardiovascular Disease: US Preventive Services Task Force Recommendation

Statement." *JAMA* 327, no. 16 (April 26, 2022): 1577–1584. https://doi.org/10.1001/jama.2022.4983.

136 **It may also effectively lower:** Sawaddiruk, P., N. Apaijai, S. Paiboonworachat, T. Kaewchur, N. Kasitanon, T. Jaiwongkam, et al. "Coenzyme Q10 Supplementation Alleviates Pain in Pregabalin-Treated Fibromyalgia Patients via Reducing Brain Activity and Mitochondrial Dysfunction." *Free Radical Research* 53, no. 8 (August 2019). https://doi.org/10.1080/10715762.2019.1645955.

136 **By blocking calcium:** Shin, Hyun-Jung, Hyo-Seok Na, and Sang-Hwan Do. "Magnesium and Pain." *Nutrients* 12, no. 8 (July 23, 2020): 2184. https://doi.org/10.3390/nu12082184.

136 **"In recent lab experiments":** Memorial Sloan Kettering Cancer Center. Turmeric." Updated March 11, 2024. https://www.mskcc.org/cancer-care/integrative-medicine/herbs/turmeric.

137 **And buy from a reputable source:** Navarro, Victor, Bharathi Avula, Ikhlas Khan, Manisha Verma, Leonard Seeff, Jose Serrano, Andrew Stolz, Robert Fontana, and Jawad Ahmad. "The Contents of Herbal and Dietary Supplements Implicated in Liver Injury in the United States Are Frequently Mislabeled." *Hepatology Communications* 3, no. 6 (June 2019): 792–794. https://doi.org/10.1002/hep4.1346.

137 **If you're sensitive to aspirin:** Therapeutic Research Center. "Willow Bark: Overview, Uses, Side Effects, Precautions, Interactions, Dosing and Reviews." WebMD. Accessed December 15, 2024. https://www.webmd.com/vitamins/ai/ingredient mono-955/willow-bark.

139 **We've seen remarkable progress:** Hodgens, Alexander, and Tariq Sharman. "Corticosteroids." In *StatPearls [Internet]*. StatPearls Publishing, 2024. http://www.ncbi.nlm.nih.gov/books/NBK554612/.

140 **The drug worked best:** Wiffen, Philip J., Sheena Derry, Rae Frances Bell, Andrew S. C. Rice, Thomas Rudolf Tölle, Tudor Phillips, et al. "Gabapentin for Chronic Neuropathic Pain in Adults." *Cochrane Database of Systematic Reviews* 2017, no. 6 (June 9, 2017): CD007938. https://doi.org/10.1002/14651858.CD007938.pub4.

140 **A 2021 systematic meta-review:** Ferreira, Giovanni E., Andrew J. McLachlan, Chung-Wei Christine Lin, Joshua R. Zadro, Christina Abdel-Shaheed, Mary O'Keeffe, and Chris G. Maher. "Efficacy and Safety of Antidepressants for the Treatment of Back Pain and Osteoarthritis: Systematic Review and Meta-Analysis." *BMJ* 372, no. 8276 (January 20, 2021): m4825. https://doi.org/10.1136/bmj.m4825.

141 **The review concluded:** Birkinshaw, Hollie, Claire M. Friedrich, Peter Cole, Christopher Eccleston, Marc Serfaty, Gavin Stewart, et al. "Antidepressants for Pain Management in Adults with Chronic Pain: A Network Meta-Analysis." *Cochrane Database of Systematic Reviews* 5, no. CD014682 (May 10, 2023). https://doi.org/10.1002/14651858.CD014682.pub2.

141 **The approval of Journavx:** US Food and Drug Administration (FDA). "FDA Approves Novel Non-Opioid Treatment for Moderate to Severe Acute Pain." News re-

lease, January 30, 2025. https://www.fda.gov/news-events/press-announcements/fda-approves-novel-non-opioid-treatment-moderate-severe-acute-pain.

141 **Both trials demonstrated:** Vertex Pharmaceuticals Incorporated. "A Phase 3, Randomized, Double-Blind, Placebo-Controlled Study Evaluating the Efficacy and Safety of VX-548 for Acute Pain After a Bunionectomy." ClinicalTrials.gov, National Library of Medicine, December 13, 2024. https://clinicaltrials.gov/study/NCT05553366; Vertex Pharmaceuticals Incorporated. "A Phase 3, Randomized, Double-Blind, Placebo-Controlled Study Evaluating the Efficacy and Safety of VX-548 for Acute Pain After an Abdominoplasty." ClinicalTrials.gov, National Library of Medicine, August 23, 2024. https://clinicaltrials.gov/study/NCT05558410.

142 **Prescription drugs approved for other conditions:** Wittich, Christopher M., Christopher M. Burkle, and William L. Lanier. "Ten Common Questions (and Their Answers) about Off-Label Drug Use." *Mayo Clinic Proceedings* 87, no. 10 (October 2012): 982–990. https://doi.org/10.1016/j.mayocp.2012.04.017.

142 **Neuromodulation, including spinal cord stimulation:** Krishna, Vibhor, and Alfonso Fasano. "Neuromodulation: Update on Current Practice and Future Developments." *Neurotherapeutics* 21, no. 3 (May 9, 2024): e00371. https://doi.org/10.1016/j.neurot.2024.e00371.

142 **Injection therapies:** Urits, Ivan, Daniel Smoots, Lekha Anantuni, Prudhvi Bandi, Katie Bring, Amnon A. Berger, Hisham Kassem, et al. "Injection Techniques for Common Chronic Pain Conditions of the Hand: A Comprehensive Review." *Pain and Therapy* 9, no. 1 (June 2020): 129–142. https://doi.org/10.1007/s40122-020-00158-4.

143 **Prolotherapy injections:** Borg Stein, Joanne. "Types of Injections That Can Help with Joint Pain." Mass General Brigham. Updated April 21, 2025. https://www.massgeneralbrigham.org/en/about/newsroom/articles/types-of-injections-that-can-help-with-joint-pain.

143 **Regenerative medicine:** Gu, Xingjian, Michelle A. Carroll Turpin, and Mario I. Romero-Ortega. "Biomaterials and Regenerative Medicine in Pain Management." *Current Pain and Headache Reports* 26, no. 7 (June 21, 2022): 533. https://doi.org/10.1007/s11916-022-01055-5.

143 **Platelet-rich plasma injections:** Gianakos, Arianna L. "Platelet-Rich Plasma (PRP) Injections in Sports." Yale Medicine. Accessed February 24, 2025. https://www.yalemedicine.org/conditions/platelet-rich-plasma-injections.

143 **Others, including: Nitrous oxide:** Cleveland Clinic. "Study Will Look at Nitrous Oxide as Complex Regional Pain Syndrome Treatment." June 24, 2020. https://consultqd.clevelandclinic.org/study-will-look-at-nitrous-oxide-as-complex-regional-pain-syndrome-treatment.

144 **Inceptiv, an implanted device:** Medtronic plc. "Medtronic Receives FDA Approval for Inceptiv™ Closed-Loop Spinal Cord Stimulator." April 26, 2024.

https://www.prnewswire.com/news-releases/medtronic-receives-fda-approval-for-inceptiv-closed-loop-spinal-cord-stimulator-302128632.html.

145 **Few pain practices:** Thomas J. Smith interview with Teresa Barker, November 14, 2023.

145 **Like many other treatments:** Johnson, Mark I., Leica S. Claydon, G. Peter Herbison, Gareth Jones, and Carole A. Paley. "Transcutaneous Electrical Nerve Stimulation (TENS) for Fibromyalgia in Adults." *Cochrane Database of Systematic Reviews* 2017, no. 10 (October 9, 2017): CD012172. https://doi.org/10.1002/14651858.CD012172.pub2.

145 **A vagus nerve stimulator:** Goggins, Eibhlin, Shuhei Mitani, and Shinji Tanaka. "Clinical Perspectives on Vagus Nerve Stimulation: Present and Future." *Clinical Science* 136, no. 9 (May 10, 2022): 695–709. https://doi.org/10.1042/CS20210507.

147 **The problem is that opioids:** Institute for Healthcare Policy and Innovation. "Unwise Opioids for Wisdom Teeth: Study Shows Link to Long-Term Use in Teens and Young Adults." University of Michigan, August 7, 2018. https://ihpi.umich.edu/news/unwise-opioids-wisdom-teeth-study-shows-link-long-term-use-teens-young-adults; American Dental Association (ADA) Media Relations. "New Guideline Details Acute Pain Management Strategies for Adolescent Adult Dental Patients." ADA, February 5, 2024. https://www.ada.org/about/press-releases/new-guideline-details-acute-pain-management-strategies-for-adolescent-adult-dental-patients.

148 **A 2024 retrospective study:** Mudumbai, Seshadri C., Han He, Ji-Qing Chen, Aditi Kapoor, Samantha Regala, Edward R. Mariano, et al. "Opioid Use in Cancer Patients Compared with Noncancer Pain Patients in a Veteran Population." *JNCI Cancer Spectrum* 8, no. 2 (February 29, 2024): pkae012. https://doi.org/10.1093/jncics/pkae012.

149 **In some treatment areas:** Dydyk, Alexander M., Nitesh K. Jain, and Mohit Gupta. "Opioid Use Disorder." In *StatPearls [Internet]*. StatPearls Publishing, 2024. http://www.ncbi.nlm.nih.gov/books/NBK553166/.

149 **The first thing is:** Staci Gruber interview with Sanjay Gupta, September 27, 2024.

151 **"Too often they're accompanied":** Perrone, Matthew. "Mind-Altering Ketamine Becomes New Pain Treatment." AP News. November 6, 2023. https://apnews.com/article/ketamine-pain-drugs-psychedelic-fda-2c67eeac1932962a7b0affc07d24c09a.

151 **"When we're talking about psychoactive drugs":** David Feifel interview with Sanjay Gupta, August 27, 2024.

151 **In 2018, the American Society:** Orhurhu, Vwaire, Jacob Roberts, Nam Ly, and Steven Cohen. "Ketamine in Acute and Chronic Pain Management." *StatPearls*, September 4, 2023. https://www.statpearls.com/ArticleLibrary/viewarticle/59718.

152 **In 2019, researchers published a systematic review:** Orhurhu, Vwaire, Mariam Salisu Orhurhu, Anuj Bhatia, and Steven P. Cohen. "Ketamine Infusions for

Chronic Pain: A Systematic Review and Meta-Analysis of Randomized Controlled Trials." *Anesthesia and Analgesia* 129, no. 1 (July 2019): 241–254. https://doi.org/10.1213/ANE.0000000000004185.

153 **Neuroscience, on the other hand:** Ricard, Matthieu, and Wolf Singer. *Beyond the Self: Conversations Between Buddhism and Neuroscience,* MIT Press, 2017.

154 **An analysis conducted by:** National Center for Complementary and Integrative Health (NCCIH). "NIH Analysis Reveals a Significant Rise in Use of Complementary Health Approaches, Especially for Pain Management." NIH. Press release, January 31, 2024. https://www.nccih.nih.gov/news/press-releases/nih-analysis-reveals-a-significant-rise-in-use-of-complementary-health-approaches-especially-for-pain-management.

155 **Yet profound cultural differences:** Terruzzi, Vittorio, Silvia Paggi, Arnaldo Amato, and Franco Radaelli. "Unsedated Colonoscopy: A Neverending Story." *World Journal of Gastrointestinal Endoscopy* 4, no. 4 (April 16, 2012): 137–141. https://doi.org/10.4253/wjge.v4.i4.137; Biggers, Larissa. "Unsedated Colonoscopy: Surely You Jest." *Colowrap Blog,* September 21, 2018. https://www.colowrap.com/blog/unsedated-colonoscopy.

156 **"We do not have that":** Harvey L. Rich email interviews with Teresa Barker, November 13, 17, 25, 2023; April 11, May 25, October 21, 2024.

157 **The exact mechanism:** Dingle, Genevieve A., Leah S. Sharman, Zoe Bauer, Emma Beckman, Mary Broughton, Emma Bunzli, et al. "How Do Music Activities Affect Health and Well-Being? A Scoping Review of Studies Examining Psychosocial Mechanisms." *Frontiers in Psychology* 12 (September 8, 2021). https://doi.org/10.3389/fpsyg.2021.713818.

Chapter 9 Brain Surgeon, Pain Surgeon

159 **That's not surprising:** Park, Rex, Mohammed Mohiuddin, Ramiro Arellano, Esther Pogatzki-Zahn, Gregory Klar, and Ian Gilron. "Prevalence of Postoperative Pain after Hospital Discharge: Systematic Review and Meta-Analysis." *Pain Reports* 8, no. 3 (May 8, 2023): e1075. https://doi.org/10.1097/PR9.0000000000001075.

159 **Even routine surgical procedures:** Dobson, Geoffrey P. "Trauma of Major Surgery: A Global Problem That Is Not Going Away." *International Journal of Surgery* 81 (September 2020): 47–54. https://doi.org/10.1016/j.ijsu.2020.07.017.

160 **For 5 percent of all surgical patients:** Bruce, Julie, and Jane Quinlan. "Chronic Post Surgical Pain." *Reviews in Pain* 5, no. 3 (September 2011): 23. https://doi.org/10.1177/204946371100500306.

162 **Writing about low back pain:** Goertz, Christine. "We're Treating Low Back Pain All Wrong." MedPage Today, April 14, 2023. https://www.medpagetoday.com/opinion/second-opinions/104026.

162 **"The problem is not the lack":** American College of Physicians. "American College of Physicians Issues Guideline for Treating Nonradicular Low Back Pain." Press release, February 15, 2017. https://www.acponline.org/acp-newsroom/american-college-of-physicians-issues-guideline-for-treating-nonradicular-low-back-pain; George, Steven Z., Christine Goertz, S. Nichole Hastings and Julie M. Fritz. "Transforming Low Back Pain Care Delivery in the United States." *Pain* 161, no. 12 (December 2020): 2667-2673. https://doi.org/10.1097/j.pain.0000000000001089.

164 **This compares with:** Nagata, Kosei, Chang Chang, Mitsuhiro Nishizawa, and Koji Yamada. "Estimated Number of Spine Surgeries and Related Deaths in Japan from 2014 to 2020." *Journal of Orthopaedic Science* 30, no. 1 (January 2025), 32–38. https://doi.org/10.1016/j.jos.2023.12.006.

164 **Interestingly, studies have found:** Maayan, Omri, Pratyush Shahi, Robert K. Merrill, Anthony Pajak, Amy Z. Lu, Yousi Oquendo, et al. "Ninety Percent of Patients Are Satisfied with Their Decision to Undergo Spine Surgery for Degenerative Conditions." *Spine* 49, no. 8 (April 15, 2024): 61–68. https://doi.org/10.1097/BRS.0000000000004714.

164 **And unsurprisingly:** Sivaganesan, A., I. Khan, J. S. Pennings, S. G. Roth, E. R. Nolan, E. R. Oleisky, et al. "Why Are Patients Dissatisfied after Spine Surgery When Improvements in Disability and Pain Are Clinically Meaningful?" *Spine Journal* 20, no. 10 (October 2020): 1535–1543. https://doi.org/10.1016/j.spinee.2020.06.008.

165 **According to a 2023 article:** Darville-Beneby, Rasheeda, Anna M. Lomanowska, Hai Chuan Yu, Parker Jobin, Brittany N. Rosenbloom, Gretchen Gabriel, Helena Daudt, et al. "The Impact of Preoperative Patient Education on Postoperative Pain, Opioid Use, and Psychological Outcomes: A Narrative Review." *Canadian Journal of Pain* 7, no. 2 (November 28, 2023). https://doi.org/10.1080/24740527.2023.2266751.

165 **Additionally, a 2025 scoping review:** Darnall, Beth D., Lauren Abshire, Rena E. Courtney, and Sara Davin. "Upskilling Pain Relief after Surgery: A Scoping Review of Perioperative Behavioral Intervention Efficacy and Practical Consideration for Implementation." *Regional Anesthesia and Pain Medicine* 50, no. 2 (2025): 93–101.

171 **1.5 fluid ounces:** Dufour, Mary C. "What Is Moderate Drinking?" *Alcohol Research and Health* 23, no. 1 (1999): 5–14.

171 **This program should aim:** Shakya, Pawan, and Sagar Poudel. "Prehabilitation in Patients before Major Surgery: A Review Article." *JNMA: Journal of the Nepal Medical Association* 60, no. 254 (October 2022): 909–915. https://doi.org/10.31729/jnma.7545.

172 **From the American College of Surgeons:** American College of Surgeons. "Strong for Surgery: Prehabilitation." Accessed December 5, 2024. https://www.facs.org/for-patients/preparing-for-surgery/strong-for-surgery/prehabilitation/.

175 **Given these numbers:** Lenza, Mario, R. Buchbinder, M. Staples, O. Dos Santos, R. Brandt, C. Lottenberg, et al. "Second Opinion for Degenerative Spinal Condi-

tions: An Option or a Necessity? A Prospective Observational Study." *BMC Musculoskeletal Disorders* 18, no. 1 (December 2017): 354. https://doi.org/10.1186/s12891-017-1712-0.

176 **A 2016 NIH evaluation:** Wu, Ming-Shun, Kee-Hsin Chen, I.-Fan Chen, Shihping Kevin Huang, Pei-Chuan Tzeng, Mei-Ling Yeh, et al. "The Efficacy of Acupuncture in Post-Operative Pain Management: A Systematic Review and Meta-Analysis." *PLoS ONE* 11, no. 3 (March 9, 2016): e0150367. https://doi.org/10.1371/journal.pone.0150367.

Chapter 10 A Powerful Pairing Against Pain: Mind and Body

180 **Garland was thrilled:** Eric L. Garland interviews with Teresa Barker, September 15, 2023; April 12, November 25, 2024, and email correspondence.

180 **In a large clinical trial:** Garland, Eric L., Adam W. Hanley, Yoshio Nakamura, John W. Barrett, Anne K. Baker, Sarah E. Reese, et al. "Mindfulness-Oriented Recovery Enhancement vs. Supportive Group Therapy for Co-Occurring Opioid Misuse and Chronic Pain in Primary Care: A Randomized Clinical Trial." *JAMA Internal Medicine* 182, no. 4 (April 1, 2022): 407–417. https://doi.org/10.1001/jamainternmed.2022.0033.

182 **In particular, it targets:** Lumley, Mark A., Howard Schubiner, Nancy A. Lockhart, Kelley M. Kidwell, Steven E. Harte, Daniel J. Clauw, et al. "Emotional Awareness and Expression Therapy, Cognitive-Behavioral Therapy, and Education for Fibromyalgia: A Cluster-Randomized Controlled Trial." *Pain* 158, no. 12 (December 2017): 2354–2363. https://doi.org/10.1097/j.pain.0000000000001036; Yarns, Brandon C., Nicholas J. Jackson, Alexander Alas, Rebecca J. Melrose, Mark A. Lumley, and David L. Sultzer. "Emotional Awareness and Expression Therapy vs. Cognitive Behavioral Therapy for Chronic Pain in Older Veterans: A Randomized Clinical Trial." *JAMA Network Open* 7, no. 6 (June 13, 2024): e2415842. https://doi.org/10.1001/jamanetworkopen.2024.15842.

182 **And still the evidence:** Driscoll, Mary A., Robert R. Edwards, William C. Becker, Ted J. Kaptchuk, and Robert D. Kerns. "Psychological Interventions for the Treatment of Chronic Pain in Adults." *Psychological Science in the Public Interest* 22, no. 2 (September 2021): 52–95. https://doi.org/10.1177/15291006211008157.

183 **"Soon I was meditating":** Vidyamala Burch interview with Teresa Barker, September 25, 2023.

183 **"The results were truly life changing":** Vidyamala Burch email interview with Teresa Barker, January 23, 2025.

184 **And you can accomplish:** Esch, Tobias, Jeremy Winkler, Volker Auwärter, Heike Gnann, Roman Huber, and Stefan Schmidt. "Neurobiological Aspects of Mindfulness in Pain Autoregulation: Unexpected Results from a Randomized-Controlled Trial and Possible Implications for Meditation Research." *Frontiers*

in Human Neuroscience 10 (January 26, 2017): 674. https://doi.org/10.3389/fnhum.2016.00674.

184 **Self-regulation involves multiple domains:** Stuart Shanker email interview with Teresa Barker, April 15, 2024; Shanker, Stuart. "Self-Regulation: 5 Domains of Self-Reg." The MEHRIT Centre, 2021. https://self-reg.ca/wp-content/uploads/2021/05/infosheet_5-Domains-of-Self-Reg.pdf.

185 **"Not the last line":** Mark Jensen interviews with Teresa Barker, September 21, 2023, January 13, 2024, and email November 26, 2024.

187 **"look beyond the pill bottle":** Darnall, Beth. "Unlocking the Medicine Box in Your Mind." Stanford Pain Medicine, September 21, 2015. https://www.youtube.com/watch?v=GeqLbJRci1Y.

187 **Among those the study identifies:** Bushnell, M. Catherine, Marta Čeko, and Lucie A. Low. "Cognitive and Emotional Control of Pain and Its Disruption in Chronic Pain." *Nature Reviews Neuroscience* 14, no. 7 (July 2013): 502–511. https://doi.org/10.1038/nrn3516.

188 **"It requires education":** Helene Langevin interview with Teresa Barker, February 21, 2024, and email May 22, 2024.

192 **" 'Oh, they think I need this' ":** Sara Davin interview with Teresa Barker, May 13, 2024.

193 **Gordon was part:** Ashar, Yoni K., Alan Gordon, Howard Schubiner, Christie Uipi, Karen Knight, Zachary Anderson, et al. "Effect of Pain Reprocessing Therapy vs. Placebo and Usual Care for Patients with Chronic Back Pain: A Randomized Clinical Trial." *JAMA Psychiatry* 79, no. 1 (January 1, 2022): 13–23. https://doi.org/10.1001/jamapsychiatry.2021.2669.

194 **"I think it made a lot of sense":** Yoni Ashar interview with Teresa Barker, January 22, 2024.

194 **"Things in your life":** Howard Schubiner interviews with Teresa Barker, January 18, March 7, May 27, 2024, and email correspondence; Lumley, Mark A., and Howard Schubiner. "Psychological Therapy for Centralized Pain: An Integrative Assessment and Treatment Model." *Psychosomatic Medicine* 81, no. 2 (2019): 114–124. https://doi.org/10.1097/PSY.0000000000000654.

195 **His 2017 *New York Times* obituary:** Conner-Simons, Adam. "Dr. John Sarno, 93, Dies; Best-Selling Author Tied Pain to Anxieties." *New York Times*, June 24, 2017. https://www.nytimes.com/2017/06/23/science/john-sarno-dead-healing-back-pain-doctor.html.

Chapter 11 Mind Your Brain

199 **In 2014, for instance, a group of US marines:** Johnson, Douglas C., Nathaniel J. Thom, Elizabeth A. Stanley, Lori Haase, Alan N. Simmons, Pei-An B. Shih, et al. "Modifying Resilience Mechanisms in At-Risk Individuals: A Controlled Study

of Mindfulness Training in Marines Preparing for Deployment." *American Journal of Psychiatry* 171, no. 8 (August 2014): 844–853. https://doi.org/10.1176/appi.ajp.2014.13040502.

200 **It too found:** Orme-Johnson, David W., and Vernon A. Barnes. "Effects of the Transcendental Meditation Technique on Trait Anxiety: A Meta-Analysis of Randomized Controlled Trials." *Journal of Alternative and Complementary Medicine* 20, no. 5 (May 2014): 330–341. https://doi.org/10.1089/acm.2013.0204.

200 **Among others, the authors:** Rodriguez-Raecke, Rea, Andreas Niemeier, Kristin Ihle, Wolfgang Ruether, and Arne May. "Brain Gray Matter Decrease in Chronic Pain Is the Consequence and Not the Cause of Pain." *Journal of Neuroscience* 29, no. 44 (November 4, 2009): 13746–13750. https://doi.org/10.1523/JNEUROSCI.3687-09.2009.

201 **Too much, too fast:** Salvati, Kathryn A., and Mark P. Beenhakker. "Out of Thin Air: Hyperventilation-Triggered Seizures." *Brain Research* 1703 (January 1, 2019): 41. https://doi.org/10.1016/j.brainres.2017.12.037; Hawkins, Selwynne M., Dominik P. Guensch, Matthias G. Friedrich, Giulia Vinco, Gobinath Nadeshalingham, et al. "Hyperventilation-Induced Heart Rate Response as a Potential Marker for Cardiovascular Disease." *Scientific Reports* 9 (2019). https://doi.org/10.1038/s41598-019-54375-9.

202 **You can adjust the length:** Norelli, Samantha K., Ashley Long, and Jeffrey M. Krepps. "Relaxation Techniques." In *StatPearls [Internet]*. StatPearls Publishing, 2024. http://www.ncbi.nlm.nih.gov/books/NBK513238/.

205 **Even doing your exact same:** Noseworthy, Matt, Luke Peddie, E. Jean Buckler, Faith Park, Margaret Pham, Spencer Pratt, et al. "The Effects of Outdoor versus Indoor Exercise on Psychological Health, Physical Health, and Physical Activity Behaviour: A Systematic Review of Longitudinal Trials." *International Journal of Environmental Research and Public Health* 20, no. 3 (January 17, 2023): 1669. https://doi.org/10.3390/ijerph20031669.

205 **In clinical trials of green light:** Kluger, Jeffrey. "Green Light Exposure May Help Reduce Pain and Headaches." *Time*, October 27, 2022. https://time.com/6225133/green-light-headaches-pain-relief/.

206 **Other research found that green light:** Martin, Laurent F., Kevin Cheng, Stephanie M. Washington, Millie Denton, Vasudha Goel, Maithili Khandekar, Tally M. Largent-Milnes, Amol Patwardhan, and Mohab M. Ibrahim. "Green Light Exposure Elicits Anti-Inflammation, Endogenous Opioid Release and Dampens Synaptic Potentiation to Relieve Post-Surgical Pain." *Journal of Pain* 24, no. 3 (March 2023). https://doi.org/10.1016/j.jpain.2022.10.011.

206 **Preclinical studies of chronic:** University of Arizona Health Sciences. "US Army Medical Research Grant Funds Study of Green Light Therapy for Postsurgical Pain." News release, September 14, 2023. https://healthsciences.arizona.edu/news/releases/us-army-medical-research-grant-funds-study-green-light-therapy-postsurgical-pain.

206 **"It's more practical":** Mohab Ibrahim interview with Teresa Barker, October 9, 2023.

207 **Drawing on her experience:** Vidyamala Burch interview with Teresa Barker, September 25, 2023.

209 **The trials found:** Martin, Laurent, Frank Porreca, Elizabeth I. Mata, Michelle Salloum, Vasudha Goel, Pooja Gunnala, et al. "Green Light Exposure Improves Pain and Quality of Life in Fibromyalgia Patients: A Preliminary One-Way Crossover Clinical Trial." *Pain Medicine* 22, no. 1 (November 6, 2020): 118–130. https://doi.org/10.1093/pm/pnaa329; De La Rosa, Jennifer S., Benjamin R. Brady, Mohab M. Ibrahim, Katherine E. Herder, Jessica S. Wallace, et al. "Co-Occurrence of Chronic Pain and Anxiety/Depression Symptoms in U.S. Adults: Prevalence, Functional Impacts, and Opportunities." *Pain* 165, no. 3 (March 2024): 666–673. https://doi.org/10.1097/j.pain.0000000000003056; Martin, Laurent F., Aubin Moutal, Kevin Cheng, Stephanie M. Washington, Hugo Calligaro, Vasudha Goel, Tracy Kranz, et al. "Green Light Antinociceptive and Reversal of Thermal and Mechanical Hypersensitivity Effects Rely on Endogenous Opioid System Stimulation." *Journal of Pain* 22, no. 12 (December 2021): P1646-1656. https://doi.org/10.1016/j.jpain.2021.05.006.

210 **In the inner dialogue about pain:** Cleveland Clinic. "Talking to Yourself: Is It Normal?" February 4, 2022. https://health.clevelandclinic.org/is-it-normal-to-talk-to-yourself; Mayo Clinic Staff. "Positive Thinking: Stop Negative Self-Talk to Reduce Stress." Mayo Clinic, November 21, 2023. https://www.mayoclinic.org/healthy-lifestyle/stress-management/in-depth/positive-thinking/art-20043950.

211 **In "Working with Pain-Related Thoughts":** US Department of Veterans Affairs. "Working with Pain-Related Thoughts." Updated March 19, 2025. https://www.va.gov/wholehealthlibrary/tools/working-with-pain-related-thoughts.asp.

214 **We ended up having a long conversation:** Rob Kyler interview with Sanjay Gupta, August 26, 2023.

215 **"Turning toward it and experiencing it":** Rob Kyler interviews with Teresa Barker, September 18, 20, 22, December 12, 2023, and email correspondence September 2023–June 2024.

215 **distraction was the most beneficial:** Baker, Nancy A., Augusta Hixon Polhemus, Emma Haan Ospina, Haley Feller, Miranda Zenni, Megan Deacon, et al. "The State of Science in the Use of Virtual Reality in the Treatment of Acute and Chronic Pain: A Systematic Scoping Review." *Clinical Journal of Pain* 38, no. 6 (June 2022): 424. https://doi.org/10.1097/AJP.0000000000001029.

215 **VR intervention reduced:** MacIntyre, Erin, Maja Sigerseth, Thomas Fiskeseth Larsen, Kjartan Vibe Fersum, Michel Meulders, Ann Meulders, et al. "Get Your Head in the Game: A Replicated Single-Case Experimental Design Evaluating the Effect of a Novel Virtual Reality Intervention in People with Chronic Low Back Pain." *Journal of Pain* 24, no. 8 (August 1, 2023): 1449–1464. https://doi.org/10.1016/j.jpain.2023.03.013.

216 **The study showed a significant:** Mohammadi, Halimeh, Javad Rasti, and Elham Ebrahimi. "Virtual Reality, Fear of Pain and Labor Pain Intensity: A Randomized Controlled Trial." *Anesthesiology and Pain Medicine* 13, no. 1 (February 6, 2023): e130387. https://doi.org/10.5812/aapm-130387.

216 **A 2023 randomized clinical trial of 149 pediatric:** Arane, Karen, Amir Behboudi, and Ran D. Goldman. "Virtual Reality for Pain and Anxiety Management in Children." *Canadian Family Physician* 63, no. 12 (December 2017): 932–934; Wong, Cho Lee, and Kai Chow Choi. "Effects of an Immersive Virtual Reality Intervention on Pain and Anxiety among Pediatric Patients Undergoing Venipuncture: A Randomized Clinical Trial." *JAMA Network Open* 6, no. 2 (February 16, 2023): e230001. https://doi.org/10.1001/jamanetworkopen.2023.0001.

216 **Hypnosis (also called hypnotherapy):** NCCIH. "Hypnosis." NIH. Accessed May 27, 2025. https://www.nccih.nih.gov/health/hypnosis.

216 **There is evidence that:** Bauzá, Margarita. "How Gut-Directed Hypnosis Helps IBS, IBD, and Other GI Disorders." Michigan Medicine. June 1, 2018. https://www.michiganmedicine.org/health-lab/how-gut-directed-hypnosis-helps-ibs-ibd-and-other-gi-disorders.

217 **We're all influenced:** Mark Jensen interview with Teresa Barker, January 13, 2024.

219 **Active Redirection:** Eleanor Stein interview with Teresa Barker, January 25, 2024, and email correspondence February 16, 2025.

Chapter 12 Befriend Your Body

223 **Buddhist monk and peace activist:** Nhat Hanh, Thich. "Body Scan." Spirituality and Practice. Accessed April 17, 2024. https://www.spiritualityandpractice.com/practices/practices/view/28468/body-scan.

224 **In medical settings:** Benson, H., M. M. Greenwood, and H. Klemchuk. "The Relaxation Response: Psychophysiologic Aspects and Clinical Applications." *International Journal of Psychiatry in Medicine* 6, no. 1–2 (1975): 87–98. https://doi.org/10.2190/376W-E4MT-QM6Q-H0UM.

227 **You can find more:** NCCIH. "Nine Things You Should Know about Chronic Pain and Complementary Health." NIH. Accessed October 21, 2024. https://www.nccih.nih.gov/health/tips/things-you-should-know-about-chronic-pain-and-complementary-health-approaches.

228 **Yet for most of her career:** Zügel, Martina, Constantinos N. Maganaris, Jan Wilke, Karin Jurkat-Rott, Werner Klingler, Scott C. Wearing, et al. "Fascial Tissue Research in Sports Medicine: From Molecules to Tissue Adaptation, Injury and Diagnostics: Consensus Statement." *British Journal of Sports Medicine* 52, no. 23 (December 2018): 1497. https://doi.org/10.1136/bjsports-2018-099308.

229 **In a study of sixty-six patients with plantar fasciitis:** Ajimsha, M. S., D. Binsu, and S. Chithra. "Effectiveness of Myofascial Release in the Management of Plantar Heel Pain: A Randomized Controlled Trial." *Foot* 24, no. 2 (June 2014): 66–71. https://doi.org/10.1016/j.foot.2014.03.005.

230 **National survey data indicate:** NCCIH. "Acupuncture: Effectiveness and Safety." NIH. Updated October 2022. https://www.nccih.nih.gov/health/acupuncture-effectiveness-and-safety.

230 **None of this surprises:** Richard Harris, interviews with Teresa Barker, February 5, 23, 2024.

231 **The needles are inserted:** Napadow, Vitaly, Richard E. Harris, and Karl G. Helmer. "Birth of the Topological Atlas and Repository for Acupoint Research." *Journal of Integrative and Complementary Medicine* 29, no. 12 (December 2023): 769–773. https://doi.org/10.1089/jicm.2023.0592.

232 **This is thought to be:** Vickers, Andrew, and Catherine Zollman. "Acupuncture." *BMJ: British Medical Journal* 319, no. 7215 (October 9, 1999): 973. https://doi.org/10.1136/bmj.319.7215.973.

235 **Be careful not to tense:** Norelli, Samantha K., Ashley Long, and Jeffrey M. Krepps. "Relaxation Techniques." In *StatPearls [Internet]*. StatPearls Publishing, 2024. http://www.ncbi.nlm.nih.gov/books/NBK513238/.

235 **Gentle stroking activates:** Reddan, Marianne C., Hannah Young, Julia Falkner, Marina López-Solà, and Tor D. Wager. "Touch and Social Support Influence Interpersonal Synchrony and Pain." *Social Cognitive and Affective Neuroscience* 15, no. 10 (April 17, 2020): 1064–1075. https://doi.org/10.1093/scan/nsaa048.

236 **It can be activated:** Meijer, Larissa L., Carla Ruis, Zoë A. Schielen, H. Chris Dijkerman, and Maarten J. van der Smagt. "CT-Optimal Touch and Chronic Pain Experience in Parkinson's Disease: An Intervention Study." *PLoS ONE* 19, no. 2 (February 23, 2024): e0298345. https://doi.org/10.1371/journal.pone.0298345.

236 **Hand-holding can increase:** Reddan, et al. "Touch and Social Support Influence Interpersonal Synchrony and Pain."

Chapter 13 Move More

241 **Think about that: prolonged sitting:** Granados, Kirsten, Brooke R. Stephens, Steven K. Malin, Theodore W. Zderic, Marc T. Hamilton, and Barry Braun. "Appetite Regulation in Response to Sitting and Energy Imbalance." *Applied Physiology, Nutrition, and Metabolism* 37, no. 2 (April 2012): 323–333. https://doi.org/10.1139/h2012-002.

242 **In her 2023 talk "Beyond Opioids":** Catherine Bushnell "Beyond Opioids: Engaging Endogenous Pain Modulation in the Brain." University of Toronto Centre for the Study of Pain, September 13, 2023. https://www.youtube.com/watch?v=Ya-6ecqgq74.

243 **Aerobic exercise:** Geneen, Louise J., R. Andrew Moore, Clare Clarke, Denis Martin, Lesley A. Colvin, and Blair H. Smith. "Physical Activity and Exercise for Chronic Pain in Adults: An Overview of Cochrane Reviews." *Cochrane Database of Systematic Reviews* 2017, no. 4 (April 24, 2017): CD011279. https://doi.org/10.1002/14651858.CD011279.pub3.

243 **Resistance exercise:** Geneen et al., "Physical Activity and Exercise for Chronic Pain in Adults."

243 **Balance and flexibility:** Geneen et al., "Physical Activity and Exercise for Chronic Pain in Adults."

243 **Motor control exercise:** Geneen et al., "Physical Activity and Exercise for Chronic Pain in Adults."

243 **Yoga:** Cronkleton, Emily, and Gregory Minnis. "The 10 Best Yoga Poses for Back Pain." Healthline. Updated August 25, 2020. https://www.healthline.com/health/fitness-exercise/yoga-for-back-pain.

244 **Stretching:** Blunk, Laurie. "How to Reduce Muscle Soreness after Exercise." *UK HealthMatters* (blog). UK HealthCare, January 5, 2023. https://ukhealthcare.uky.edu/wellness-community/blog-health-information/how-reduce-muscle-soreness-after-exercise.

244 **Tai chi:** NCCIH. "Tai Chi: What You Need to Know." NIH. Updated December 2023. https://www.nccih.nih.gov/health/tai-chi-what-you-need-to-know.

244 **Dance and creative movement:** Shim, Minjung, R. Burke Johnson, Susan Gasson, Sherry Goodill, Richard Jermyn, and Joke Bradt. "A Model of Dance/Movement Therapy for Resilience-Building in People Living with Chronic Pain." *European Journal of Integrative Medicine* 9 (January 1, 2017): 27–40. https://doi.org/10.1016/j.eujim.2017.01.011.

244 **Has been shown to improve pain coping:** Hickman, Benjamin, Fereshteh Pourkazemi, Roxanna N. Pebdani, Claire E. Hiller, and Alycia Fong Yan. "Dance for Chronic Pain Conditions: A Systematic Review." *Pain Medicine* 23, no. 12 (December 1, 2022): 2022–2041. https://doi.org/10.1093/pm/pnac092.

244 **To add somatic:** Karadag, Paige, and Jenna Gillett. "Keep On Moving: How Somatic Practice Can Effect Living Well with Chronic Pain." *WITHIN Blog.* Warwick Sleep and Pain Laboratory, January 27, 2021. https://warwick.ac.uk/fac/sci/psych/research/lifespan/sleeplab/projects/within/blog/january2021/.

244 **Notice where in your body:** Warren, Sarah. "How to Approach Exercise When You're in Pain." *The Somatics Blog.* Somatic Movement Center, June 16, 2022. https://somaticmovementcenter.com/how-to-approach-exercise-when-youre-in-pain/.

244 **The goal is not to go for the burn:** Karadag and Gillett. "Keep On Moving."

244 **Whatever exercise plan you choose:** Sluka, Kathleen. "Exercise Can Change Everything for Pain." *One Thing,* season 2, episode 8. https://www.youtube.com/watch?v=cHPI2PAZAhw; University of Iowa Health Care. "Exercise to

Treat Chronic Pain." March 1, 2018. https://uihc.org/health-topics/exercise-treat-chronic-pain; Kathleen Sluka interview with Teresa Barker, February 20, 2024.

245 **An Action Plan:** Office of Disease Prevention and Health Promotion. "Prevent Back Pain." US Department of Health and Human Services. Updated March 21, 2024. https://odphp.health.gov/myhealthfinder/healthy-living/safety/prevent-back-pain#take-action-tab.

246 **Steady and sane:** Aluko Hope interview with Teresa Barker, September 16, 2023.

248 **Time your exercise and meals:** American Heart Association. "Food as Fuel before, during and after Workouts." July 31, 2024. https://www.heart.org/en/healthy-living/healthy-eating/eat-smart/nutrition-basics/food-as-fuel-before-during-and-after-workouts.

Chapter 14 Sleep Well

249 **"A robust body of research":** Carla York email interview with Teresa Barker, Feb 23, 2024.

250 **"Sleep deprivation is an even greater issue":** Dedhia, Param, and Robert Maurer. "Sleep and Health: A Lifestyle Medicine Approach." *Journal of Family Practice* 71, Supplement 1 (January 2022): S30–S34. https://doi.org/10.12788/jfp.0295.

251 **At the same time:** National Sleep Foundation. *2015 Sleep in America Poll: Sleep and Pain.* March 2015. https://www.thensf.org/wp-content/uploads/2021/03/2015-SIA-Sleep-and-Pain.pdf.

252 **Consuming high-glycemic:** Cleveland Clinic. "What Is the Glycemic Index?" Updated April 15, 2025. https://health.clevelandclinic.org/glycemic-index.

254 **should check for sleep specialists:** American Academy of Sleep Medicine. "Requirements for the American Board of Sleep Medicine Behavioral Sleep Medicine Certification Examinations." Accessed May 23, 2025. https://www.aasm.org/resources/pdf/bsmguidelines.pdf; American Board of Medical Specialists. "Specialty and Subspecialty Certificates." https://www.abms.org/member-boards/specialty-subspecialty-certificates.

254 **If waking up:** Maldonado, Michelle. "How to Calm Racing Thoughts at Bedtime." Mindful. January 19, 2021. https://www.mindful.org/how-to-calm-racing-thoughts-at-bedtime/.

254 **Help make bedtime sleep time:** Gupta, Charlotte C., Madeline Sprajcer, Colleen Johnston-Devin, and Sally A. Ferguson. "Sleep Hygiene Strategies for Individuals with Chronic Pain: A Scoping Review." *BMJ Open* 13, no. 2 (February 2, 2023): e060401. https://doi.org/10.1136/bmjopen-2021-060401.

254 **Experts recommend:** National Heart, Lung, and Blood Institute. How Much Sleep Is Enough?." NIH. Updated March 24, 2022. https://www.nhlbi.nih.gov/health/sleep/how-much-sleep.

255 **The best room temperature:** Pacheco, Danielle, and David Rosen. "Best Temperature for Sleep." Sleep Foundation. Updated March 7, 2024. https://www.sleepfoundation.org/bedroom-environment/best-temperature-for-sleep.

255 **It's well established that mindfulness:** Pacheco, Danielle, and Anis Rehman. "Meditation for Sleep." Sleep Foundation. Updated February 26, 2024. https://www.sleepfoundation.org/meditation-for-sleep.

256 **A Sample Meditation for Sleep:** Pacheco and Rehman. "Meditation for Sleep."

Chapter 15 Eat Well

259 **Nutrition is considered:** Elma, Ömer, Katherine Brain, and Huan-Ji Dong. "The Importance of Nutrition as a Lifestyle Factor in Chronic Pain Management: A Narrative Review." *Journal of Clinical Medicine* 11, no. 19 (October 9, 2022): 5950. https://doi.org/10.3390/jcm11195950.

260 **According to the authors of a 2020 study:** Hendrix, Jolien, Jo Nijs, Kelly Ickmans, Lode Godderis, Manosij Ghosh, and Andrea Polli. "The Interplay Between Oxidative Stress, Exercise, and Pain in Health and Disease: Potential Role of Autonomic Regulation and Epigenetic Mechanisms." *Antioxidants* 9, no. 11 (November 23, 2020): 1166. https://doi.org/10.3390/antiox9111166.

260 **Healthy diets:** Jiang, Shuai, Hui Liu, and Chunbao Li. "Dietary Regulation of Oxidative Stress in Chronic Metabolic Diseases." *Foods* 10, no. 8 (August 11, 2021): 1854. https://doi.org/10.3390/foods10081854.

261 **The Mediterranean diet:** National Heart, Lung, and Blood Institute. "DASH Eating Plan." NIH. Updated January 10, 2025. https://www.nhlbi.nih.gov/education/dash-eating-plan.

261 **which has a low fat content:** Critselis, Elena, Meropi D. Kontogianni, Ekavi Georgousopoulou, Christina Chrysohoou, Dimitrios Tousoulis, Christos Pitsavos, et al. "Comparison of the Mediterranean Diet and the Dietary Approach Stop Hypertension in Reducing the Risk of 10-Year Fatal and Non-Fatal CVD Events in Healthy Adults: The ATTICA Study (2002–2012)." *Public Health Nutrition* 24, no. 9 (August 3, 2020): 2746. https://doi.org/10.1017/S136898002000230X.

263 **She encourages all of us:** Ring, Melinda. "What If You Could Be Your Own, Best, First Doctor?" TEDxChicago, January 25, 2022. https://www.youtube.com/watch?v=G5CpG5l3qy0.

265 **Although individual factors:** News in Health. "Hydrating for Health." NIH, May 2023. https://newsinhealth.nih.gov/2023/05/hydrating-health.

268 **One study found:** Rindfleisch, J. Adam. "Eating to Reduce Inflammation." Whole Health Library. US Department of Veterans Affairs, July 27, 2018. https://www.va.gov/WHOLEHEALTHLIBRARY/tools/Eating_to_Reduce_Inflammation.asp.

270 **It has been shown:** Caron, Jesse P., Margaret Ann Kreher, Angela M. Mickle, Stanley Wu, Rene Przkora, Irene M. Estores, and Kimberly T. Sibille. "Intermittent Fasting:

Potential Utility in the Treatment of Chronic Pain across the Clinical Spectrum." *Nutrients* 14, no. 12 (June 2022): 2536. https://doi.org/10.3390/nu14122536.

271 **As Harvard Health explains:** Harvard Health Publishing. "Quick-Start Guide to an Anti-Inflammation Diet." Harvard Medical School, April 15, 2023. https://www.health.harvard.edu/staying-healthy/quick-start-guide-to-an-antiinflammation-diet.

271 **Its "One Meal at a Time":** Johns Hopkins Medicine. "Anti Inflammatory Diet." Accessed February 20, 2024. https://www.hopkinsmedicine.org/health/wellness-and-prevention/anti-inflammatory-diet.

Chapter 16 Cultivate Connection

273 **People with chronic pain:** Bannon, Sarah, Jonathan Greenberg, Ryan A. Mace, Joseph J. Locascio, and Ana-Maria Vranceanu. "The Role of Social Isolation in Physical and Emotional Outcomes among Patients with Chronic Pain." *General Hospital Psychiatry* 69 (March–April 2021): 50–54. https://doi.org/10.1016/j.genhosppsych.2021.01.009.

273 **the experience of rejection:** Baumgartner, Jennifer N., Michael R. Haupt, and Laura K. Case. "Chronic Pain Patients Low in Social Connectedness Report Higher Pain and Need Deeper Pressure for Pain Relief." *Emotion* 23, no. 8 (2023): 2156–2168. https://doi.org/10.1037/emo0001228.

275 **Living It: Marsha Garcia:** Marsha Garcia interviews with Teresa Barker, January 16, June 11, April 23, 2024; February 12, 2025.

277 **"We intuitively believe":** Lieberman, Matthew D. *Social: Why Our Brains Are Wired to Connect.* (Crown Publishers, 2014), 5.

278 **Simply put, humans are social:** Stuart Shanker interview and email correspondence with Teresa Barker, April 15, 2024; Shanker, Stuart. "Self-Regulation: 5 Domains of Self-Reg." The MEHRIT Centre, 2021. https://self-reg.ca/wp-content/uploads /2021/05/infosheet_5-Domains-of-Self-Reg.pdf.

278 **A remarkable study:** University of California–Los Angeles. "Rejection Really Hurts, UCLA Psychologists Find." *ScienceDaily*, October 10, 2003. https://www.sciencedaily.com/releases/2003/10/031010074045.htm.

278 **Though it might not leave a mark:** Eisenberger, et al. "Does Rejection Hurt?"

279 **A wave of new research:** Powell, Victoria D., Navasuja Kumar, Andrzej T. Galecki, Mohammed Kabeto, Daniel J. Clauw, David A. Williams, et al. "Bad Company: Loneliness Longitudinally Predicts the Symptom Cluster of Pain, Fatigue, and Depression in Older Adults." *Journal of the American Geriatrics Society* 70, no. 8 (2022): 2225–2234. https://doi.org/10.1111/jgs.17796.

280 **During one of my:** Murthy, Vivek H. "Surgeon General: We Have Become a Lonely Nation. It's Time to Fix That." Opinion, *New York Times*, April 30, 2023. https://www.nytimes.com/2023/04/30/opinion/loneliness-epidemic-america.html.

280 **The dawning recognition:** "Loneliness as a Health Issue." Editorial, *Lancet* 402, no. 10396 (July 8, 2023): 79. https://doi.org/10.1016/S0140-6736(23)01411-3.

281 **As the work of Eisenberger:** Sturgeon, John A., and Alex J. Zautra. "Social Pain and Physical Pain: Shared Paths to Resilience." *Pain Management* 6, no. 1 (January 2016): 63–74. https://doi.org/10.2217/pmt.15.56.

Chapter 17 Savor Moments and Memories

285 ***Carpe diem:*** Britannica. "Carpe Diem." Accessed February 23, 2025. https://www.britannica.com/topic/carpe-diem.

285 ***Carpe Diem Regained:*** Krznaric, Roman. *Carpe Diem Regained: The Vanishing Art of Seizing the Day*. Unbound, 2017, 10.

286 **I'm reminded:** Theodore Roosevelt National Park. "What Are the Badlands?" US National Park Service. Updated August 19, 2015. https://www.nps.gov/thro/learn/kidsyouth/whatarebadlands.htm.

286 **As adults, we have:** Science Direct. "Metacognitive Awareness." Accessed October 25, 2024. https://www.sciencedirect.com/topics/medicine-and-dentistry/metacognitive-awareness.

287 **Bryant himself shared:** Bryant, Fred B. "Current Progress and Future Directions for Theory and Research on Savoring." *Frontiers in Psychology* 12 (December 14, 2021): 771698. https://doi.org/10.3389/fpsyg.2021.771698.

289 **Psychologists and others:** Garland, Eric. "Restructuring Reward Processing with Mindfulness-Oriented Recovery Enhancement: Novel Therapeutic Mechanisms to Remediate Hedonic Dysregulation in Addiction, Stress, and Pain." *Annals of the New York Academy of Sciences* 1373, no. 1 (June 2016): 25–37. https://doi.org/10.1111/nyas.13034.

289 **The 2023 randomized, controlled trial:** Finan, Patrick H., Carly Hunt, Michael L. Keaser, Katie Smith, Sheera Lerman, Clifton O. Bingham, et al. "Effects of Savoring Meditation on Positive Emotions and Pain-Related Brain Function: A Mechanistic Randomized Controlled Trial in People with Rheumatoid Arthritis." Preprint, medRxiv, September 8, 2023. https://doi.org/10.1101/2023.09.07.23294949.

292 **The poet and author:** Gay, Ross. *Inciting Joy: Essays*. (Algonquin Books of Chapel Hill, 2022), 8.

292 **"But what happens":** Gay, Ross. *Inciting Joy*. 4.

Index

Page numbers in italics refer to illustrations.

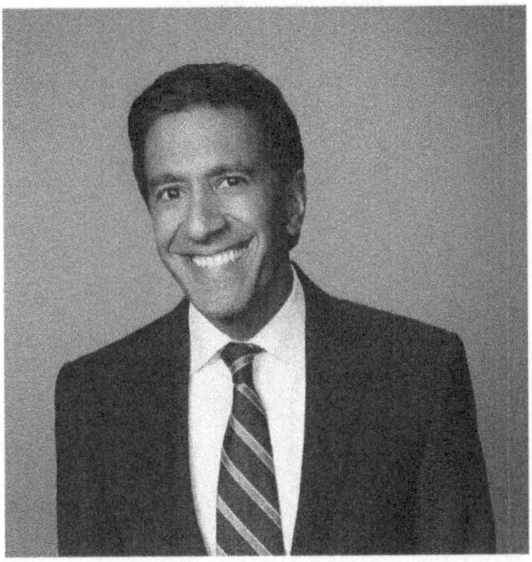

Jeremy Freeman/CNN

Dr Sanjay Gupta is CNN's Emmy Award–winning chief medical correspondent and the host of the acclaimed podcast *Chasing Life* (formerly *Coronavirus: Fact vs. Fiction*), America's go-to resource for expert advice on how to stay healthy and safe. The #1 *New York Times* bestselling author of *Chasing Life, Cheating Death, Monday Mornings,* and *Keep Sharp,* Dr Gupta lives in Atlanta, where he works as an associate professor of neurosurgery at the Emory University School of Medicine.

RAISING READERS

Books Build Bright Futures

Dear Reader,

We'd love your attention for one more page to tell you about the crisis in children's reading, and what we can all do.

Studies have shown that reading for fun is the **single biggest predictor of a child's future success** – more than family circumstance, parents' educational background or income. It improves academic results, mental health, wealth, communication skills and ambition.

The number of children reading for fun is in rapid decline. Young people have a lot of competition for their time, and a worryingly high number do not have a single book at home.

Our business works extensively with schools, libraries and literacy charities, but here are some ways we can all raise more readers:

- Reading to children for just 10 minutes a day makes a difference
- Don't give up if your children aren't regular readers – there will be books for them!
- Visit bookshops and libraries to get recommendations
- Encourage them to listen to audiobooks
- Support school libraries
- Give books as gifts

Thank you for reading.
www.JoinRaisingReaders.com